ENTITLEMENT POLITICS

SOCIAL INSTITUTIONS AND SOCIAL CHANGE
An Aldine de Gruyter Series of Texts and Monographs
SERIES EDITOR
James D. Wright, *Tulane University*

ENTITLEMENT POLITICS

Medicare and Medicaid
1995–2001

DAVID G. SMITH

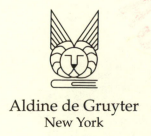

Aldine de Gruyter
New York

ABOUT THE AUTHOR

David G. Smith is Richter Professor Emeritus of Political Science at Swarthmore College and has been a student of health policy since 1965. His primary teaching areas are constitutional law and jurisprudence; health policy; and American government and public policy. Among his books is an earlier study of health policy, *Paying for Medicare: The Politics of Reform* (Aldine, 1992).

ALDINE DE GRUYTER
A division of Walter de Gruyter, Inc.
200 Saw Mill River Road
Hawthorne, New York 10532

This publication is printed on acid free paper ∞

Library of Congress Cataloging-in-Publication Data
Smith, David G., 1926–
    Entitlement politics : medicare and medicaid, 1995–2001 / David G. Smith.
        p. cm. — (Social institutions and social change)
    Includes bibliographical references and index.
    ISBN 0-202-30718-2 — ISBN 0-202-30719-0 (pbk.)
    1. Medicare. 2. Medicaid. 3. Medical policy—United States. I. Title. II. Series.
    RA412.3 .S635 2002
    368.4′26′00973—dc21
                                  2002001111

Manufactured in the United States of America
10 9 8 7 6 5 4 3 2 1

Contents

Acknowledgments

This book could not have been written without the help of many generous, informed, and perceptive individuals. It is a pleasure to acknowledge some of their contributions.

I am grateful to the Robert Wood Johnson Foundation for its expeditious and generous financial support to meet travel and research expenses. By acting quickly, the foundation made interviews possible while key participants were still readily available. Though the foundation supported this research, it did not sponsor it and bears no responsibility for the contents or conclusions of this book.

This book relies heavily upon interviews. I owe a great debt to the many individuals who gave of their time, shared their insights and knowledge, and trusted me to represent their views fairly and with discretion. I have tried to honor that trust. I hope that what I have said in this book can serve as a small payment on the debt I owe.

Many of the people I interviewed—especially from congressional staff, HCFA and other government agencies, and advocacy and research groups—were busy and committed people. I am grateful for the time they gave, as well as for their considered opinions. Among those who were especially generous and helpful were Sheila Burke, Kathy Buto, Debbie Chang, Gary Christoph, Gary Claxton, Howard Cohen, Janet Corrigan, Nancy-Ann deParle, Jack Ebeler, Judith Feder, Bruce Fried, George Greenberg, Dick Hegner, Chris Jennings, Chip Kahn, Jeff Kang, Julie James, Jeanne Lambrew, Lisa Layman, Lauren LeRoy, Bob Moffit, Marilyn Moon, Judy Moore, Lee Partridge, Robert Reischauer, William Scanlon, Andy Schneider, Bill Vaughan, Bruce Vladeck, Dan Waldo, Barbara Wynn, Don Young.

Several individuals read and commented upon parts or all of the manuscript: Lynn Etheredge, Chuck Gilbert, Dick Hegner, and Hillard Pouncy. I am grateful for their interest and their help.

I would like to acknowledge separately and especially the contributions of Lynn Etheredge, who mentored this work from beginning to end, read and commented upon the entire manuscript, contributed materials and e-mail updates, and offered friendly encouragement and thoughtful suggestions along the way.

This book is dedicated to my wife, Eleanor, who also offered friendly encouragement, was patient with my impatience, and carried more than her share of the household and family obligations while this work was in progress.

1

Introduction

Medicare and Medicaid politics have seldom been dramatic. Along with Social Security, they are the biggest entitlement programs and, as such, are generally regarded as established institutions. They are vitally important to their beneficiaries and other stakeholders. As programs, they are technical, multilayered, and complex. Because of these characteristics, both Medicare and Medicaid have, for the most part, developed incrementally, along lines established by the original legislation, and with few surprises or major changes. The year 1965, when Medicare and Medicaid were first enacted was, by contrast, a year of major change and of drama. Thirty years later, in 1995, when the Republican party took over both the House and the Senate and challenged settled presumptions about the role of government in society, they brought high drama to their campaign against entitlements.

With budget balancing and reducing or eliminating entitlements key to the Republican strategy, the Medicare and Medicare programs were hauled on stage, so to speak, and became reluctant participants in a drama that led in December and January to the shutdown of the federal government and a constitutional crisis (Drew 1996:Chs. 17, 18).

The constitutional crisis was resolved for a time, and Republicans and Democrats shifted to more traditional modes of legislative behavior, passing a genuinely bipartisan though relatively minor health care bill in 1996.[1] In 1997, Congress and the president negotiated a critical summit agreement, after which they enacted the Balanced Budget Act of 1997 (BBA 97), the legislative vehicle for a huge and dense body of amendments, entitled "The Medicare, Medicaid, and Children's Health Provisions."[2] These amendments were strongly supported by the president and bipartisan majorities in both the House and Senate. They have been described as a major victory for bipartisanship and as the most fundamental changes in the Medicare and Medicaid programs since their inception. Yet change does not always solve underlying problems or achieve lasting agreements. In fact, the preliminary summit

agreement took issues of entitlement and fundamental structure off the table
for consideration as part of the budget reconciliation. For Medicare, especially,
BBA 97 postponed these issues rather than resolving them. Medicaid is a different story, and provides an instructive contrast—but more of that later. Had
a Democrat won the presidential election of 2000, then BBA 97 might have
become the more or less settled program structure, to be modified over the
years, by cycles and epicycles of incremental change.

The election of November 2000 put the Republican party in power for the
first time in nearly fifty years, though with a minority president, lack of a popular mandate, a Senate divided 50–50, and a majority of only five in the
House. Declining invitations to form a peacetime "national unity" government, the Republicans decided that they would govern and that to govern
they needed their conservative base. They affirmed again the conservative
Republican goals of the first Reagan administration and the 104th Congress:
cutting taxes and the budget; reducing the size of the central government; and
decentralizing or privatizing government programs. For now, specific intentions with respect to entitlements remain in doubt, though governors have
renewed protests against Medicaid restrictions,[3] and both President Bush and
Republicans in Congress have said on several occasions that they would
"reform" Medicare, along lines recommended by the Bipartisan Commission.[4]
Despite campaign rhetoric of "compassionate conservatism," many Republicans spoke of continuing the "revolution" that Ronald Reagan began in 1980
and that they failed to complete in 1995. And the Bush administration and
the Republican Congress committed themselves to a tax and budget-cutting
strategy that seems likely to revive, sooner or later, the central controversy
over Medicare/Medicaid entitlements.

Developments since the terrorist attacks of September 11 do not seem
likely to end the conflict over these entitlements. The stimulus package that
ultimately failed to pass the Senate, late in December 2001, did so in part over
an entitlement issue: whether health benefits for unemployed workers should
take the form of tax credits or premium subsidies and Medicaid expansion
(Toner 2001b). In the coming months, a potent combination of rising health
care costs and recession will increase the strains upon private insurance, the
health care entitlements, and federal and state budgets. Politically, Democrats
will have strong incentives to defend and extend these entitlements and
Republicans to curb or transform them.

If the Republicans succeed in their long-term strategy of transforming
Medicare and Medicaid, then—counting welfare—they will have radically
changed entitlements in the United States.[5] An achievement of this magnitude, without some major crisis driving it, would be remarkable under any
circumstances, and seems even more so because, at no time—including the
first Reagan administration—have the Republicans had full control of both
Congress and the presidency. Divided government, bare majorities, and lack

of a popular mandate for change have characterized the politics of entitlement from the first Reagan administration to the present. But Republicans have managed, then as now, to mobilize, leverage, and use the political power they did have. The account in subsequent chapters explores the meaning of this statement in detail, and what this kind of mobilization politics has meant for Medicare and Medicaid politics and policy.

As noted, the larger issue has been not budget reduction or entitlements as such, but the role and size of the federal government and the balance between public and private responsibilities. Medicare and Medicaid were targeted in 1995 because of their size and because they were more vulnerable than Social Security. As they were central to much of domestic politics, especially between 1995 and 1997, the controversy over them provides a good illustration of policymaking in this era of high political and partisan mobilization. The complement of this proposition is even more important for students of Medicare and Medicaid politics and policy, for Medicaid and Medicare have been swept into the turmoil of national politics, and what has happened and is happening to these programs cannot be understood without taking into account the larger context of national politics.

To say that Republicans deliberately used a strategy of political and partisan mobilization in their attack on entitlements is not to suggest that this approach was confined to Medicare and Medicaid nor used by Republicans alone. In the 104th Congress, the new speaker of the House, Newt Gingrich, and the House conservative leadership launched their campaign with the Contract with America and moved from that to welfare reform before settling on an omnibus reconciliation bill with Medicare and Medicare specially featured. Before the 104th Congress, a mobilization strategy had some precedents in President Clinton's campaign for health care reform in 1993–94; and much of the response by the Clinton administration to the Republican's initiatives in 1995 and beyond was to counter with a strategy and tactics similar to those employed by the Republicans.

The Bush administration and the congressional Republicans seem deeply committed to completing the conservative revolution begun in 1981 and renewed in 1995, combining goals common to each of these episodes with a strategy and tactics of political mobilization resembling in important ways that of Newt Gingrich and the House Republicans of 1995. This time, the Republican party controls the presidency, which makes an enormous difference. But the earlier history of BBA 95, which was vetoed, and of BBA 97, which passed, are important for understanding this relatively new game of high political and partisan mobilization, the moves and countermoves that characterize it, and the consequences it has for Medicare and Medicaid policy.

The Republican party has been systematic and more successful in adapting to and taking advantage of this mobilization style of politics and, as noted, has used it to make the most of its narrow majorities. In Medicare and Medicaid politics since 1994, four elements or constituents seem to be most important: (1) commitment to a long-term strategy; (2) enforcing party discipline; (3) combining tax cuts and budget reduction; and (4) employing a campaign mode of legislation. Some comment on each of these will help to illustrate their use and importance.

One notable characteristic of the contemporary Republican party has been the time and effort it puts into developing long-term strategies and goals— much more, for instance, than the Democratic party.[6] This commitment to a long-term strategy helps the national party leadership raise money, recruit candidates, fund conferences and research, and center its energies on a few critical messages and policy options. Strategy also guides tactics, which can be important—in war or politics—especially if the opponent fails to see the relationship between them or lacks an effective response. We can leave aside the philosophical issue of whether it is good for national parties to have long-term strategies. However, the amount of strategizing and counterstrategizing over the Medicare and Medicaid entitlements has increased deception, maneuvering for strategic advantage, and the use of tactical ploys, leaving residues of anger, cynicism, and mutual distrust.

Strengthened congressional party leadership and party discipline have been other factors enhancing Republican legislative effectiveness. This development was historically complex but the House reorganization of 1994–95, led by Speaker Newt Gingrich, institutionalized the transformation, affected the Senate in turn, and continues to shape Medicare and Medicaid policy today. Leaving the details aside for now (see pp. 32–34) this change shifted much of the control over the legislative process in the House from the regular legislative committees to the speaker, the party leadership institutions, and the chairs of some key committees. It also tightened party control over the legislative agenda and over the membership and staffing of the committees. The Senate did not go so far, but has still moved in this direction. An important point is that most of these changes have lasted and continue to affect the policy process throughout the continuing entitlement disputes.

Shifting power toward the party leadership can promote strategic and tactical effectiveness and may help overcome the particularism and snail-paced incrementalism of the legislative committees. But this kind of partisan mobilization also generates important tensions when directed toward programs like Medicare and Medicare. These programs are technical in nature, affect beneficiaries' lives and the livelihoods of powerful providers, and are invested with both mystique and pathos. Much of the book is about what occurs under such conditions.

Budget discipline and tax reduction are important in themselves, as direct expressions of a long-term Republican commitment to reduce the size and reach of the federal government. One powerful method of enforcing fiscal discipline is through the budget reconciliation process. Following this procedure, House and Senate first agree upon a budget resolution, setting budget targets (with savings) in broad categorical terms. This is followed by a reconciliation bill in the process of which legislative and tax committees recommend changes to bring authorizations and revenues into conformity with the budget resolution. Reconciliation does not by itself shrink the budget or reduce deficits, but when backed by a strong resolve to achieve these ends and additional mechanisms such as CBO scoring, offsetting requirements, and sequester procedures,[7] it can be enormously powerful.

The reconciliation process has been important for Medicare and Medicaid for two paramount reasons. One is that reconciliation provides a sensitive and comprehensive method for reducing budget outlays. Medicare and Medicaid are perennial drivers of budget increments; and they are complex and technical. The reconciliation process was not specifically designed for this kind of challenge, but it might well have been since it combines great coordinative power with the capacity for fine adjustment. In addition, Medicare and Medicaid require a lot of tinkering—for which the reconciliation procedure is well suited since it brings together budget constraints with legislative amendment. Since increments for one activity may be offset with reductions from another, reconciliation can be readily adapted for program enhancements as well as for cuts in authorizations or outlays. As a consequence, the budget reconciliation process has been uniquely important for the Medicare and Medicaid programs. In fact, most major changes in Medicare or Medicaid from 1982 to the present[8] have been made, or sought, through a series of omnibus budget reconciliation acts (OBRAs), including the vetoed BBA of 1995 and the BBA of 1997, which passed.

The budget reconciliation process is highly adaptable and, in addition to budget reduction and incremental program changes, can be used for major restructuring or combined with other strategies, such as cutting taxes. In the first Reagan administration, for instance, budget reconciliation was combined with a tax-cutting strategy and used to initiate a major campaign against entitlements (Jones 1988:37ff.). This is a precedent that worries Democrats as they contemplate President Bush's ten-year $1.6 trillion tax cut. Reconciliation can also be used in combination with other legislative strategies to restructure programs comprehensively. At one point, the Clinton administration briefly considered, though later abandoned, a proposal to make the monster Health Security Act of 1993 part of a reconciliation bill. And the Republican Congress, both in 1995 and 1997, chose the budget reconciliation procedure as a vehicle for comprehensive restructuring of Medicare and Medicaid, a project almost as daunting in its complexity and difficulty as Clinton's health care reform.

As the Reagan example suggests, some of the less manifest objectives of the budget reconciliation process may be as much sought after or even more important than the declared ones (Jones 1988:38). In a word, budget reconciliation can be a way of mobilizing collective energy and getting a lot done in a hurry. For an item, it sets common goals and a series of deadlines. It puts a premium on overall strategy and coordination and tends to legitimate centralization of power in the leadership and key committee chairs. Finally, it brings together budgeting, taxation, and authorization in a way that facilitates high-level negotiation and sends the message that policy will be primarily leadership driven rather than "bubbling up" from the authorizing committees in the time-honored, traditional fashion.

The centralizing of leadership initiative and the pursuit of long-term strategic goals provide incentives to use and to strengthen the reconciliation process. In general, though, budget reconciliation tends to be relatively undisciplined and ineffective, especially as a way of cutting the budget or reducing program outlays, without some major impelling force such as rapidly escalating program costs or yawning budget deficits. One way of supplying this external impetus, especially when deficits are relatively small or nonexistent—as in a period of budget surplus—is with a large tax cut, which can be used either to discourage additional spending or to create a sense of fiscal stringency. This was a strategy pursued by the first Reagan administration and one that seems to have commended itself to the present Bush administration as well.

Another practice that has grown over the last decade has been to treat legislation more and more like a campaign. The first Reagan administration and President Clinton's health care reform were precedents for this kind of behavior. More recent instances have been the Republican Contract with America of 1994–95 and the BBAs of 1995 and 1997. Despite the Medicare and Medicaid reforms of 1997—which were generally seen as a major settlement and a triumph of bipartisan politics—this approach to legislating has carried over into subsequent debates over additional Medicare coverage, a pharmaceutical benefit, and a patients' bill of rights. Given the narrow margins in Congress, which have put a premium upon mobilization tactics, the campaign mode of legislating is likely to be a lasting phenomenon.

"Campaign mode" is an ambiguous term, intended to suggest resemblances to both political and military campaigns. This complex of activities developed especially from a history of divided government, the growing importance of campaign finance, the Clinton administration, and the 104th Congress. Divided government or even weak majorities encourage strategic moves to maximize a political advantage: for instance, the self-declared mandate and "seize and hold" strategy of the first Reagan administration. In addition, divided government tends to encourage a continual campaign, with both sides seeking to bolster their power by appealing to a present public or future majority. Modern elections require almost continuous campaigning, especially to raise money, even with pseudoevents, and to hold together labile electoral support (Dionne 1998). In the first Clinton administration, health care reform especially took on the intensity and nationwide appeal of a plebiscite. And the 104th Congress, with the House under Speaker Gingrich's leadership, continued the campaign style, adding a great deal of military rhetoric and tactics. It is dangerous behavior because it incites response in kind and tends to escalate out of control. Unfortunately, it is much like war: seeking surprise and strategic advantage; mandating secrecy and "nonfraternization" with the "enemy." mounting propaganda and "disinformation" campaigns; and putting electoral victory above legislative achievement or ultimate reconciliation.

As popular and well-entrenched entitlements, Medicare and Medicaid were strategically and symbolically important to both Republicans and Democrats. Changing them radically would require a major political effort—so that mobilization techniques such as those described were seen as necessary, especially for winning on some of the big issues such as entitlement status, size of tax cuts, or restructuring the programs. At the same time, coordinated mobilization efforts were combined with or alternated with other, more traditional approaches. For instance, even in 1995, when the political and partisan mobilization was at a peak, a number of related health care bills were considered as part of a separate "incremental" strategy. A health insurance bill that passed in 1996,[9] and that contained a number of major provisions that had been part of the vetoed BBA 95, was incremental in nature and remarkably bipartisan. BBA 97 also began in a campaign mode but—following a strategic summit agreement—was concluded as bipartisan legislation both in spirit and substantive content.

Yet political and partisan mobilization seem likely to continue for the indefinite future as part of Medicare and Medicaid politics and policy: as a dominant influence, a latent threat, a partial manifestation, or a residue of distrust and bitterness. The design and packaging of incremental legislation, for instance, will likely be shaped by the overriding aims and methods associated with mobilization strategies. Genuine bipartisan collaboration with respect to Medicare and Medicaid policy may occur as a welcome relief but generally as an exception to the prevailing expectation. And the campaign mode of legislation persists, like an incubus moving to another habitat: for instance, in the perennial or eternal debate over patients' bills of rights (see pp. 334ff.).

One unhealthy consequence of the politicizing of Medicare and Medicaid policy has been to separate the rhetoric and ideology of the public debates from the technical and organizational realities underlying issues of cost containment or program structure. This development is unfortunate since it leaves even informed citizens at a loss in evaluating the claims being made. Because of the technical nature of these programs, though, a second line of defense has been the expert review and comment of administrative and congressional staff and outside specialists or advocacy groups that are adept at pointing out glitches in program design, numbers that do not add up, or inequities in treatment or payment formulas and making their views known where they will have an impact. This kind of critical activity has been a powerful protection against mistakes, excess, or undue influence, especially when the policy or legislative process was structured so as to hear and take advantage of such contributions.[10] Of course, as Medicare and Medicaid politics have become more ideological and divisive, this kind of potentially constructive activity has less purchase or leverage. But it remains effective, sometimes surprisingly so and in ways that often represent creative adaptations to new political realities that can serve as useful precedents for confronting an unknown future.

Another important moderating influence upon Medicare and Medicaid politics has been the long-standing presumption that policy for these programs should be largely bipartisan, both in its making and substantive content. With high levels of political mobilization, that particular restraint ceases to be effective. In default of this moderating influence on party politics, a kind of "constitutional politics" has gained renewed significance—a development that reminds us that the federal system of government was originally designed to combat factions, immoderate majorities, or political tendencies to an extreme. James Madison, in describing his "compound Republick" (*Federalist* No. 10) stressed especially the protections afforded by federalism, bicameralism, the separation of powers, and their attendant checks and balances. In the context of this study, it is reassuring that these constitutional restraints continue to serve as protections and enlightening to observe how often they do so in ways that Madison and other drafters of the Constitution seem to have anticipated.

In dealing with the politics of entitlements, this account intentionally goes at some length into the substance of the programs, the policies that are involved, and the views of different protagonists about the major issues in dispute. It is worth mentioning several reasons for this emphasis, since they will signal in advance some of the important themes that run through the book.

Medicare and Medicaid are technical fields in which data, scientifically based argument, and professional opinion play a major role. These programs are also well-established—so that their history and administrative culture affect both policy and politics. Program history and technical policy considerations figure prominently in debates and often affect political outcomes. Getting familiar with the language of discourse (including the myriad acronyms) and learning about specific programs and the underlying policy issues not only helps to understand what is going on but also to anticipate policy and political outcomes.

Understanding what is going on has acquired a new significance in this era of mobilization politics, campaign-style legislation, and PR "spin" applied to almost everything political. It was critical, for instance, in the 1995 controversy over how to "save" Medicare to understand whether proposals driven by strategic political goals had a sound basis in policy. The obverse can be equally important: political success can sometimes depend on having the best policy argument and knowing when and under what circumstances it can get "traction," to use the current lingo. In the same vein, the more recent strife over a patients' bill of rights seems best understood not as policy, but as campaign-style rhetoric, often separated from critical thought about underlying policy or attempts to reach a politically negotiated solution.

Getting fairly deeply into program history and policy has another virtue: helping to understand different points of view. A successful lawyer said that he never felt ready for trial until he had prepared the best brief he could for the opponent's side. That way, he understood the strengths and weaknesses of both sides. The perspective gained enabled him to see why particular points were vital and had to be defended even at great cost, and why others were less so and could be considered negotiable. Not only is this lawyer's perspective vital to defend or attack a particular policy initiative, it is equally important in reaching lasting, bipartisan compromises.

The legal analogy is useful for making a further observation about the design and feasibility of major program changes or restructuring. One of the most powerful restraints upon a judge, in our system of jurisprudence, is the requirement of writing an opinion that will address the issues, articulate a solution, and then defend that decision with a coherent argument. Not infrequently, judges attempt decisions that simply "won't write." They may find a different and more successful rhetoric; but they have also been known to change their minds about the merits of the case. Because of its technical nature and the weight of various "authorities," Medicare and Medicaid policy is somewhat similar. A strong showing that the program will not work as designed, that the budget numbers do not add up, or that the impact data are worse than supposed can sometimes stop or deflect a political initiative. Also, Medicare and Medicaid are unusual for the number of individuals, committees, and staff agencies set to monitor their activities. Such oversight can be effective on occasion in pushing for program modification or in tempering political initiatives.

Paying close attention to the phenomenology of policy development can help anticipate whether an initiative is likely to succeed. For instance, with important proposals, key staff would often think in terms of the requisite elements that must be developed and working together for an initiative to have a good chance of success: ideology or "message," along with a powerful "mantra";[11] a plausible political strategy and tactics; and a proposal design with supporting expertise and numbers. The list is striking for its recognition of realities in an era of mobilization politics. It does not predict, except that it can help to construct plausible "scenarios" and foretell some failures, function pretty well to increase chances for success, and help adjust to a changing environment.

This book provides (Chapter 7) a rather comprehensive account of implementation, which includes both rule-making and program design as well as later experience with some of the most important statutory provisions. One reason for this inclusion is that implementation is part of policy and politics and, for that reason, vital for an understanding of the policy process. Another reason is that to be significantly engaged with Medicare or Medicaid policy, a knowledge of implementation and how HCFA (CMS) operates is important. Perhaps the most important reason—at least in the author's view—is that implementation says so much about what is feasible and prudent to do. For that reason, a knowledge of implementation—rather like the role of autopsies at an earlier stage in medical history—is indispensable for seeing how policy works out in practice and for learning how to evaluate and, at times, to discount some of the claims of politicians and policy experts.

The main purpose of this book is to provide an overview of the Medicare and Medicaid programs and an account of recent political and policy developments that will help the reader to interpret these events, evaluate the process and some of its outcomes, and acquire a sense of how to proceed independently to learn more or do more about these programs.

This book is also about American government and politics. Beginning with 1995 and the 104th Congress, the Medicare and Medicaid programs have been caught up in wider struggles over the size of the federal government, the status of entitlements, and the restructuring of domestic programs. Conservative Republicans have boasted about "finishing the Reagan Revolution," both in 1995 and 2001. Of course, they may yet succeed. Their success so far has been astounding—without a domestic crisis, a popular majority, or a mandate impelling them, relying on will, discipline, planning, and skillful exploitation of discontent and weaknesses in the political system. As an example of the deliberate engineering of political change within a constitutional democracy it is unusual, even unique. Medicare and Medicaid are useful as case studies of this saga because they provide a variety of illustrations of a semirevolutionary process and of ways in which it has been augmented but also diverted, "cooled out," or checked.

The struggle over entitlements and the future of Medicare and Medicaid is likely to continue; and this account is intended to provide guidance in anticipating the forms it may take. The bipartisan compromise over Medicaid reached in 1997 may prove to be durable, at least in its general outlines and principles. No similar compromise has been reached with respect to Medicare, although there is some sentiment for "declaring a victory and going home,"[12] by adopting the 1999 proposal of the Bipartisan Commission. In the author's view, that would be a "nonsolution." One of the ironies of recent history is that partisan strife over Medicare has so complicated the political and policy issues that only a serious and genuine bipartisan effort bringing forth the best efforts of both Democrats and Republicans—and some of the best industry leaders and policy experts in the field—is likely to achieve genuine reform. Judging from our past history, another likely path would be to try patching and mend-ing until a major economic or health care crisis creates the collective sense of urgency to do something in a hurry. Either way, the more interested parties know about the history, politics, and policies of these programs, the better our prospects for devising workable, equitable, and lasting solutions.

NOTES

[1] Health Insurance Portability and Accountability Act of 1996 (HIPAA) P.L. 104-191.

[2] P.L. 105-33, August 5, 1997.

[3] *Westside Mothers v. Haveman*, 133 F. Supp. 2d 549, Mar. 26, 2001, holding that private parties could not sue the State of Michigan over Medicaid EPSDT requirements, is an example of how an unexpected court ruling could revive a fundamental controversy over Medicaid policy.

[4] The National Bipartisan Commission on the Future of Medicare, which reported in March 1999, recommended that Medicare be restructured along lines of the Federal Employee Health Benefits Plan and "premium support" used as the method of financing.

[5] Even Social Security would be partially privatized by allowing some of the payroll tax to be individually invested in private accounts.

[6] Whether it is desirable for American national parties to have long-term strategic goals is an interesting question. For instance, one might doubt the value of long-term goals as such in a marriage or in the judging of law cases. For political parties, devotion to such goals can result in the sacrifice of important substantive or procedural objectives. Yet in the current party competition, the Democratic party may be handicapped by a lack of long-term goals.

[7] The Budget Enforcement Act of 1990 requires that legislation reducing revenues or increasing expenditures be completely "offset" by other revenue increases of expenditure reductions; if offsets do not occur, a sequester mechanism can be invoked to make the requisite changes.

[8] The Prospective Payment System was enacted as part of the Social Security Amendments of 1983, P.L. 98-21, April 20, 1983. But even that was hooked up to a legislative vehicle, i.e., the Social Security Amendments, "must pass" legislation because of the individuals dependent on their Social Security checks.

[9] The Health Insurance Portability and Accountability Act (HIPAA).

[10] Such activities can strengthen other influences such as "neutral competence" and "institutional memory" within the civil service. Another relevant comparison would be the German ideal of a *Rechtsstaat,* within which a professional civil service and public attitudes support rationality and restraint.

[11] Meaning here not a mystical formula or incantation but a political slogan, such as "reforming Medicare in order to save it" or "slashing Medicare to provide tax breaks for the rich." Whether true or even credible, the mantra works to reinforce the larger message.

[12] This was Senator George Aiken's formula for getting out of Vietnam.

2

Historical Background

Medicare and Medicaid are among the most important institutions of our society and deeply rooted in tradition and law. As with other great institutions, for example, the Constitution, origins and historic development are important for establishing precedents and legitimating interpretations. Historic accounts provide clues for understanding the dynamics and prospects for change. And a record of experimentation may turn up ideas for change or caution restraint.

At the same time, both Medicare and Medicaid have been criticized for being too bound to past practices and policies. It has been observed that victors in war study how the most recent war was won—with the implication that the losers are learning how to win the next one. This saying may be true, in fact, with respect to Medicare and Medicaid. It also suggests that one problem with a historic perspective, just as with "institutional memory" within the civil service or Congress, is that it can be used too much to defend what has worked in the past and not enough to facilitate change. But that need not be true. A vitally important reason for studying the historic background of these programs is that such knowledge can be used to adapt to emerging needs as well as understand what should be preserved.

I. MEDICARE AND MEDICAID—INITIAL LEGISLATION

Medicare and Medicaid—Titles 18 and 19 of the Social Security Amendments of 1965, were landmark achievements of the Kennedy-Johnson administrations. The legislation was passed, after President Kennedy's assassination and the 1964 elections, by a heavily Democratic Congress that saw this legislation as redeeming a promise to the American people.[1] In recognition of the occasion, President Johnson flew to Independence, Missouri, to sign the legislation in the presence of Harry S. Truman who, as president in 1950, had suffered a humiliating defeat in an earlier attempt to enact a program of national health insurance.

One reason for the congratulatory mood was that Medicare–Medicaid was a greater achievement than even its principal supporters had expected. It was passed after a series of defeats in the Kennedy administration and despite the opposition of the American Medical Association. Moreover, it included not one initiative, as originally planned, but three. The legislation began with the King–Anderson bill, backed by the administration, which would have extended the social security benefit to cover hospital and nursing home costs. Not covered were medical and surgical benefits or care for the poor not entitled to Social Security. However, two alternative proposals were being considered along with King–Anderson. One was the AMA-sponsored "Eldercare," an expanded version of the Kerr–Mills program, which was a grant-in-aid scheme to provide medical assistance for the aged poor. The other was the Byrnes bill, similar to the federal employees' health program, for a contributory plan covering medical and surgical benefits (Marmor 2000:118). Making the most of an opportunity, Congress combined all three into what Wilbur Mills, Chairman of the House Ways and Means Committee called a "three-layer cake." With modifications, the King–Anderson bill became Part A of Title 18, a hospital insurance benefit. The Byrnes bill became part B of Title 18, a voluntary and contributory medical-surgical benefit, without coverage for drugs. And the AMA version of Kerr–Mills became Title 19, or Medicaid, added with little discussion and almost as an afterthought (Friedman 1995).[2]

There was cause for celebration in the passage, finally, of national legislation dealing with universal categories of need—the elderly and the indigent. But the analogy of a three-layer cake is useful to call attention to the historic fact that Medicare–Medicaid was from the beginning a joining of separate parts, never an integrated system. Medicare Part A (the hospital insurance) grew out of a tradition of social insurance. Payroll taxes were contributed to a trust fund and there was a strong sense of entitlement to the same medical care that everyone else got. Medicaid, by contrast, built upon public assistance theory and practice. Recipients had to establish "eligibility" and they often got welfare medicine from underpaid "vendors." From the beginning, then, the program established a two-tiered system of mainstream medicine and care for the poor. Moreover, it covered a small minority of the poor: only those with "categorical" eligibility,[3] excluding many, especially the "working poor" who were in need but with incomes above state poverty lines. Because Medicaid was chronically underfunded and covered only a minority of the poor, many went without health care or the costs of uncompensated care were shifted to Medicare providers, insurance companies, other payers, or local charities.

Medicare itself was divided between Part A and Part B, establishing hospital and physician benefits, respectively. This dualism helped to gain provider support and eased the pinch for beneficiaries, especially for expensive hospital stays. But it built in two different forms of payment: cost reimbursement for hospitals and payment of charges for physicians. This difference in payment methods created incentives to overutilize hospital care and underutilize less expensive physician services. It worked against some approaches to change, for instance, capitation. Moreover, reforms directed at Part A or Part B have developed separately and at different times, almost never as combined parts of a comprehensive strategy.

Another important feature of the original Medicare–Medicaid legislation was the way in which it approached cost containment: putting much of the burden on beneficiaries rather than providers. Medicare provided for reimbursement of hospitals' "reasonable costs" and for payment of physicians' "reasonable charges," language that appeared to contemplate stringent cost containment, but left much to interpretation. The statute also specified that claims processing would be handled by "fiscal intermediaries" and "carriers," pretty much the same private insurance agencies that providers had dealt with before Medicare (Myers 1970:178ff.). In practice, many of the early administrative decisions implementing Medicare were permissive and conceded much with respect to accounting practices and allowances on claims (Feder 1977:Ch. 6). At the same time, the legislation came down heavily on the beneficiary and the demand side. Medicare had numerous exclusions, deductibles, and copays intended to limit utilization. Physicians (though not hospitals) could bill for additional payments, over and above the amount allowed by Medicare. Medicaid, like the earlier Kerr–Mills program, continued to be a grant-in-aid entitlement in which the states paid up to half of the total costs, sometimes taxing the resources of the poorer ones and leading them to raise eligibility requirements and cut funds for care. In summary, cost containment features were weak, and much of the incentive for restraint in utilization was put on the beneficiary, not the provider.

Despite their limitations, Medicare and Medicaid have stood as peculiarly American approaches toward nationally sponsored health insurance—unlike any system anywhere else in the world. Medicare brought much greater income security and "mainstream" medicine to the elderly; and Medicaid made a meager down payment on health care for the poor. Their separate existence has divided reform efforts between advocacy of more comprehensive schemes of health insurance and Medicare–Medicaid-only strategies aimed at improving or extending these programs. Indeed, much of the history of health policy since 1965 can be described as an alternation between these two strategies: campaigns for national health insurance followed by or in competition with attempts to reform Medicare and Medicaid. This dualism continues, energizing much of the politics of health care. However the tension is ultimately resolved, both perspectives of Medicare–Medicaid politics are important: the continuing reform of specific programs versus involvement in larger agendas, whether health related or not.

II. MEDICARE: REFORM EFFORTS

Medicare has been a popular and successful program, from the perspective of both beneficiaries and providers. Programmatically, Medicare achieved its primary aims: to increase security for the elderly and provide them with access to mainstream medical care. Polls commonly show high approval ratings among beneficiaries, with almost all segments of opinion ranking it among our most essential domestic programs. It got nearly universal participation by providers and, generally, a high level of continuing satisfaction despite a long history of increasingly intrusive regulatory reforms. Politically, Medicare has proven almost unassailable, except with strategies alleging to "save" or improve it.

Much of the support for Medicare results from the original "social contract" created by the legislation itself.[4] In that original contract there were two elements: a guaranteed benefit for the elderly, and assurance of protection for provider interests. In the words of Robert Ball, "We proposed assuring the same level of care for the elderly as was then enjoyed by paying and insured patients: otherwise, we did not intend to disrupt the status quo" (1995:67). It was a "strategy of acceptability," not a scheme to reform the health care system. Health care providers and insurance companies got assured protection and the elderly got an entitlement. These two elements of guaranteed benefit and provider protection are not merely an implicit understanding, but are prominently written into the statute, a circumstance that has important consequences politically and especially for any reform schemes. In fact, the two elements most responsible for the success of the program have also been the main obstacles to its reform.

Title 18—the Medicare title—is strong on a philosophy of entitlement. Throughout, it speaks in terms of universality and equality, often using such language as "any person entitled" and "any eligible beneficiary."[5] Section 1802, the second paragraph under Title 18, assures beneficiaries "free choice" of provider and access on equal terms. In a larger context, an important reason for associating Medicare with social insurance was to increase the sense of entitlement and distance the program from the welfare tradition of alms and charity (Marmor 2000:16). Similarly, establishing Hospital and Supplementary Medical Insurance "trust funds" added to the symbolism of entitlement as well as suggesting that those responsible for administering the program have a fiduciary responsibility—are charged with a trust (Myers 1970:Ch. 2).

Along with the specifically defined and broadly available benefit established by Medicare for beneficiaries, there was a complementary protectiveness of and deference to providers, beginning with the first section of Title 18, which categorically prohibits any interference with the practice of medicine. In the same spirit, the Medicare statute delegated much of the implementation of the statutory provisions to physicians and other providers, to private bodies, or to agencies other than the federal government. Consistent with this approach, the statute adopted the "reasonable costs" and "reasonable charges" familiar to and preferred by providers and the insurance companies. Claims were to be paid and audited, and disputes settled by nominated "intermediaries" and "carriers," which were required to be insurance companies (typically the claims-paying agencies already familiar to the providers). The statute also encouraged extensive consultation with state and local accrediting agencies in determining the "conditions of participation" for Medicare and in making the specific determinations that providers had met those conditions.[6] Already noted was that much of the burden of cost containment was put, not on the providers, but upon the beneficiaries in the form of deductibles, copayments, and limits upon coverage.

A number of the key provisions in the statute and many steps taken in the early implementation are to be explained by a desire to forestall crippling opposition and to get a huge and complex program up and running. For its time, Medicare was a "reach" and it is still inspiring to read the history of these early days (Ball 1993; see also Feder 1977). At the same time, Medicare was viewed with ambivalence, not least within the Department of Health, Education, and Welfare (DHEW)and among others who helped create the program and were engaged in its implementation. Early on, officials within the Social Security Administration (SSA) and members of the Health Insurance Benefits Advisory Council (HIBAC)[7] puzzled over how much to indulge providers in order to get the program firmly established and over how many of the concessions already made to try to win back. As provider fees and aggregate program costs rose, a number of concerned administrators and congressional staff began thinking about what could be done.

Until the 1980s, changes in Medicare were largely incremental in nature, aimed at perfecting in detail and following the basic philosophy of the statute rather than changing it. For instance, the development of the "customary, prevailing, and reasonable" (CPR) limits on physician payment, the provisions for taking assignment[8] by physicians, and even the Medicare Economic Index were largely adapted from private sector practices and consistent with a fee for service (FFS) approach. Cost reimbursement for hospital per diems and "ancillaries"[9] were adapted to fit Medicare patients but otherwise followed accepted industry practices. The Professional Standards Review Organizations (PSROs) were extensions of utilization review mandated by the Medicare statute. During the 1970s there were also various experiments with payment methodology, such as incentive reimbursement for hospitals and attempts at bundling or discounting ancillaries, but none of these produced lasting or significant change.

A notable exception to this pattern was the Social Security Amendments of 1972.[10] Title II of this compendious statute included over ninety different sections dealing with Medicare and Medicaid. A landmark piece of legislation, the 1972 amendments laid out two different paths for tackling reform. One was regulatory: the creation of agencies and authorities such as the PSROs, the Sec. 1122 constraints on hospital capital expenditure for Medicare, and the Medical Economic Index for limiting increases in physician payments.[11] The other was to move toward alternative payment systems with an authorization for research and demonstrations, provisions for "waivered"[12] experiments, and encouragement for Medicare HMOs. In principle, the legislation looked beyond the underlying Medicare FFS method of payment to include and encourage alternative approaches; and many of the most significant Medicare reforms began with or were strongly influenced by research and demonstrations authorized by Secs. 222 and 223 of the amendments of 1972.

The HMO Act of 1973 was not intended as a reform of Medicare but became important over time because of the appeal of managed care and an alternative method of payment. In the early years, most Medicare administrators were fully occupied with nurturing a new program and paid little attention to an option that would affect at most 2–3 percent of the beneficiaries. Largely through the efforts of a few DHEW officials and private sector enthusiasts, a Part C HMO alternative was included in the Social Security Amendments of 1972.[13] The larger importance of the HMO Act, passed in 1973, lay in the capitation approach to payment and the policy and political appeals of this device. For capitation not only helps to contain costs, it shifts risk to the provider and encourages competition and cost-saving innovation. It also frees providers and insurers to manage more freely by getting rid of regulations associated with cost reimbursement and FFS payment. On doctrinal grounds, such an approach was appealing to economists, to those skeptical of regulation and preferring private sector approaches, and to for-profit enterprises. Neither HMOs nor an HMO option for Medicare gained much support in the 1970s. But as health care costs continued to rise and many became disillusioned with regulatory approaches, the HMO option for Medicare grew in appeal—not so much for beneficiaries as for policymakers—especially after 1980.

The Nixon–Ford Economic Stabilization Program (ESP), which lasted from 1971 until discontinued under the Ford administration in 1974, was important less for any lasting legislation than for a bold attempt at price control and the lessons drawn from that initiative. ESP began with a general price freeze in 1972. Under Phase II, which also began in 1972, physicians and hospitals got a separate price control regime that was not notably successful but was important for learning about the theoretical and practical difficulties in developing such a program. Some of the most significant research and experiments in cost containment began then, and much was learned about approaches that would not work (Zubkoff 1976).

Sustained efforts to amend Medicare began after the Carter presidency, and the failure during that administration of efforts at hospital cost containment. One consequence of that failure was to turn attention toward more limited goals: from National Health Insurance [NHI] and attempts to contain hospital costs in general toward "Medicare only" approaches. The prolonged controversy over hospital costs mobilized the hospital constituency and got it thinking in terms of national health policy. And it educated the Congress and left it with a sense of unfinished business. With both general inflation and medical care costs continuing to rise, cost containment became increasingly the central problem of Medicare, while issues of access, beneficiary liability, and quality of care became secondary in importance.

The first major health legislation of the Reagan era was the Tax Equity and Fiscal Responsibility Act of 1982, or TEFRA,[14] which was part of the reconciliation package of 1982. It included three major health care reforms: a hospital cost containment scheme that anticipated the Prospective Payment System (PPS) of 1983; the Professional Review Organizations (PROs), a restructuring of the PSROs established by the Social Security Amendments of 1972; and the authorizing of risk-based Medicare HMOs. Including three different approaches to Medicare cost containment, TEFRA was a remarkable expression of bipartisan resolve. It was notable for two other reasons: the moving cause or occasion for the legislation—distress over the rapidly rising budget deficit; and the first use of budget reconciliation as a vehicle for major health care legislation.

Probably the most important single Medicare reform since the program began in 1966 was the PPS enacted in 1983.[15] It was based upon diagnosis related groups (DRGs) a refined and much researched system for predicting inpatient hospital resource use for particular diagnoses or procedures, such as a kidney infection or a hip replacement. This system made it possible to pay prospectively for a bundle of hospital services and in this respect was a marked departure from the previous cost reimbursement method. The successful enactment of PPS also showed that something of this magnitude could be done, both technically and politically.

With hospital costs addressed—for the time, at least—attention shifted quickly to physician payment as the next likely target. Under consideration as policy vehicles were three approaches. One was "physician DRGs," to extend the PPS approach to cover inpatient physician costs, with the hope of later developing an outpatient methodology. A second option, especially favored by the Reagan administration in keeping with its "procompetition" theme, was capitation, implemented as a payment mechanism through vouchers or some variety of government approved HMO.[16] The third, favored in Congress, was to develop some form of physician fee schedule. None of these approaches seemed initially to offer a solution. The physician DRG approach faded rapidly for technical reasons (Smith 1992:139ff.) Vouchers were anathema to the Democratic Congress; a physician fee schedule was equally unacceptable to the Reagan administration. It took six years to achieve a resolution.

This long period of controversy was notable on two accounts. One was the sharpening of procompetition and proregulation alternatives, so that "fee schedule" and "capitation," by themselves only technical devices, were wrapped in ideology and made part of opposing worldviews. The other was the way in which Congress, relying upon the reconciliation process, moved steadily to regulate physicians' fees anyway, encouraging physician "participation," tinkering with the Medicare Economic Index and "fee freezes," limiting balance billing, and even establishing criteria for "unreasonable charges." Then, in 1986, Congress created the Physician Payment Review Commission, a main purpose of which was to provide technical advice for Congress as it proceeded to develop a physician fee schedule independently of the administration.

Six years after PPS, the Medicare Fee Schedule (MFS) was enacted as part of the Omnibus Budget Reconciliation Act (OBRA) of 1989,[17] with a target date of January 1, 1992, set for implementation. This amendment of Medicare was a technical feat comparable in magnitude to PPS, though less of a departure from the existing payment method. Payment under the MFS was based on "work" and "resources" rather than the "charges" of the existing CPR system, but otherwise followed the FFS approach. A major reason for choosing a "resource-based" approach was to make payment adjustments "fair" for individual physicians, specialties, and regions. An important innovation was to put in place a global restraint on total increases in payment. Its name, "volume performance standard," implicitly recognizes the special weakness of fee schedules: the difficulty of controlling "volume," or increases in number and intensity of services to offset fixed fees. Also significant was the prominence given to research on "appropriateness" of various services and procedures, and using the results of this research to establish practice guidelines, clinical standards, and review criteria.

The MFS was the last major reform prior to the Clinton administration. After 1992, the focus of attention shifted dramatically from Medicare and Medicaid to President Clinton's (and other) proposals for national health insurance. After these initiatives had failed, it was a new world for health policy both because much had changed and, even more, because people perceived reality differently—developments important for understanding Medicare policy during the Clinton administration.

III. MEDICARE AND THE CONTEMPORARY WORLD

One comment by critics of Medicare policy is that too much effort is spent on fixing a 1965 Cadillac. Apt or not, the comparison nicely captures a number of the main grounds for criticism: that the Medicare program is outdated, hard to fix, needlessly expensive, and might be better traded for a new or more suitable model. The alternative suggested is usually some variant of managed care.

In truth, the original designers didn't want "Cadillac" medicine, only care as good as other people got. But they did make it hard to change models, especially by guaranteeing free choice of physician and professional autonomy. These guarantees presumed FFS medicine and a limited range of experimentation. And with the one exception of risk-based Medicare HMOs, all major reforms have assumed the basic FFS model and have built upon that with various schemes of regulation or administered pricing. Not surprisingly, in a consumer, market-oriented environment, more people have begun to question the regulatory emphasis of Medicare and HCFA and to urge that procompetition or private sector remedies be considered more seriously.

Some of their arguments are long-standing. Others date from much more recent experience. But they have in common a theme that the administration of Medicare needs to be "modernized" or brought in line with best practices elsewhere, especially in the private sector.[18]

One persistent complaint is about the "regulatory burden" of FFS Medicare: the general "hassle factor" for providers and the costs and inefficiencies of administering such a program. Unfortunately, this is one of those areas where it is difficult to separate volume of complaint from seriousness of injury, but it is a continuing problem. Important in the present context is the widespread antiregulatory mood and the added fact that health care providers in particular, are heavily burdened by paperwork and regulations. Many people in the government, the provider community, and the private sector believe that the regulatory burden in health care might be eased, made friendlier, or even reduced by methods that rely more on market incentives or private institutions. In this connection, it is perhaps worth recalling that much of the early push that developed in Congress for HMOs and "voucher" type approaches arose as much from a distaste for regulation and the kind of politics it produced as it did from a concern about cost containment.[19]

Another perennial concern that has grown dramatically since 1992 is fraud, waste, and abuse in the Medicare program. One fundamental problem with rules and regulations, especially administered pricing, is their induced effect: people find ways around them. The persistence of fraud, waste, and abuse along with the growth of a whole industry devoted to techniques of gaming the Medicare payment system has been disquieting to various agencies as well as to Congress. Estimates of the losses have ranged from a low of 5 to a high of 20 percent of total program costs. Either figure represents a serious amount of money. The General Accounting Office and the Congress would often exhort HCFA to "modernize" its methods of oversight and, generally, to police the intermediaries and carriers more effectively. But HCFA, which was limited by statute to contracting with insurance companies—practically speaking, the same intermediaries already in place—could do little more than exhort them in turn. Eventually, this pathology was broadly addressed by reforms in 1996 and 1997. Before that, however, it added to a widespread perception that FFS Medicare was generative of fraud, waste, and abuse and that HCFA was lax in seeking to control it.

During this same period of time, doubts grew that Medicare costs could be adequately constrained with the existing institutional arrangements. The Prospective Payment System, for instance, proved good for setting a prospective price and ratcheting down on annual updates, but not easy to extend to cover hospital costs as they were shifted from an inpatient site and "ballooned" outside the hospital (Smith 1992: 115). The Medicare Fee Schedule, good for setting value-based fees and rectifying some inequities in provider payment, has not been equally successful in controlling volume. Meanwhile, Medicare—which from 1984 to 1993 did better than the private sector, in 1994 showed an annual rate of increase substantially higher than the private sector. There are technical issues about how to interpret this development (cf. Levitt, Lazenby, and Sivarajan 1996), but there was justifiable skepticism, on several accounts, about the existing regulatory approach to cost containment and grounds for thinking that the limits of regulatory action may have been reached.

Rising health care prices were also a powerful driving force in the private sector, setting off a series of continuing transformations, beginning in the mid-1980s, that have been variously described as a "minor revolution" or a "new paradigm" (cf. Zelman 1995:5; Etheredge 1995b).

While difficult to characterize or explain adequately, several trends were cooperating and converging. One was a business movement: Fortune 500 corporations and business purchasing alliances, increasingly proactive, often displaced insurance companies, and negotiated with providers for price discounts as well as deciding what health plans employees would be offered. In this market environment, HMOs and other managed care organizations had both incentive and opportunity to innovate, with more effective methods of cost containment and with new and attractive offerings such as preferred provider organizations and "point-of-service" options for employees, and with utilization review and claims auditing services for self-insurers. Closely related was a "quality movement" concerned broadly with quality of care: how to determine appropriate care, how to measure outcomes, and beyond that how to purchase prudently or "buy right." This was a transforming process that, along with the stimulus of rising prices, may well have powered the real "take-off" for managed care.

In any event, perceptions in politics are often more important than reality. And the comparison of traditional FFS Medicare with private sector efforts seemed to be unfavorable. In the private health care market, with traditional indemnity plans becoming prohibitively expensive, private sector employers began to get rid of the FFS plans or reduce them to residual offerings, provide a number of new and attractive choices, and shift a part of the burden of choice and payment to the employees. By such measures, they substantially reduced overall costs. With this kind of comparison, many knowledgeable people—and not just conservative Republicans—thought that maybe the private sector had provided a model worth emulating or, at least, mining for some ideas.

Also important for Medicare policy was the belief that HCFA had acquired over the years an anti-HMO "mind-set," making adaptation to managed care and contemporary trends difficult. Some alleged that HCFA "hates HMOs." More charitably, others said that HCFA was doing what it did well, which was to administer a traditional FFS program, and that it looked benignly upon HMOs but did not push them, since they represented (then) a small fraction of the total number of Medicare beneficiaries.[20] Under the Clinton administration, moreover, HCFA strongly encouraged a number of managed care options. But the conviction that HCFA did better by the FFS program than it did for managed care was hard to dispel and led many both in the health care industry and in Congress to feel that HCFA was not the best agency to lead the Medicare program into the future.

Looking more toward the future, one adaptive challenge for the Medicare program will be covering the costs associated with technological advances—biomedical discoveries, drugs and tools of the medical trade, and new practice applications. Some believe that we are on the threshold of another great wave of technological innovation—a belief made credible to many by the surge in new pharmaceutical products (Schwartz 1994; Goldsmith 1994:80–81). Particular innovations might not cost more and might even save money by substituting drugs or noninvasive exploration for surgical procedures. Capturing those savings, though, would probably require hard choices, imposing management, and educating beneficiaries about their interests and obligations (Goldsmith 1994). Furthermore, the Medicare program is not organized to pursue such activities aggressively, with the delegation of initial coverage decisions to the carriers and a presumption of covering all approved, nonexperimental procedures.

For the longer term, demography will become one of the most powerful forces shaping Medicare policy. We have now had thirty-five years of Medicare. Thirty more years will bring us to the year 2030, when the "baby boomers" will have retired. By then, the changes in age distribution of the population will be quite dramatic, even frightening. In 1995, there were 33.5 million Americans over sixty-five or 12.4 percent of the population. By 2030, that number will have risen to seventy million or 20 percent of the population, and the "very old" (those over eighty-five) will have doubled. Meanwhile, the number of active workers contributing to the trust funds will have dropped from 3.3 to 2 workers per beneficiary (Moon and Davis 1995:31; Waite 1996:220). These demographic numbers pose not so much a problem of management as one of how Medicare fits within a total program of elder care and how to apportion costs between generations.

In the decade from 1985 to 1995, much thought was being given to the future of Medicare, ways to protect the budget and save money, "modernize" the program and take advantage of private sector innovations, and even explore radically different alternatives, such as an FEHBP defined contribution option. Against this were the facts that the standard FFS Medicare continued to be enormously popular with the beneficiaries, who overwhelmingly chose this option—with its gaps in coverage, deductibles and copays—rather than managed care. The FFS program was also preferred by providers, especially physicians and hospitals. Over time, moreover, it did as well on costs as managed care, in spite of large subsidies for special groups such as primary care physicians, "disproportionate share" hospitals, and medical schools, as well as a considerable amount of fraud, waste, and abuse. In sum, there were many problems with the Medicare program, but it was not "broke" and among beneficiaries and providers there was little will to fix it.

IV. MEDICAID—PERENNIAL ISSUES AND REFORM EFFORTS

Title 19 of the Social Security Amendments of 1965 bears the caption, "Grants to the States for Programs of Medical Assistance," a heading expressive of the basic features of the Medicaid program. It grew out of some thirty years of experience with federal and state public assistance activities,[21] which funded limited amounts of medical care for various categories of needy people, either through direct (cash) or vendor payments. Medicaid support was largely confined to categories eligible for matching under the Social Security Act: families with children (typically single-parent) and the aged, blind, and disabled. Recipients were "means-tested"—they had to meet income and resource standards, though states could also qualify the "medically needy," those whose medical expenditures would put them within state eligibility limits. Those enrolled for public assistance under one of these categories qualified automatically for Medicaid. But the determination of categorical eligibility, the administration of the Medicaid program, and the provision of medical services beyond a federally mandated minimum were up to the individual states so long as they conformed with broad federal guidelines, designated a single state agency, and submitted an approved plan. Federal matching support varied for each state, from a minimum of 50 to a maximum of 83 percent, according to per capita income within the particular state.

From the beginning the Medicaid program was both popular and problematic. Thirty-seven of forty-eight states joined in the first eighteen months, some of them opting for the full range of optional services and increasing eligibility with liberal definitions of "medically needy" (U.S. Congress, Senate 1970:esp. Ch. 2; see also U.S. Congress 1993:26–37). Initially Medicaid was more expensive than anticipated and, generally, has continued to be so. Like most categorical programs, there was steady pressure to add to or broaden categories, to expand coverage and improve services, and to maintain balance or equity between groups. At the same time, there was great variation in services provided and in state standards for eligibility and allowable maximum income and resource retention.

Early on, several persistent themes emerged in the evolution of the Medicaid program. One was to complete an unfinished work: adding details of implementation, setting standards of care or categorical limits to eligibility, and giving substance to established benefits. A second theme was to expand eligibility and coverage beyond that established in the original statute: for instance, including pregnant mothers or nursing home residents; adding preventive benefits or posthospital care; and selectively extending federal matching. Both for the federal and the state governments, cost containment was a perennial issue, rising at times to crisis levels, especially in times of recession or fiscal stringency. Add to this that the Medicaid program covered eventually all the states and four territories with their variations of local culture, population groups, economic circumstance, and administrative competence and it is easy to see why Medicaid officials describe the program as "complicated."

When initially passed, the Medicaid title was a much less finished statutory product than Medicare. Even as implementation of the program began, the House was holding hearings on amendments and additions needed immediately or in the near future. Meanwhile, state and federal officials, governors, and members of Congress were concerned both about rapidly increasing costs and about the quality of nursing home care.[22] Both these issues were addressed in the Social Security Amendments of 1967.[23] Rising program costs were dealt with primarily by limiting eligibility for the medically needy. According to the new legislation, states could not set upper income limits higher than 133 percent of their own AFDC standard for a family of four. Practically, states could still raise limits for the medically needy, but only by increasing their own cash assistance programs. With respect to long-term care, federal standards were established for skilled nursing homes and states mandated to license programs for training nursing home administrators.

Two other provisions of the 1967 Amendments broadened or improved benefits. One was a "free choice" option, stating that beneficiaries could get covered services from any qualified provider that "undertakes" to provide that service, freeing beneficiaries from dependence on the states' traditional vendor payment arrangements. The second, Early and Periodic Screening, Diagnosis and Treatment (EPSDT), mandated state programs under which eligible children, up to the age of twenty-one, could be screened for medical deficiencies or chronic conditions and referred for treatment for those conditions discovered.

The Social Security Amendments of 1972 were of considerable importance for Medicaid, although their unintended consequences proved, eventually, to be more important than the intended ones. One category of amendments addressed the problem of rising costs, especially by adapting for Medicaid sev-

eral measures that applied mainly to the Medicare program: directing states
to make use of the PSROs and to develop utilization control programs of their
own; subjecting Medicaid facilities to regional comprehensive health planning; and authorizing start-up funds for Medicaid HMOs in hopes that managed care would control costs (U.S. Congress 1993:31). The amendments also
included steps to ease some of the cost pressures on the states. A mandate that
states move toward increasingly comprehensive programs by broadening the
scope of services and liberalizing eligibility requirements was completely
revoked. Also terminated was a "maintenance of effort" requirement prohibiting states from reducing aggregate expenditure for their share of a supported program. With the exception of health planning, which did slow the
increase in nursing home beds, most of these measures had little short-term
effect on Medicaid program costs.

Of much greater consequence was the impact of the 1972 amendments on
long-term institutional care. The amendments created the Supplemental
Security Income (SSI) program, which "federalized" the adult welfare categories of aged, blind, and disabled, leaving AFDC with the states. The federal
poverty level then became the test for eligibility, including Medicaid. Meanwhile, in 1971 and 1972, Congress added optional services and coverage for
"intermediate care facilities,"[24] first for the elderly and then for long-term psychiatric patients and persons who were mentally retarded. The cumulative
effect of these changes was to add to Medicaid a large number of long-term,
costly patients, increasing total program costs and dramatically shifting the
balance of expenditures between the elderly and disabled and other Medicaid
beneficiaries. By 1987, for instance, this population, which represented 28
percent of recipients, generated 73 percent of Medicaid expenditures, while
the AFCD population, which was 66 percent of Medicaid recipients, used only
25 percent of the services (Oberg and Polich 1988:87).

Program spending during the 1970s rose at an annual rate of 17.3 percent
(U.S. Congress 1993:32), more than quadrupling in a decade. Most of this
growth resulted from general inflation and rising medical costs rather than
increased services per beneficiary (ibid.). But the mood in Congress, especially
in the latter half of the decade, was more that of cost containment than of program enhancement, and two of the approaches encouraged during this period
were, ultimately, to be of great consequence.

One such approach was to attack fraud and abuse, always good in principle,
and acquiring political visibility from several scandals especially relating to
Medicaid HMOs. During the Carter administration, the topic gained added
prominence as a preliminary to a national health insurance initiative. The legislation that resulted, the Medicare–Medicaid Anti-Fraud and Abuse Amendments of 1977[25] were more bark than bite—announcing penalties but
making little provision for enforcement. The legislation did introduce many
of the concepts and established precedents for the future. It also authorized
funding for state Medicaid fraud control units. A companion measure required

states to develop computerized Medicaid management information systems. Though initially the impact of this legislation was small, some twenty-odd years later the fraud and abuse program appears to have become remarkably effective.

Another approach gaining favor was the use of alternative payment systems, especially capitation and HMOs. While the intent of the Medicaid law was that hospital and nursing home providers be paid their full cost, some states from the beginning had contracted with managed care plans. Also, payment methods for the "medically needy" allowed for some variation. At the same time, there had been HMO scandals in the 1970s, especially in California and Florida, some involving organized crime. Moreover, capitation for a Medicaid population seemed inherently prone to abuse because of the incentives to "underserve." Initially, the federal approach was incremental and gingerly: supporting some demonstrations in the states and establishing a limited option in the HMO amendments of 1976, which restricted beneficiaries to federally qualified HMOs with not more than 50 percent Medicaid enrollees.[26]

A novel and not entirely successful attempt to encourage modifications of reimbursement methodology was the Boren Amendment, part of the Omnibus Reconciliation Act of 1980[27] This legislation provided that states could set rates for SNFs and ICFs, independently of the prescribed cost-reimbursement methods, so long as the rates were "reasonable and adequate to meet the costs" of "effective and economic" operation in conformity with relevant laws, regulations, and safety and quality standards. The states had to file a plan with the secretary of DHHS and make assurances and "findings" that the plan would fulfill such requirements. Within these limits, they could operate with considerable freedom, both from existing cost-reimbursement methods and from the secretary's guidelines. In the following year the same concepts were applied to hospitals, adding that the rates established had to take into account the needs of hospitals serving a "disproportionate share" of poor or special needs patients and to assure that "individuals eligible for medical assistance" would have access to inpatient services of "adequate quality."

The Boren Amendment did encourage experimentation, most states adopting various alternative payment methods, especially for nursing homes. Yet language like "reasonable and adequate" and "findings" resonates in the law, and the Boren Amendments were highly productive of lawsuits by institutional providers, with the somewhat paradoxical result that legislation intended to free the states made some of them timid in their experimentation and a proviso designed, at least in part, to protect beneficiaries has diverted funds to institutional providers and away from community-based practitioners and their patients. In 1990, the U.S. Supreme Court in a 5–4 decision upheld federal jurisdiction over such law suits under 42 U.S.C. 1983, prompting derisive comment about the civil rights of hospitals.[28] In any event, the Boren Amendment was repealed by BBA 97.

The Omnibus Budget Reconciliation Act of 1981[29] swept Medicaid into the grand strategies of the first Reagan administration, one of which was to use budget reconciliation to shrink and restructure domestic programs. As part of a package of domestic cuts, Medicaid increases would be capped at the rate of growth of the gross domestic product (GDP), a drastic reduction that was modified by the House.[30] To enable states to meet this target, they were allowed more freedom in restructuring their programs: by extending the Boren amendment to hospitals, and by creating new 1915 (b) and 1915 (c) waivers for managed care and home and community-based experiments. Penalties for failure to implement the EPSDT program were abolished; and states were given added freedom to reduce coverage for "medically needy" beneficiaries (U.S. Congress 1993:35).

The combined efforts of the federal government and the states had a profound impact on the Medicaid program, especially between 1981 and 1984. Factors other than Medicaid program changes were at work: a decline in both general and medical inflation; and changes in AFDC and SSDI eligibility rules. But there was real and drastic program shrinkage. Spending for FY 1981 through FY 1984 dropped to a 7 percent annual rate of increase from a previous average of 17 percent. Relative to those living in poverty, the number of Medicaid beneficiaries also dropped to a historic low in 1983 (ibid.:37); and Medicaid spending for AFDC children in poverty, relative to other Medicaid recipients, hit another low in 1984 (Oberg and Polich 1988:87). In other words, reduction was both shrinking total expenditures and moving the program farther from its original mission of providing medical care for welfare recipients, especially families with dependent children.

But 1984 marked a turning point and the beginning of a remarkable transformation of the Medicaid program through a steady accumulation of incremental changes that started in that year and extended through 1990. For the most part, these changes originated in the House Commerce Committee and were enacted through a series of budget reconciliations. In sum, they slowed the momentum and reversed the direction of change initiated by the Reagan administration. They also shifted Medicaid program emphasis away from welfare categorical eligibility toward the health needs of people—especially women, children, and the aged—who lived below the federal poverty line, gradually broadening eligibility, increasing coverage, and raising quality.

The Deficit Reduction Act of 1984[31] began the process by requiring states to cover pregnant women who met income standards for AFDC but were not for various reasons—such as not already being a mother—receiving welfare payments. Thereafter, eligibility was broadened in stepwise fashion, setting new requirements but allowing states to go higher with a federal match, then once again raising the mandated levels. In this manner, coverage for pregnant women and children was extended up to 133 percent of the federal poverty line with optional limits raised to 185 percent of poverty. Mandates for children living in poverty began with birth to age one, then crept up to five and six, and eventually to nineteen years of age. States were also permitted to extend Medicaid coverage to the elderly and disabled with incomes too high for SSI but below the federal poverty line.

Along with this extension of coverage, Congress moved in a similar fashion to increase or enhance benefits for the Medicaid beneficiaries. The list of required benefits was increased, especially to meet the needs of underserved or remote populations.[32] In OBRA 89, EPSDT was revitalized and states were required not only to provide screening and diagnosis for children under twelve living in poverty, but to treat any physical or mental deficiencies found, even though the services required were not covered by the state Medicaid program. Other benefits were made eligible for optional coverage, such as case management, hospice for the terminally ill, and home and community-based services for the frail elderly. And states were required to cover premiums and cost sharing for the elderly poor, up to and eventually beyond the federal poverty line.[33]

Congress acted in a variety of ways to assure more acceptable levels of quality for Medicaid services generally. States were required to pay rates sufficient to attract providers and maintain adequate access to care, and to make payments to disproportionate-share institutions. Medicaid HMOs were subjected to independent audits and made liable to civil monetary penalties for underserving beneficiaries. Most comprehensive were the nursing home reforms of 1987,[34] which established standards for scope of services, levels and quality of staffing, residents' rights, and physical facilities. These were sufficiently elaborate that Congress required the states to make additional payments to the nursing facilities to offset the expense.

These congressional reforms, seen by many in Washington as a great legislative achievement, were not unanimously acclaimed in the states, where Medicaid had once again become a large and rapidly growing budget item (Rowland, Feder, and Salganicoff 1993:Ch. 7). Aside from the "out-of-control" finances of Medicaid, state officials had, by 1990, real and important complaints. One was, simply, that too much was dictated by Washington or HCFA without enough intergovernmental collaboration. Many who had supported and welcomed the severing of Medicaid from welfare categories were unhappy at the number of options turned into mandates and the "strings" that accompanied federal funds.[35] They felt both harassed and fiscally damaged by provider lawsuits, increasing rapidly as a result of court interpretations of the Boren Amendment, and they were squeezed by a deteriorating economy, swelling welfare rolls, and rising medical costs. Governors, legislators, and officials who had worked long years to improve the Medicaid program in their own states and who had supported many of the federal changes felt ill-used and complained of both injury and insult.[36]

These state and Medicaid officials responded to the rising program costs in a number of ways. One was to protest, with increasing stridency, the number of mandates from Congress. Reluctant to decrease Medicaid, both because of its popularity and its draw on federal dollars, some states raised taxes. A number also cut discretionary items in the budget, such as higher education and welfare. Cost containment was not an especially effective alternative, in part because of existing mandates and the prospect of Boren amendment lawsuits, but states were able to realize some incremental savings through reducing physician payments, cutting optional services and introducing copays, and expanding the use of managed care. By far the most lucrative recourse was to draw down more federal money through various schemes to increase matching funds—getting the federal government to share more of their common burden (Rowland, Feder, and Salganicoff 1993:34ff.).

One popular strategy was to use provider taxes or donations—from hospitals, nursing homes, or other providers—to finance some part of a state's Medicaid program and count these amounts as state program expenses toward the federal match. The additional federal payments could then be used either to fund the state Medicaid program generally, as "enhanced" payments to specific providers, or as part of a disproportionate share pool.[37] This practice, which the federal government had earlier condoned or encouraged on a small scale, grew rapidly after 1987, reaching dramatic proportions by 1991. In that year, the Congressional Research Service estimated that payments for disproportionate-share and provider tax and donation schemes would reach a total of between $23 and $25 billion, roughly 34 percent of total projected Medicaid expenditures. Late in 1991, though, Congress acted to curb these practices. Provider taxes were limited to 25 percent as contributions to a state match, and donations could not be counted. DSH funds were capped at 12 percent of total Medicaid expenditures, with individual state limits to be set in 1992. The loophole was reduced in diameter, though not closed and states have continued to devise similar schemes to increase their Medicaid funding.

By 1992, the Medicaid program had been greatly transformed and enhanced, with increased benefits for women and children, the elderly and disabled, and ties to welfare eligibility loosened, it had become in many ways a national program for the poor and medically needy. Yet great inequities remained, and the states grumbled at mandates, fiscal burdens, and outdated matching formulas. Meanwhile, Medicaid expenditures continued to rise—by 11.9 percent in 1990, 30.1 percent in 1991, and 30 percent in 1992, reaching $114 billion in that year (Rowland et al. 1993:23).

Health Care Reform and Aftermath

From 1992 though 1994 the debate over national health insurance (NHI), or "health care reform," dominated federal health policy. It was a central issue during the 1992 presidential campaign, and within the Clinton administration the main agenda item once deficit reduction legislation passed.[38]

Medicare and Medicaid, which were to have been folded into the Health Security Act, figured only incidentally in the debates.

This is not the place to rehearse in detail the problems with the various NHI proposals, but some of the observations about the administration's "Health Security Act" are pertinent to later health policy developments. Of the administration plan, its advocates and its opponents alike said that the administration "tried to go too far, too fast, and without explaining it to the American people." Other observations were that it was "too big and complicated," that the "numbers never added up," that it misjudged opinion about health insurance, and that the timing was bad. One comprehensive account blamed the American political system (Johnson and Broder 1996) and another the legacy of the Reagan era (Skocpol 1996). The demise of the Health Security Act and the general failure of health care reform were probably "overdetermined" outcomes for which there was, without much doubt, plenty of blame to apportion. However one sees this history, many who participated in this experience were also involved in the later controversies over Medicare and Medicaid. The health care reform episode affected these later events in various ways—a carryover of participants and policy options, attitudes and tactics, and political backlash with its electoral consequences.

Health care reform relied heavily upon a campaign mode of policymaking, with most of what that entails. In the first and most obvious sense, it grew out of a presidential campaign and was both promoted and attacked with the broad ideological appeals, mobilization strategies, and the zeal that goes into such campaigns. Health care reform also resembled a military campaign, with emphasis upon strategy and tactics, secrecy and noncollaboration, and plotting for the ultimate destruction of an adversary. Not surprisingly, the campaign wore people out and spent their reserves of energy and morale.

Collegiality and institutional values suffered. The administration developed its proposal through a large, secret task force, working outside the Congress. Separate committees in the House and Senate, groups, and even individual legislators worked on reform proposals of their own. Partisanship, factionalism, and individualism all increased during this episode. Within the House, health care reform helped unify opposition under the leadership of Newt Gingrich and the conservatives. Among members departing the Senate—some of whom were strongly bipartisan in health policy—a common complaint was loss of collegiality and the rise of incivility and partisanship. A big loser was the tradition of bipartisan collaboration in health policy.

One positive contribution of health care reform is that it canvassed the policy options and put many of them on the public agenda for the first time. Managed competition was extensively debated along with "single-payer" schemes and "vouchers." Various combinations of taxes and mandates were explored. Adaptations of existing programs that were considered then figured prominently in later debates over Medicare. One such proposal was to adopt the Federal Employee Health Benefits Program as a model for national health insurance.[39] Another was to use Medicare as a basis for a comprehensive national program by expanding Part C.[40] Medical savings accounts were discussed as an option especially suitable for an individual mandate. The Health Security Act included prescription drugs and increased benefits for mental health and for women and children—all items for later agendas. It also contained provisions for malpractice and antitrust reform and a strengthened fraud and abuse program.

Like campaigns generally—political or military—health care reform produced its veterans: those who lived through it and remembered. From both sides of this struggle, there were cadres remaining with a knowledge of the issues, with official and political lines of communication, and with experience in the tactics and strategy of this kind of campaign. This may have been a factor that worked, later, to the advantage of the Democrats. A number of their veterans, having come to Washington for the big event, were unusually talented and energetic. They learned about operating in the campaign mode of policymaking during health care reform. And some of them were not entirely unhappy, later on, at the development of a "payback" opportunity.

Health care reform was also a contributing factor in the midterm election of 1994—a sweeping victory for the Republicans. How much of this dramatic shift was attributable to health care reform is debatable.[41] But a number of Republican leaders treated the election as a plebiscite on "big government" and the administration's "failed" domestic policies, of which health care reform was a prime example. So it was effective in helping Republicans to unite and mobilize partisan energy. And the inglorious demise of health care reform just before the election seemed significant as well as leaving the Democrats divided and low in spirit.

Just prior to the midterm election of 1994, over three hundred House Republican candidates and incumbents signed a Contract with America designed to "change the nation" (Gillespie and Schellhas 1994; see also Gingrich 1995). In the ensuing election, the Republicans won decisively in every region except the Northeast—a victory that could plausibly be seen as a mandate on the order of the New Deal election of 1932 or the Great Society election of 1964. Republicans retook the House after forty years, adding fifty-three seats. In the Senate, which Republicans had held only twice in sixty years, they won all the open seats and defeated two incumbent Democrats for a gain of eight. No Republican incumbent, either in the House or Senate, was defeated. In the popular vote, Republicans gained nine million over their 1990 vote while Democrats lost one million. Certainly, there was a message here.

Whether or not the election represented a mandate for fundamental change, the newly elected House majority, led by Newt Gingrich, acted as though it did and began organizing with that aim in mind. Meeting in Washington, December 5–7, the House Republican conference elected Gingrich as speaker, followed by Dick Armey (Tex.) as majority leader and Tom Delay (Tex.) as chief whip. Seniority was overridden in chairmanships for three key committees: Robert Livingston (La.) for Appropriations, Thomas Bliley (Va.) for Commerce, and Henry Hyde (Ill.) for Judiciary. Freshmen were given a large number of seats on these committees and on Budget and Rules, and several named as subcommittee chairmen. These and various procedural changes strengthened both party leadership and the position of the Speaker.

On January 4, the first day of the new Congress, Speaker Gingrich held the House in session until 2:24 the next morning—an unprecedented but carefully rehearsed scenario—while the Republicans made a down payment on the Contract with America by amending many of the rules and procedures of the House. They ratified nominations of the earlier caucus. Changes were made in committee jurisdiction and a number of committees and subcommittees abolished—especially patronage committees favored by Democrats. Committee staffs—seen as distracting sources of unwanted policy proposals—were cut by one-third, a move later to hurt the Republicans themselves.[42] Term limits were imposed upon committee chairmen, subcommittee chairmen, and the speaker—six years for them and eight for the speaker. After fourteen and a half hours, eight roll call votes, and over two hundred resolutions, the speaker banged his gavel, closing the first day. Most of these changes were minor, but some—such as term limits for chairmen and a three-fifths majority to raise taxes—were of grave import. Not a single Republican voted against any of the resolutions—displaying a discipline and resolution described by Democrats as "awesome."

For the next hundred days, the House agenda was the Contract with America. The ten articles in the Contract—selected largely for their vote-getting appeal—contained scores of provisions ranging from a balanced budget amendment and congressional term limits to tax cuts and entitlements, regulatory reform, crime prevention, and national security. At the one hundred–day mark, the House had passed all of the Contract items except term limits,[43] again displaying almost flawless discipline. Yet little of this ever became law, either as part of the Contract or as separate bills. The most important provisions—such as the Balanced Budget Amendment, a middle-class tax cut, product liability, welfare block grants, and the missile defense—either lost in the Senate or because of presidential intervention (Drew 1996:363, 364). And the biggest substantive change—the line item veto—was of little benefit to Republicans.

At the same time, the Contract with America did serve admirably its main political objective, which was to mobilize and unify Republicans in support of the campaign-style politics adopted by the Republican House leadership, Newt Gingrich in particular. A major reason for promoting the Contract idea, according to Gingrich,[44] was to nationalize the midterm elections and turn them into a plebiscite: the Clinton administration or the Republicans (Gingrich 1995). The Contract items grew out of a Republican agenda, but they were also chosen for their popularity and their unambiguous appeal to conservatives and disaffected voters. Once in power, these Contract items had strong appeal to the huge and largely conservative cohort of House freshmen Republicans. Also, for a party long in opposition, it was a ready agenda and a mobilizing and unifying device—like a short and splendid war. And the aura of invincibility impressed both Republicans and Democrats—perhaps too much in both instances.

With benefit of hindsight, there were a number of reasons to believe that the new Republican majority was less than invincible. For an item, the majorities were not overwhelming. In the House, even with enormous electoral gains and five postelection Democratic defections, the Republicans had a majority of only thirty-six—too small to survive significant defections and far from enough to override a veto. Of that majority, seventy-four were freshmen, long on conservative ideology and agenda, but short on experience or institutional wisdom. Moreover, the Senate never underwent a comparable "revolution." Even with the addition of two Democratic defections, the Republicans had only fifty-four Senate seats, a number of them held by moderates or relatively liberal Senators. And in the Senate, there was no major organizational change, overriding of seniority, or strengthening of the leadership. Indeed, the biggest change of this sort was to elect Trent Lott as chief whip rather than Alan Simpson, intentionally weakening Robert Dole, the new majority leader.[45] Despite urging from House leadership, the Senate refused to sign the Contract with America. Instead, Senate Republicans developed a seven-point "Advertisement," an "Agenda for the Republican Majority"—by comparison, a "political dwarf"—and passed some proposals of their own.[46] Several of the most important House bills stalled in the Senate, and a number of Senators allowed that they had never signed any contract and looked with disdain upon the freshmen and the "Newtoids" in the House.

Medicare was specifically omitted from the Contract with America, recognizing the size and complexity of the program and reserving it for the coming and decisive struggle over the budget (Drew 1996:138). Nevertheless, the Contract was important for the future of both Medicare and Medicaid. The first items in the Contract were the Balanced Budget Amendment and the line item veto, important tools for deficit reduction. And the block grant proposal for welfare would have ended one entitlement: a way to save money and to begin dismantling the welfare state. Including these items in the Contract imputed to them some elements of legitimacy as the fulfillment of promises made to the American people. It also tended to associate expenditure reduction and restructuring of these programs, especially in the House, with a campaign mode style of legislation, helping to sustain and direct the mobilized energy. These were good tactics, recalling Nietzsche's aphorism about the good fight that justifies any cause.[47] But they may be better for a coordinated assault than for a continuing struggle.

NOTES

[1] "Medicare" had also been used as the title for Truman's ill-fated national health insurance proposal in 1950.

[2] With acknowledgments to my good friend, Dick Hegner, for calling this article to my attention.

[3] Initially states covered four historic "cash assistance" categories of Families with Dependent Children, Old-Age Assistance, the Blind, and the Permanently and Totally Disabled, plus an optional category of the "medically indigent," those whose medical expenses would put them under a state-determined poverty line (Myers 1970:268).

[4] Cf. Social Security Amendments of 1965, P.L. 39-97, esp. Sec. 1801 and Sec. 1802.

[5] The civil rights struggle was in full course at the time and steps to assure equal access for poor and elderly blacks was one of the nobler battles fought in the implementation of Medicare and Medicaid.

[6] I. S. Falk, an important figure in the genesis and implementation of Medicare is reported to have described Medicare as "the only legislation, the details of which were entirely designed by its enemies." Karl Yordy, Institute of Medicine. Interview, September 9, 1987.

[7] HIBAC was appointed from groups affected by Medicare to advise the Social Security Administration on the implementation of Medicare. Its role was especially important on such key issues as conditions of participation, utilization review and cost control, and payment and accounting practices. It was abolished in 1983 when the Prospective Payment System was established.

[8] Agreement by a physician to payment allowed by a third party as payment in full, i.e., to forgo balance billing.

[9] Ancillaries were hospital services or supplies provided in addition to the standard per diem charges for the room, food, nursing, and some routine services. Ancillaries were a particular problem because, like an a la carte menu, the number of items or their individual prices could be easily increased by the provider and billed to the patient or insurer.

[10] P.L. 92-60 (Oct. 30, 1972).

[11] An index of physician inputs and expenses constructed by the government and used since 1973 as an aide in controlling Medicare cost increases.

[12] The secretary of the Department of Health and Human Services (DHHS) may waive various statutory requirements in order to allow states to experiment with innovative Medicaid programs.

[13] Sec. 1876, added to Title XVII. Included in the initiating group were John Veneman, a Nixon political appointee; Tom Joe, a welfare policy specialist; and Paul Ellwood MD, then executive director of the American Rehabilitation Foundation (Brown 1983:205, 206).

[14] P.L. 97-248 (1982).

[15] Social Security Amendments of 1983, P.L. 98-21 (Smith 1992).

[16] For example, the TEFRA "competitive medical plans" (CMPs)—health plans that did not meet the standards for federally qualified HMOs but were allowed to enter into Medicare risk contracts.

[17] P.L. 101-239.

[18] Many GAO reports have dealt with this topic, but see in particular U.S. General Accounting Office (1996b). See also Reischauer, Butler, and Lave (1998).

[19] Including, for example, both David Stockman and Richard Gephardt.

[20] Peter Bouxsein, Institute of Medicine. Former deputy director of Office of Managed Care, HCFA. Interview, August 1, 1996.

[21] Beginning with the Federal Emergency Relief Administration, 1933–35.

[22] Cf. Myers's (1970) description of Medicaid administration in New York State, esp. Ch. 13.

[23] P.L. 90-248.

[24] Intermediate Care Facilities (ICFs) were first established by the Social Security Amendments of 1967 as a less expensive (and less regulated) alternative for persons not needing full nursing care. (Stevens and Stevens 1974:120).

[25] P.L. 95-142.

[26] The 50 percent requirement was intended to protect quality. To attract at least 50 percent of non-Medicaid enrollees, the HMO would, presumably, have to be of reasonably high quality.

[27] P.L. 96-499.

[28] Sec. 1983 suits derive, remotely, from the Civil Rights Act of 1871, which was intended originally to reach "night riders" such as members of the Ku Klux Klan. Wilder v. Virginia Hospital Association, 110 S.Ct. 2510 (1990). On the Boren amendments generally, see Rowland, Feder, and Salganicoff (1993:Ch. 4).

[29] P.L. 97-35, Aug. 13, 1981.

[30] Changed to three years at the medical CPI with penalties for exceeding that rate of growth.

[31] DEFRA, P.L. 98-369.

[32] For example, creating the Federally Qualified Health Centers (1989), which considerably enhanced existing efforts in poor and rural areas.

[33] Under the Qualified Medicare Beneficiary (QMB) program, which was mandated by the Medicare Catastrophic Coverage Act of 1988. The QMB program was continued and expanded, even though the MCCA was repealed.

[34] In the Omnibus Budget Reconciliation Act of 1987, P.L. 100-203.

[35] There was much talk at the time about "unfunded mandates," but these applied mostly to environment, disability, and fair labor standards. Medicaid mandates were "funded" in the sense that a match accompanied most of them; but there were regulations and many of the mandates were federal requirements that states would have preferred to decide for themselves.

[36] Ray Sheppach, National Governors' Association. Interview, June 16, 1999.

[37] Disproportionate-share payments for hospitals serving a "disproportionate" number of Medicaid patients originated in 1981. The use of DSH pools as a way of maximizing Medicaid payments became a major problem in 1990 and beyond.

[38] Omnibus Budget Reconciliation Act of 1993, P.L. 103-96.

[39] Proposed by the Heritage Foundation and sponsored in the Senate by Don Nickles (R., Okla.) (Johnson and Broder 1996:365).

[40] HR 3600, the Stark-Gibbons bill. It was reported out of committee by a narrow 20–18 margin but never debated on the floor.

[41] Behind the Republican victory in 1994 was a long history of cultivating attractive candidates and nursing key constituencies. By November 1994, a number of issues also favored Republicans (e.g., the crime bill, taxes) and Democrats had lost some of their core support over NAFTA and the tax legislation of 1993. Also, Republicans mobilized their base by hitting hard some hot issues while Democratic turnout was low. Cf. "Rare Combination of Forces Makes '94 Vote Historic," Congressional Quarterly Almanac (1994), p. 561.

[42] Another reason was to curb the power of committee and subcommittee chairmen. Personal staffs were not touched.

[43] The House passed the Balanced Budget Amendment, but lacked the two-thirds necessary to send it to the states.

[44] Especially Reagan Democrats and Ross Perot supporters.

[45] A move attributable in large measure to Phil Gramm's presidential aspirations and desire to weaken Dole's support.

[46] *Congressional Quarterly,* September 24, 1994, p. 2712, and February 25, 1995, p. 578.

[47] "Ye say it is the good cause which halloweth even war? I say unto you: it is the good war which halloweth every cause." Thus Spake Zarathustra, I, Ch. 10.

3

Medicaid and the
Balanced Budget Act of 1995

Those who were there, in the House of Representatives early in 1995, comment upon the revolutionary mood and expectations of Republicans and the demoralization and lack of direction on the part of the Democrats. By the same time the following year, the situation was much changed—with Democrats mobilized and, for them, relatively united and with Republicans in disarray and low in morale. The large and visible reason for this reversal of fortunes was President Clinton's vetoes, the winter shutdown of the federal government, and the Republican failure to prevail in the confrontation. In the final showdown, deficit reduction numbers, a tax cut, and Medicare were the big issues. But Medicaid politics and the opposition to block-granting and cutting the program by $184 billion over seven years helped rally the Democrats, develop strategies, win some early victories, and sustain the resolve to fight.

An important, even fateful, Republican decision was to schedule Medicaid before Medicare on the House agenda, largely because it seemed an easier target. This ordering meant taking up Medicaid at a time when House Democrats were still disunited and struggling to organize and agree on their own set of priorities. As one result, Democratic party leadership played less of a role. Absent a strong party voice, though, the constitutional checks of federalism, bicameralism, and separation of power still operated, much as Madison originally thought they would in his "compound Republick."[1] In fact, they seemed especially effective for policies involving Medicaid, which were technical and largely nonpartisan in nature but touched upon fundamental values such as entitlement and the constitutional politics of federal-state relations. Also, having controlled the Congress for most of the past forty years, the Democrats had valuable experience in how these institutions could be used to advantage.

Taking on Medicaid first had a further advantage for the Democrats of allowing them to regroup, devise ways to counter or contain Republican initiatives, and put in place the key elements of an overall strategy. When the Republicans began putting together their 1995 budget resolution, early in March, neither the congressional Democrats nor the Clinton administration had decided whether or how to save Medicaid. By November, both the president and the Democrats in Congress were united on a do-or-die defense of both the Medicare and Medicaid entitlements. Along this path, successes in fighting for Medicaid helped unify the Democrats, improve their strategy, and strengthen their resolve. Moreover, this particular battle persuaded many Republicans that doing away with the Medicaid entitlement might not be worth the effort and political costs. The episode permanently removed the luster associated with this particular initiative.

I. BACKGROUND AND EARLY MOVES

The Medicaid entitlement, though vital to its beneficiaries and important for this account, was one relatively small part of the budget reconciliation, otherwise known as the Balanced Budget Act (BBA) of 1995. This was a huge undertaking, the centerpiece for the 1995 session of Congress. But that act was itself only a vehicle for larger goals shared by many Republicans, especially those associated with Newt Gingrich, the new speaker. Moved by this shared vision, the legislative process in the House took on qualities of a campaignlike mobilization. A sense of the dynamics of this mobilization helps to understand both the behavior of the legislators and the importance of the struggle over the Medicaid entitlement.

The charismatic, revolutionary leadership of Newt Gingrich provided much of the direction and energy for the supercharged House agenda of 1995. He spoke often of revolution and of transforming America.[2] To do that he would rebuild the Republican party and make the House and its speaker once more the energetic center of government, challenging the presidency.[3] And like great leaders, he had both vision and the ability to translate that vision into compelling strategies and practical institutional forms.[4] He planned for and, more than any other man, brought about the Republican House victory of 1994. He remade the Republican House leadership and the office of speaker, pushed through the Contract with America, and took full charge of the House legislative agenda.[5] He not only rivaled the president, he seemed the more powerful figure. At times he stumbled, even blundered,[6] but for much of the year he seemed invincible. And Democrats were uncertain whether to fight, strike a deal, or flee for cover.

An important resource for the leadership program was the freshman Republican class—long on enthusiasm and short on experience. They arrived boasting about cutting the federal government down to size, completing the Reagan revolution, and doing away with entitlements, the Great Society, and even the New Deal. Almost every member of this group was indebted to Gingrich, either for personal assistance or support from GOPAC.[7] Among the seventy-three freshmen Republicans, sixty-five were challengers who had unseated Democrats—and felt especially called upon to make a difference (Fenno 1997:29ff.). Less than half of them had any previous electoral experience and only seven had ever served in a governing legislative majority. In comparison with other freshmen cohorts, there were fewer graduate degrees, fewer lawyers, and many more representatives of small business. Many thought of themselves as "citizen representatives," there to get the job done and then return home (ibid.:26). As a group, they were a source of enormous energy—useful if channeled, but destructive if not.

A major factor in consolidating leadership was the accession to power, along with Gingrich, of House Republican members who had long opposed the "accommodationist," go-along philosophy of the Republican minority, in favor of an openly confrontational style and contesting with the Democrats for power (ibid.:9). A number from this group, elected to key party posts or appointed by the speaker to strategic committee chairs, provided a cadre of energetic leaders. At the same time, the unprecedented number of freshmen given important committee posts, even subcommittee chairs, increased support for conservative policy goals and, for the most part, the speaker's agenda as well.

In retrospect, the Republican Contract with America was a brilliant strategy and had a major influence upon subsequent developments. As a policy proposal, most of its elements were either trivial or ill-conceived, chosen because of their popularity and prospects for easy passage. But as an agency for change, as a means to promote a continuing revolution, the contract was hugely successful. Not only did it help produce the Republican majority, it provided "daily successes" for the newly elected freshmen while the leaders prepared for the main events. Other contributions were to socialize and train inexperienced legislators as well as to ginger up some of the veterans. And it added legitimacy to several of the leadership's most important agenda items—such as balancing the budget and a middle-class tax cut. In setting one hundred days for completion, Gingrich and others likened enactment of the contract to the famous hundred days of the New Deal—an unprecedented feat of legislative creation. From one perspective, the comparison is preposterous, but from another it is not: for the Contract with America provided some of the same experience and psychic and social benefits without the historic occasion of a genuine crisis.

Language like "revolution" or "coup" needs to be used cautiously, if at all. But it is important to be aware that Gingrich, many of the House leaders, and the members of the freshman class often spoke in terms of sweeping change and shared a vision of transforming American federal government and many established programs much more fundamentally than merely reducing a few entitlements and cutting taxes. The Contract with America included, for instance, term limits, a balanced budget amendment, and an item veto—legitimate enough, but with constitutional importance and ramifications little understood by the American people or, for that matter, many of the new representatives supporting its articles. A view widely shared was that the federal government needed to be reduced in size and responsibility, with functions delegated or privatized where possible. Growing out of the Contract with America and actively promoted by the chief whip, Tom DeLay, one agenda item was systematically cutting the appropriations of regulatory agencies, such as the Environmental Protection Agency or the Department of Agriculture (Drew 1996:257) and using appropriations "riders"[8] to block enforcement of existing regulations. Another, seemingly innocuous provision, known as the Istook amendment, would have prohibited private groups that received any federal funds from lobbying—a measure aimed at "liberal" organizations such as universities and foundations as well as federally funded agencies such as legal services, the Corporation for Public Broadcasting, the National Endowment for the Arts, and the National Endowment for the Humanities (ibid.:267). More is involved in these proposals than changes of domestic policy. They go to the nature of government itself and its relation to society. As a close friend of Speaker Gingrich said, "He wants to change the way people think about government."[9] And many of the House Republican majority shared that aim.

The magnitude of the budget reductions was one indication of the sweeping change being contemplated. Over seven years the House Republicans proposed $894 billion in spending cuts. This was to be achieved with over half the budget—social security, defense, and interest on the national debt—exempted or "off the table." Of the savings, nearly three-fourths ($627 billion) was to come from entitlement programs, especially Medicare, Medicaid, education, and welfare. Another objective, included in the Contract with America, was to cut taxes by $353 billion over the seven-year period—a fateful linkage. No reductions of this size had ever been attempted.[10] Moreover, it was to be combined with efforts to restructure many of these programs. Dick Armey, the majority leader, predicted that "knees will buckle" at the magnitude of the task and some members said that it seemed like "walking off a cliff." On the Democratic side, many feared that it would be the end of Medicare and Medicaid as they had known them; others, that a coup or revolution was under way.

From the beginning, Republican leaders in both the House and Senate assumed that the budget and a reconciliation bill would be the most important work of the 1995 term. The reconciliation technique was, by itself, another important resource. Budget reconciliation is, of course, a useful and even essential method of bringing appropriations and revenues into line and handy, by the way, for amending entitlement programs. In the present context, it had another potential advantage of great importance: as a powerful device for mobilizing and concentrating collective energies. Within the House, it was an adult and serious follow-on to the Contract with America. It set a clear target with a deadline. It brought effectively together goals of deficit reduction, tax cuts, and program amendment. It would expedite or bypass ordinary committee procedures so that years of ordinary work could be compressed into one term. Though not usually perceived that way,[11] budget reconciliation lent itself handily to a campaign mode of legislation prevalent in the House of 1995, facilitating and reinforcing an all-or-nothing strategy that helped create the high-stakes showdown at the end of the year.[12]

Even if fresh and well-organized, the House Democrats would have been awed by the mobilization of the Republicans, their unity, and the speed with which they moved through the contract articles. As it was, in January and February of 1995, House Democrats were close to exhaustion from the struggle over health care reform and depressed, even in shock, over their crushing defeat in the November election.[13] They were also disunited, without a message or agreed-upon priorities of their own, and uncertain about how to proceed.

In the House, the Democrats did not mount an effective defense and did relatively little to oppose the rapid passage of the Contract with America, article after article. They sought to tighten some provisions—for instance, with respect to unfunded mandates and environmental protection. They looked to the Senate for an effective opposition to the Balanced Budget Amendment, and they attempted to delay passage with a laundry list of fifty amendments. None of this was of much avail: the contract passed easily. The only article that failed in the House was the term limit amendment. For most votes, the Republicans maintained near-perfect discipline, voting unanimously for the article or with one or two crossing the aisle. By contrast, Democratic defections were frequent and large, often a quarter to a third of their party.

The House Democrats' behavior could be ascribed in part to their despondent state. But they also faced a strategic dilemma that often afflicts the minority party in the House—deciding whether to compromise or to fight. For Medicaid, especially at this juncture, the issue was either to compromise and save what they could of the entitlement or stand on principle, build the best case they could, and hope either to win in the Senate or persuade the president to veto. Some downside risks of standing on principle would be defection of conservative Democrats and losses on other issues, and saving nothing if they failed in the Senate and the president decided not to veto.

Time would not wait. Strategic choices had to be made facing critical uncertainties: whether the House Democrats could hold together enough to sustain a veto; what to expect from a Senate with fewer seasoned Democratic leaders or Republican health liberals; and whether Clinton, who had yet to veto a bill, would come to the defense of Medicaid, a program he had not loved. These decisions all had to be made in "real time,"[14] that is, in haste, under stress, and lacking knowledge about critical variables and who could be counted on.

II. BUDGET RESOLUTION

On April 7, one week before the one-hundred-day deadline, the House completed its work on the Contract with America. In an unprecedented nationwide television address, the speaker celebrated the victory, but reminded weary[15] House Republicans of the tasks confronting them upon their return from the spring recess. On the agenda were significant changes in almost every area of federal domestic policy, including such contentious items as immigration, school prayer, and abortion, and complex ones like income tax overhaul, banking legislation, health insurance portability, and restructuring Medicare.[16] Dominating all other items was the goal of balancing the budget in seven years.

To make a beginning on deficit reduction, the House Republicans moved swiftly, initiating a number of measures in February. One early step was to require "offsets"[17] for supplemental appropriations requested by the president for defense and flood relief.[18] Meanwhile, in a manner reminiscent of the first Reagan administration, the Appropriations Committee began assembling a major rescissions[19] bill with $17.4 billion in cuts from already existing authorizations: including veterans' medical care, home heating, summer jobs for youth, adult literacy education, and public broadcasting. At about this time, John Kasich, concerned about paying for tax reductions promised by the contract, announced a five-year plan to take $100 billion from discretionary spending and another $90 billion from federal pensions, Medicare, welfare, and food stamps. He promised deeper cuts when the Budget Committee produced its 1996 budget resolution, boasting, "You ain't seen nothing yet."[20]

A Republican strategy that was to prove hazardous was to combine budget cutting with the pursuit of collateral, sometimes ideological goals. The rescissions bill, for instance, included a large number of legislative "riders" directed at environmental programs, including the elimination of specific functions, barring program activities, and blocking implementation of rules mainly to the benefit, according to Democrats, of loggers, polluters, and Republican governors.[21] Another example was the addition by the Economic and Educational Opportunities Committee, to a House welfare bill, of a provision converting the school lunch program into a block grant. The first of these sallies created an enormous controversy and led to a defection by Republicans moderates—one of the first major defeats for the majority (Drew 1996:259ff.). The second, along with other cuts in the rescissions bill, enabled the Democrats to play the "Grinch" or "Scrooge" card: blame the Republicans for cutting school lunches for poor children, and taking away popular PBS programs like Big Bird and Barney (ibid.:264) in order to provide tax cuts for the wealthy.[22]

In themselves, these episodes had little significance for the coming battle of the budget or for Medicare or Medicaid,[23] but they helped rally the Democrats, gave them issues they could articulate effectively, and enabled them to go on the offensive to a limited extent. They also suggested to Democrats two winning strategies. One was to let the opposition overextend itself on the Democrats' own familiar turf—which was entitlements and grants programs. The other was to attack by linking tax cuts for the rich with cutting entitlements for the elderly, the children, and the poor. Republicans countered by denying they were "cutting" programs, only slowing their growth. But this message was somewhat less compelling than the images of hungry school children and needy old folk.

A major step taken by the House Republicans was to adopt the goal of balancing the budget by 2002, and combine this with substantial tax cuts. This development owed much to the Contract with America, which showcased both a balanced budget and a number of tax benefits, especially a tax credit of $500 per child, aimed at the middle class. Debates over a balanced budget amendment, the first article in the contract, helped to commit the House Republicans to the idea—both more definite and more ambitious than the pallid objective of deficit reduction. Meanwhile, John Kasich, the Budget Committee chairman, was looking for $200 billion in budget cuts to cover costs—mostly tax reductions—of the Contract with America. He had also been asked by Gingrich to put the deficit on a "glide path," aiming at a balance by 2002.[24] The notion of a balance in seven years was then hardened into a definite objective at a leadership meeting on February 15.

In contrast to the rather casual development of the first objective of a balance by 2002, tax reductions were a hotly disputed topic, with many Republicans aware of how politically dangerous the issue might be. But tax reduction was a long-standing staple of Republican policy and a campaign pledge with intense support from conservatives in Congress, the Christian Coalition, and small business. Moreover, the House Republicans had gotten themselves deeply committed to tax cuts as part of the Contract with America and backing off seemed certain to be politically costly if not impossible.

During this period, budget issues were being widely discussed, both in the House and Senate. Debate over the Balanced Budget Amendment raised awareness of what balancing the budget would mean in fiscal and programmatic terms. With as much as $1.6 trillion in deficit reduction[25] being projected over seven years, it was understood from the beginning in the House that 1995 would be a year in which the budget would be a "leadership" issue, engaging party and committee leaders at the highest level, and that the budget would drive policy in other, substantive areas. John Kasich, aware of the amount of persuasion and arm-twisting needed to reach that number, set up working groups to bring together important members of the budget, the authorizing, and the appropriations committees in an effort to promote specific commitments. Both Kasich and Robert Livingston, chairman of the

Appropriations Committee, exhorted members to think beyond the usual kind of budget trimming to include major changes such as eliminating, privatizing, or restructuring programs.[26]

From the beginning, Republican leaders in the House and the Senate assumed that entitlements would be considered for the cuts needed to balance the budget, but were understandably reluctant to discuss publicly the specific programs and how much would be taken from them. Yet Robert Dole, the majority leader, said as early as mid-February that balancing the budget within seven years would require savings of at least $146 billion from Medicare and another $75 billion from Medicaid (Johnson and Broder 1996: 573). And the Senate—moving ahead of the House—was contemplating by April a budget resolution that would take $250 billion from Medicare and $160 from Medicaid, with no tax cut.[27] The House, already committed to large tax reductions, would perforce have to exact even bigger "savings" from these entitlements.

Medicaid in the House of Representatives

Though seen as less important and less difficult than Medicare, Medicaid went first in the new Congress for a number of reasons. One was that more time was needed for the staff work and policy discussions on Medicare—for comprehensive assessment, a major restructuring, new payment systems, and an enormous amount of data and calculations. Talks with Republican governors about Medicaid policy had gained momentum and seemed to be moving in a favorable direction. Going first with Medicaid also seemed like it might be a way to "steal a march" on Democrats and score an early victory.[28] The last calculation in particular turned out to be wrong.

In 1994, the Republicans not only captured both houses of Congress, they won thirty of the governorships, for a gain of eleven. This majority included eight of the nine most populous states and a number of governors who had been actively experimenting with tax reduction, reform of welfare programs, and the Medicaid entitlement. This group, and especially the Republican Governors' Association, would have to be consulted and be, at the least, acquiescent in the ultimate Medicaid proposals. But in the overwhelming electoral endorsement these governors had received, the Republican leadership in Congress sensed a historic opportunity and decided, even prior to the new Congress, to give Republican governors a prominent role in entitlement reform (Drew 1996:81).

After the election, the Republican governors' annual conference was held in Williamsburg, Virginia. This meeting was important to strengthen affinities among the Republican governors and House Republicans and to promote block grants as a preferred Republican policy option. One message brought to this meeting, especially by some of the more vocal and enterprising gover-

nors—such as Tommy Thompson of Wisconsin and John Engler of Michigan—was the desirability of turning the welfare program into a block grant
and giving the states much greater freedom to manage for themselves. At the
time, the House Republican leadership had no expressed intention of block-
granting welfare. The Contract with America proposed reform, but not a
block grant. For Medicaid, Republicans in Congress were considering only
incremental changes and $10 billion in savings.[29] But a vocal group within
the Republican Governors' Association was eager to get rid of federal restrictions and "strings," saying that it was willing to accept more responsibility
and receive less money in exchange for greater freedom to manage welfare
programs in their own states. For Newt Gingrich, this was an unexpected but
welcome development; and he agreed to the concept, saying "Let's do it"
(ibid.:85).

What was agreed upon with respect to Medicaid is less clear, but it seems
probable that a restructuring was at least tacitly accepted at the same time.[30]
Newt Gingrich proceeded as though it were, discussing with Governor
Tommy Thompson (Wisc., R), the vice-chairman of the National Governors
Association (NGA), and Howard Dean (Vt., D), the NGA chairman, his own
proposal to give states more control in exchange for less money. At the time,
he said that Medicaid growth could be capped at 5 percent a year just by eliminating inefficiencies.[31] Not at all new, the same idea had been proposed in the
first Reagan administration but failed to pass a Democratic House.

At the NGA January conference in Washington, a number of Republican
House and Senate committee chairmen met with Republican governors to discuss Medicaid policy, including transforming the program into block
grants.[32] As for block-granting Medicaid, the conference was not of one mind.
Some said that a "hit" of $10 billion would be worth it to be free of the man-
dates and regulations. There was almost unanimous support for the proposition that spending cuts of the magnitude proposed by Congress without
greater program flexibility would be the worst of all possibilities. The conference adopted a policy resolution that recommended against any "unilateral"
caps on federal spending for Medicaid. Growing out of this meeting, though,
was a task force of the sort favored by Speaker Newt Gingrich: a group of
Republican governors charged to work with high-level Republican congressional leaders on proposals for Medicaid reform.[33]

For several reasons, the congressional Republicans might have been wise
not to start with Medicaid. For one thing, the Medicaid growth rate had
dropped sharply—from a high of 28.8 percent in 1992 to 8 percent in
1994. Much of this change was attributable to federal legislation limiting
DSH payments, a decline in medical inflation, and an upturn in the business
cycle. Numbers like these make a goal such as capping the federal contribution at a 5 percent annual increase seem more attainable, yet can also make the
capping itself seem less vital. Among experienced governors thinking about

demographics and fiscal politics, they could also raise an issue of *cui bono*: who is really benefiting from the capping of this entitlement? And who will bear the costs, down the road?

When it came to block granting, moreover, Medicaid was quite a different story from welfare. Collectively, Medicaid was huge—over seven times the size of the minuscule welfare program. Over time, unlike welfare, Medicaid had become increasingly "mainstream," providing services for pregnant mothers and children, many of the uninsured and working poor, indigent parents of the middle class, and the mentally ill and disabled. Medicaid providers were increasingly well-established community institutions and known to individual congressmen who had served on county councils or hospital boards. Furthermore, there was no great movement for "Medicaid reform" as there was for "welfare reform." Even had there been, Medicaid was enormously complex, with fifty states and four territories and their program adaptations, layered one on top of another, for more than thirty years.

The governors still had a number of grievances and desired program changes. High on the list was "unfunded mandates," especially directives that expanded coverage without additional funds.[34] Even more important for some was the need to revisit the federal funding formula (Federal Medical Assistance Percentage), which was narrowly based on each state's personal per capita income and locked in a number of historic inequities. In addition, there was displeasure at being micromanaged from a distance with the various "strings" attached to grants, such as nursing home standards or reimbursement floors. "Waivers" were another source of complaint, especially the time and difficulty required to get one from HCFA; and there was the Boren Amendment, which allowed nursing homes and hospitals to sue if payments fell below the standard of "reasonable and adequate" for "effective and economic operation."

House Budget Resolution

Much of the critical discussion about a basic strategy for Medicaid was taking place in February and March as the House pushed ahead on the Contract with America. Welfare reform passed the House on a partisan vote of 234 to 199 on March 24, using block granting as an instrument of change.[35] It is worth noting, in passing, that welfare reform did not pass the Senate until September 19 and then only after a number of bipartisan compromises. Meanwhile, Medicaid was swept along in the House by the budget resolution process. By mid-February, House Republican leadership and the RGA task force of governors had agreed upon their basic formula for Medicaid: a capped entitlement with reduced annual increments, the most commonly mentioned number being 5 percent.[36] A "capped entitlement" meant that Medicaid would stay in the entitlement column and be a predictable item that individual states could count on year by year; but the cap would be real enough and would entail far-reaching programmatic changes, driven mainly by funding cuts. To emphasize this point, John Kasich, the chairman of the House Budget Committee, said that strict spending targets would be set to restrain entitlement programs such as Medicare and Medicaid, and that authorizing committees should be "creative" in how they met their global targets.

The budget resolution passed by the House on May 18 was a major achievement, and could even be called revolutionary in scope, since House Republicans meant it to be a vehicle for sweeping policy changes going far beyond deficit reduction and incremental tinkering with programs. Like most budget resolutions, this one came down to a few pages and numbers—establishing overall revenue, spending, and deficit totals, limits for functional budget categories, and reconciliation instructions for the authorizing committees.[37] But it involved four months of intense effort: developing numbers and forecasts, lobbying the appropriations and authorizing committees, dealing with hardships and equities, mobilizing party resources, and coordinating with and seeking to persuade the Senate.[38] It took an "enormous amount of physical energy, intellectual effort, and political chips."[39] It also took on momentum, so that members found themselves, as Newt Gingrich said, "growing into the revolution" (Drew 1996:209–10). The resolution[40] called for a deficit reduction of $1.04 trillion, spending cuts of $948 billion, with reductions of $288 billion in Medicare spending over seven years and $184 billion from Medicaid—numbers many Republican members had scarcely thought possible when this process began. Not to be missed was a tax cut of $358 billion and the fact that nearly half of the total budget reductions came from Medicare and Medicaid alone.

Revolutionary or not, some experienced observers thought even at this stage that the Republicans and the Budget Committee might have overreached. Howard Cohen, the lead Commerce Committee staffer for Medicaid, said when he heard $184 billion was to be taken from Medicaid, he "wanted to quit" and went to John Kasich to plead that "we can't do it." Karen Nelson, one of the two or three most experienced staff persons in Congress, said that even though many Democrats feared Medicaid might be lost, she knew from the beginning that the numbers were too high and that the savings would get harder as the reconciliation process moved forward.[41] Ray Sheppach, the executive director of the NGA, observed that the NCA was too pluralistic for block grants to be attractive with savings of that magnitude.[42]

At a press conference the next day, Gingrich remarked that the budget resolution was not the end of the reconciliation process, but the beginning of six months of hard work (ibid.:211). Authorizing committees generally were to have until July 14, about two months, to report out changes. An extra two months were allowed for Medicare reforms, which would be developed initially in the speaker's task force and then sent to Ways and Means and Commerce for markup. For Medicaid, both House Commerce and Senate Finance were expected to hold hearings in June and to report markup legislation before July 14. As events developed, Medicaid took over two months longer, neither House Commerce nor Senate Finance reporting until late September.

Senate Budget Resolution

Though beginning from a very different position than the House, the Senate eventually passed a budget resolution fairly close to the House version. The Senate never signed the Contract with America, did not share Newt Gingrich's enthusiasm for "transformational" strategies, and began with moderate interest in deficit reduction and almost none for tax cuts. Bringing the Senate along owed much, of course, to the conviction and energy of the House Republicans; but it also involved an interplay of such factors as the shared fate of partisans, spill-over effects of the campaign mode of legislation, and the influence of presidential aspirations.

For the budget generally, and especially with a reconciliation, the House normally begins and does most of the heavy lifting, with the Senate often following that lead and modifying rather than substituting—especially when the same party controls both houses. In 1995, this presumption was further strengthened by the House victory and the sense of mandate that it conveyed, so that senators sometimes went along even when prudence counseled otherwise.

In the Senate, two principals were Pete Domenici (NM), chairman of the Senate Budget Committee, and Bob Packwood (Ore.), chairman of the Senate Finance Committee, the authorizing committee for both Medicare and Medicaid. Both men favored deficit reduction in principle. Domenici had, just the previous year, developed a robust Republican minority version that failed to pass. But Packwood was more in favor, generally, of deficit reduction at the expense of the military not Medicare and Medicaid beneficiaries, and Domenici, at least initially, thought in terms of a relatively modest "down payment" on the deficit—nothing so grand as eliminating it.[43] Neither of them wanted a tax cut, especially one that would be paid for by entitlements.

Even though the Senate never developed any genuine enthusiasm for the Contract with America and a number of its provisions died there, one effect the contract did have on the Senate was to get it more involved than usual in the politics of the budget—including the Balanced Budget Amendment, the rescissions bill, and, ultimately, the goal of balancing the budget in seven years. The Balanced Budget Amendment, passed by the House on January 26, occasioned a lively debate and got quite a bit of bipartisan support in the Senate, but on March 2 failed by one vote to reach the necessary two-thirds.[44] When the amendment failed, the goal of deficit reduction became even more important in order not to falter (or appear to falter), and to save something from the defeat.[45] As one result, Domenici was under more pressure from Dole and party leaders to fall in with the deficit reduction goal (Drew 1996:204). With reluctance and still not conceding, he began briefing key Republicans on what balancing the budget would entail.

The president's first budget, which appeared on February 6, was a precipitating event of an interesting sort. The budget itself, brief and scanty of detail or numbers, was clearly a "placeholder" and an invitation to the Republicans to "go first." It served up some moderate spending cuts of $144 billion with a middle-class tax cut of $65 billion over five years for a total deficit reduction of $81 billion—less than one-fifth of President Clinton's own deficit reduction package for 1993.[46] Among Democrats, there were differing views about this strategy. Some thought that the Republicans were hanging themselves and did not want to get in the way of that process. Others believed that more detail in a Democratic budget would only facilitate Republican budget slashing and were reluctant on that score. Either way, there was no disposition to cooperate by offering a serious budget at that point.

Republicans in both House and Senate were deeply disappointed for several reasons. Going it alone meant taking all the blame, while if the Democrats would come part of the way it would be easier and less risky to argue for more of a good thing. "Coming to the table" by Democrats would also promote well-targeted cuts obviating use of the budget meat axe, which, aside from collateral damage, earns opprobrium for its crudity. And unilaterally revealing your own numbers (and detailed plans) would make it easier for the opposition to identify who gets hurt and mobilize an effective protest.

The Senate Republicans faced a difficult situation. They felt a strong obligation to support their House colleagues, and not leave them politically exposed when fighting a good fight and taking heavy fire. Moreover, some Senators wanted to win big—either because of a conservative agenda or because of their own presidential ambitions. But the Senate as a whole had never signed on for the Contract with America or balancing the budget. There would be serious opposition to cutting Medicare or Medicaid entitlements for a tax cut or even to balance the budget. And Pete Domenici had a good sense for the difficulty involved in a deficit reduction that took on entitlements without bipartisan support. So it was rhetoric—but more than that—when he said he "didn't know how to get this done" without a forthcoming proposal from the administration.[47] In effect, the administration's stance made compromise more difficult. Moreover, the debate over the Balanced Budget Amendment and responding to Democratic taunts about the impossible dream of reaching a balance had gotten Republicans so extended that to back off now would have entailed symbolic loss and political damage. The administration's reticence protected Democrats, but it also tended to close the door on compromise.

As the budget resolution moved forward, various savings formulas for

Medicaid were proposed. In the House, Gingrich's formula of a block grant with a 5 percent cap on annual increase had been generally accepted, though with little debate on its implications. Late in February, Senator Packwood, chairman of the Finance Committee, said that he thought both Medicare and Medicaid could be held at a 5 percent annual growth rate, rather than the current projection of about 10 percent.[48] No mention was made of a block grant. A week later, Senator Judd, reporting on entitlements for the Republican Health Care Task Force, recommended savings for Medicare of $100 billion to $120 billion over five years and for Medicaid, savings of $115 billion. For Medicaid, the Task Force recommended an annual cap on growth of 4 percent. About then, Pete Domenici was developing a budget resolution with Medicare reductions of $250 billion and, for Medicaid, $160 billion over seven years. This figure for Medicaid would require shrinking the program from its then current 11 percent annual increase to 4 percent. These numbers were comfortably close to the House totals of $288 billion for Medicare and $184 billion for Medicaid. According to an aide, Domenici decided on this course because it made little sense to take the pain of deficit reduction without getting the payoff that would come from going all the way to a balance.[49]

Still, there was no support for a tax cut despite a bill passed by the House on April 5 (HR 1215), reducing taxes for families and businesses by $189 billion over five years. This bill, a last installment on the Contract with America, got the votes of twenty-seven Democrats who crossed party lines to support it. The Senate indicated that it would not consider the bill; and Senator Domenici, once again, made it clear that he would not use Medicare or Medicaid to provide a tax cut.

At the same time, with the House bill and the president offering his own version, there was strong support for tax reduction in the Senate—especially from Sen. Phil Gramm (R., Tex.), who was running for president as the only "true conservative," and who had with him a bloc of twenty conservative Senators, plus an unknown number of liberal Republicans and Democrats. Robert Dole, the majority leader, supported tax cutting more for tactical than policy reasons. As majority leader, his approach was to move in concert, to "allow no light" between himself and Newt Gingrich,[50] and as a presidential aspirant he could ill afford to be flanked on the right by Phil Gramm. In addition, some Democrats were beginning to think that a tax cut might be politically expedient.

Despite this kind of pressure, the most Domenici would concede was to allow the use of $170 billion paid for by lower debt interest and higher tax revenues *only if* CBO would certify that the deficit reduction plan put in place would actually achieve a balance by 2002.[51] This formula was changed after a floor fight, led by Phil Gramm, and some overnight brokering by Robert Dole to provide that Congress "shall" rather than "may" cut taxes if the budget is in balance (Drew 1996:212). In this form, the budget resolution was passed by the Senate on the next day, May 25, by a vote of 54–45.

Since the implications of this formula were that a tax cut would be considered only if the budget was certifiably going to be in balance, Republican senators could argue that they were not slashing Medicare and Medicaid to provide tax cuts for the wealthy and middle class, and they seem to have made genuine efforts not to do that. In any event, $170 billion was considerably less than the House proposed tax cut of $358 billion. Still, the Senate's tax cut decision had important consequences for the budget reconciliation that lay ahead: by dividing Republicans, undermining their appeals for bipartisan collaboration, and giving Senate Democrats an opening for an effective counterattack.

III. BUDGET RECONCILIATION

From a political perspective, the prognosis for Medicaid did not look good. For one item, Medicaid recipients—single mothers and children, the disabled, and the elderly poor—are not a cohesive or articulate constituency. Moreover, at this point welfare reform seemed almost a certainty and Medicaid was regarded by many—both governors and members of Congress—as a "welfare" kind of entitlement and not likely to be strongly defended. Democrats were disorganized and without a comprehensive strategy; and the momentum was with the Republican majority. A good many participants and observers, both Democrat and Republican, thought that Medicaid would be "block granted" and its status as an entitlement ended.[52]

Nevertheless, it is worth noting that some were skeptical, even then, that Medicaid would be an easy target. Various members of this group observed that the support for Medicaid was complex and pervasive,[53] that bipartisanship was a requisite for reform of a major entitlement, including Medicaid,[54] that the governors' association was pluralistic and unlikely to buy any simple formula,[55] and that Congress would not "give away" that kind of money without "strings" attached.[56] Though resembling Edmund Burke in their appreciation of entrenched institutions, these were mostly individuals with no particular ideological bent, who had been around for some time and had a rich experience with the institutions they were observing.

In 1995, reconciliation[57] was to be the critical phase of the budget cycle. It was central to the "transformational" strategy promoted by Newt Gingrich and the House Republican majority and accepted, if not enthusiastically endorsed, by the Senate Republicans. In this process—which is vast and complex, reconciling taxes and revenues, authorizations and appropriations in the budget cycle—Medicaid was a relatively minor part and was expected to be dealt with handily. In both House and Senate, the budget resolutions allowed just under two months for the authorizing committees to hold hearings, mark up, and report back the program changes that would produce the requisite savings. Medicaid dragged on over two months longer. It proved to be much more controversial and less "transformable" than anticipated.

Two factors were especially important in accounting for this particular and rather unexpected outcome. One was the nature of the Medicaid program itself: both its complexity and its increasingly "mainstream" characteristics. The other was the checks on the majority traditionally associated with federalism and bicameralism, especially the states' diverse program interests and the role of the Senate and a few senators. In this respect, Medicaid is a particularly interesting example of a kind of entitlement politics, in which a seemingly powerless constituency gets defended by some predictable friends and some rather unexpected champions.

There was, potentially at least, considerable bipartisan consensus on some of the Medicaid features that should be changed. Most agreed that the payment formula needed "modernizing"; that Sec. 1915 waivers should be modified so as to encourage Medicaid managed care options; and that fraud and abuse and "disproportionate share" scams should be addressed. Most would probably go along with repeal of the Boren Amendment and with some relaxing of nursing home standards. But one effect of putting block grants and budgetary reductions first and making them central was to sharpen disagreement and minimize the possibility of such collaboration.

The notion of a block grant for Medicaid with a 5 percent cap on annual growth dated back at least to 1982 and the first Reagan administration. It surfaced again early in 1995. But it seemed to generate relatively little enthusiasm except among a small group of Republican governors and leadership Republicans in Congress strongly committed to a budget-cutting formula. The 5 percent was generally seen as too procrustean and the block grant as one—but not necessarily the best or only—way to achieve greater flexibility and responsiveness to local needs. Moreover, neither idea addressed the need for a more demographically and geographically sensitive payment formula.

Since the block grant (more narrowly, a "capped entitlement") was well advertised in advance, objections were registered and modifications were proposed considerably before the budget reconciliation, beginning with the first week of the new Congress and continuing thereafter. Individual governors objected that a "one-size-fits-all" 5 percent solution did not speak to their particular condition and that it would, for example, punish high growth as well as some "waiver" states. Carl Volpe,[58] though avowing the NGA's willingness to consider such formulae, warned prophetically that a 5 percent cap would provoke a "formula fight" among the states. In the Senate, liberal Republicans from the beginning suggested that another idea entirely would be better: such as encouraging managed care for women and children and the Medicaid acute care population (Chafee) or a "swap" in which the federal government would be responsible for the elderly and disabled and states would take over welfare and acute care for AFDC recipients (Kassebaum). Paradoxically, the House Republicans, especially in the Commerce Committee, found themselves for a time considering not just one but two or even three block grants to cover, separately, acute and long-term care or, in one version, the disabled, long-term care, and low-income women and children—and explaining to some of the more zealous governors that "block grants" did not really mean "no strings" or no protections for vulnerable populations.[59]

Despite these significant portents, Republican leadership and the budget committees in both House and Senate pressed for a cap. In the Senate, Pete Domenici put the case forcefully and cogently, arguing that "we are absolutely wasting our money" by granting waivers and encouraging states to experiment without capping their funds.[60] In the House, the Budget Committee persisted with its formulaic 5 percent, and Republican leadership also pressed Michael Bilirakis, chairman of the authorizing Commerce Committee, to continue support for the 5 percent cap even though his own state, Florida, would lose money.[61] Meanwhile, with the expected "formula fight"[62] beginning, GOP leaders were recognizing that a flat 5 percent cap was not likely to work and were seeking a more responsive formula that would take into account poverty rates and projected Medicaid growth.

Large amounts of money and big swings in payment depended on both the visible and less visible aspects of the formula itself: what the cap on growth would be; what year would be set as a baseline and what could be included in the base; how large the federal match would be, and what variables would determine how it was apportioned among the states. Moreover, the 5 percent cap represented a drastic reduction in total funds available, so that the formula determined, in effect, how a shrinking amount would be divided, setting one state against another. Ray Sheppach, chief executive of the National Governors Association, estimated that $50 billion was at stake in the formula variations. Observing that he had seen huge formula fights over a $15 billion highway construction bill, he added that Medicaid payment would have a major impact not just on state budgets but upon providers, beneficiaries, and major industries within the states.[63]

Fixing the distribution formula—which no one denied needed doing—proved almost impossible, especially in a manner that was both rational and acceptable. Considering the sources of grievance, it was like asking for a poultice for whatever ailed state governments. A short list of relevant variables included program history, poverty percentages, demographics and case mix; provider resources, attitudes, and local ecology; state tax base and fiscal politics; local recession vulnerability; and immigration of elderly and/or aliens, legal and illegal.[64] New York, for instance, spending more per Medicaid recipient than any other state, was proud of its beneficence and wanted to maintain it. High growth states, including seventeen in the "Sunbelt" region, feared a cap on growth, especially a low one. Texas and California, hard pressed by unpaid care for illegal aliens, thought they deserved help on that account. Florida had these problems in addition to a continuing influx of elderly, many of them Medicaid beneficiaries. High-DSH states had a good thing going and wanted to keep it. Waivered states like Oregon and Tennessee did not want to be penalized for being venturesome or cost-effective. And recession-sensitive states feared the cumulative impact of an economic downturn and a capped federal contribution—reduced tax revenues and surging numbers of unemployed and Medicaid recipients with no additional federal dollars.

Much of the negotiation over the distribution formula fell to a relatively few members of the Commerce Committee and especially the staff.[65] Even veteran staffers, inured to complexity and detail, were awed by the intricate rules, the program variations, and the difficulty of finding common ground. The negotiations took a little over four months, endless hours on the telephone or in meetings with governors, and over 1400 computer runs.[66] Even as the House Commerce Committee prepared to mark up its own version on September 20, the Republican governors were still unable to agree on a distribution formula.[67] Before that, on September 15, President Clinton had pledged to veto any bill with reductions of the size projected by the GOP Medicare/Medicaid proposals. In the intervening months, the opposition had organized, gained confidence, and found its voice.

During the first months of 1995, Democrats and Medicaid advocacy groups were trying to organize and develop a strategy. Like an army after a defeat, some battle-scarred veterans and centers of opposition remained, but with no general strategy, a lack of organization, and a foreboding sense that the cause was probably lost. Many said they believed that welfare and Medicaid would almost surely be block granted. One Medicaid veteran said that his group hoped for a formula fight since they thought there was little chance of prevailing on the merits.[68] Major interest groups, such as the American Association of Retired Persons (AARP) and the hospital associations, were watching and waiting. And Democrats in Congress and the administration either had no strategy or were divided about what it should be. They could complain that the cuts were excessive, but that lacked force without dramatic particulars. As late as March, according to one official, "we were dying on Medicaid—with no clue that we could win."[69]

A critically important group for both Medicaid and Medicare was an informal task force that had developed during health care reform and began meeting again in the aftermath of the 1994 election. Initially, almost all were prominent actors in health care reform, so that they were experienced and had extensive knowledge of specific programs, such as Medicaid. They knew each other well and had established channels of communication. Though in no sense a superdepartmental task force—all of its members reported to their own superiors as before—it was a counterpart to the Medicare task force that Newt Gingrich had appointed in the House. They brought to bear a formidable amount of political and technical expertise themselves and had ready access to in-depth resources. As a group, they were particularly well adapted to brief administration officials, help develop strategy and message, or shape actionable policy alternatives for approval at the highest level—for instance, an alternative to Medicaid block grants or a deficit reduction budget.

The membership varied over time and by task, but meetings were frequent—weekly and sometimes daily, especially during 1995. Almost always present were Bruce Vladeck, HCFA administrator, who supplied programmatic expertise; Judith Feder (replaced by Jack Ebeler), deputy assistant secretary for planning and evaluation; Nancy-Ann Min (de Parle) an associate director from the Office of Management and Budget, and Christopher Jennings, health adviser to the president with appointments to the Domestic Council and the National Economic Council. Supporting this group was a small number of technical people: Ira Burney from the Office of the Secretary, with a legendary knowledge of program detail; Peter Hickman from HCFA's Office of Legislation; Jeanne Lambrew, a "numbers" person and special assistant to the assistant secretary; and Mark Miller, chief of the Health Finance Division in the Office of Management and Budget.

One of the early challenges for this group was to develop an effective response to Republican Medicaid proposals. Since there was, for the moment, no comprehensive strategy—even on Medicaid—the only plausible approach was to attack the size of the cuts and point out their impact upon Medicaid beneficiaries, providers, and state and local governments. All the group had at that time were the global figures being talked about, not detailed budget numbers. Absent that, they resorted to OMB options papers, CBO figures, and whatever they could glean, largely speculating about more specific program numbers and, drawing upon the expertise of Ira Burney and others, trying to develop a sense for who would be hurt and how badly.[70] What they developed from this process would then be turned into "talking points" for briefing officials, sharing with congressional committee staff, or passed up to the White House Office as suggestions. According to report, Jack Ebeler—who replaced Feder—had a particular gift for converting such fugitive data and weak inferences into striking illustrations and stinging "talking points."

Another important resource was the minority staff of the Commerce Committee and the personal staff of Henry Waxman and John Dingell, both iconic figures in health affairs. Although drastically reduced in numbers, the remaining staff[71] was a repository of thirty years of institutional memory and had assembled a vast store of policy expertise and specific knowledge about who had what interests at stake, and who could be counted on to stir the grass roots—or "grass tops" in the descriptive current lingo. Such expertise and contacts were useful in many ways during these critical months: to provide apt and timely information to the ranking members during committee negotiations; to develop tactical "message" amendments for committee markups and floor debates; to alert, energize, and coordinate advocacy groups; and to leverage the administration's efforts.[72]

How effective such countering activities were is hard to say. The House

Republicans took precautions: doing away with subcommittee hearings and keeping the legislative details secret until immediately before the markup.[73] During the markup, the majority seemed little deterred, and some knowledgeable observers dismissed the Democrats' efforts as annoyances but not of serious consequence.[74] But several of the ways in which observers and participants thought these activities were effective provide important insights into the legislative process. One observer believed the "message" amendments were useful for raising the morale of the Democrats and their Medicaid advocacy group allies.[75] A majority staffer said that the amendments, "any one of which could have cost an election," were useful in educating Republican members, especially freshmen, about Medicaid and the people who depended on it, and in making these same members realize that they might need some political cover. According to a Democrat, one tangible effect in the Commerce Committee markup was to revive set-asides and other protections for vulnerable populations.[76] Several Democrats spoke about the effect the debates and amendment votes had upon governors, who were hearing in their own states not just about the poor, but about nursing homes and the middle-class families of their residents, and from hospitals and other health care providers.[77] Scores of amendments and votes with messages to groups within the states, coming at the time of the formula fight, helped make governors aware that Medicaid reform was full of thorns and not an unqualified benefit.

Mounting a credible defense of Medicare in the House may have influenced the president as well. The June budget, signaling the administration's battle plan, included Medicaid as one of its top priorities.[78] When the budget resolution was adopted, Clinton threatened to veto the reconciliation if it cut Medicare and Medicaid deeply; but he also threatened to veto other bills. Many Democrats, especially in the House, were not confident he would make good on such threats. As for contributions of advocacy group and committee activities, Democrats said they got the president to care more about Medicaid,[79] may have kept him from wavering,[80] and helped convince him there was enough support to sustain a veto.[81]

One salient aspect of the Medicaid defense was the absence of powerful interest group support—not surprising since the poor are seldom effectively mobilized or well represented. Most noticeable for its absence was the AARP, an enormously powerful lobby and advocacy group, pretty much sitting this one out.[82] Other groups that were active, such as Families, USA, the National Council on the Aging, or the Catholic Health Association, were small, spread thin, or marginally interested. An exception was the hospitals, especially those serving Medicaid patients, providing a striking illustration of a convergence of interest producing a "virtual representation" of the poor by some powerful patrons.

The American Hospital Association (AHA)—along with the American Medical Association (AMA) and the AARP—was among the groups whose views and support had been solicited by Newt Gingrich and the House

Republicans after the election. Responses among the hospital group were mixed. The AHA and the Federation of American Health Systems, for instance, while working with House leadership on restructuring Medicare, were concerned about the size of the budget cuts. Late in January, the AHA organized a task force that was to report on the impact of the reductions being considered. AHA leadership also expressed concern about Medicaid and the regional swings in payment that a block grant would produce. [83] Increasingly at issue, especially for the AHA and hospitals treating the poor, were reductions in hospital subsidies such as the Medicaid DSH allowance and payments for direct and indirect medical education expenses.

These hospitals, with their clinics, emergency rooms, and indigent patients, saw these payments—especially the Medicaid DSH—as an essential part of the system of subsidies and cross-subsidies that enabled them to treat the poor and no-pay patients and still stay in business. With the variations in patient population, local ecology, financial structuring, and public-private relations, moreover, drastic reductions or anything beyond a cautious incrementalism risked serious dislocation or even collapse. The issue was important for the poor—but also for almost every local hospital, for the hospitals' allies and dependents, local governments, state hospital associations, and, of course, their political representatives. As one AHA official put it, "There are some breezes that set all the wind-chimes tinkling"—and this was one of them.[84]

The House budget resolution of May 18—with the size of its Medicare and Medicaid reductions—was an important triggering event for the hospital constituency, leading over a period of weeks to sharp exchanges with the House leadership and negative advertising in the media.[85] Just before the Memorial Day recess, the AHA, abetted by various other hospital groups and state hospital associations, launched a major campaign replete with national TV ads, videos and information kits for individual hospitals, and local visitations upon the representatives.[86] House Republicans responded in kind, with action kits for their members, advice on how to counter the "Astro-Turf" (phony grass roots) assault, and some veiled threats about what such activities might cost the hospitals.[87]

How significant this episode was is debatable. The AHA was the first major provider group to come out in opposition to the House Republican proposals. Medicaid was in part defended because of other larger reductions in Medicare hospital payments. At the same time, AHA leadership said that Medicaid and especially the DSH payments were vital for them and that they put even more effort into campaigning for Medicaid than they did for Medicare.[88] Medicaid DSH payments were at least important in leading a major group to make a determined stand on the wider issue of hospital payments. In the Medicare Preservation Act, as passed by the House, Medicaid DSH payments survived, though in modified form, by allowing the existing payments to be folded into the state's baseline.

By this time, the governors had largely endorsed a block grant but remained divided over the funding formula for distributing dollars among the states. One proposal, which appeared as part of the Clinton administration's June 13 budget, was for per capita caps (PCCs). These became the most important and sustained effort to provide an alternative to block grants. The idea behind this proposal[89] was to limit the growth in expenditure per individual Medicaid recipient. Since this approach would let dollars follow the individual, it would help the high-growth states. PCCs would work better in a recession. They could also be segmented by beneficiary group and adjusted to case mix differences among states. Since they avoided explicit redistribution by state they provided a way out of the formula fight. Not least, they retained the concept of an entitlement.[90]

This option was apparently offered in good faith as a compromise solution by the Clinton administration[91] and was seriously considered in the Senate, especially by Bob Graham (Fla.), who led a major campaign in support of PCCs. But the proposal gained little support from the governors, many of whom saw it as a "wedge" issue and/or a booby trap. It was a wedge issue because it set states that were well off under Medicaid formulas against those that were not. It was a booby trap because it would be easy for OMB or the Congress to ratchet down on such caps—leaving the states with clamorous and underserved but still entitled Medicaid recipients. As one astute observer said, for governors, "Things can be legal but not politically optional."[92] In other words, governors could legally reduce benefits for the elderly, disabled, and women and children but at enormous political costs. They saw PCCs as the "worst of all possible worlds" and, most likely, a powerful device to shift costs from Washington to the states.

Ultimately, the best compromise—assuming some form of cap combined with increased flexibility for the states and substantial protection for Medicaid recipients—may have been one that some of the Republican committee members and the staff had supported from the beginning. This was to have separate categories of funding for the poor, the elderly, and the disabled; Medicare premium assistance; and mandatory set-asides equal to 85 to 90 percent of the expenditures between FY 1992 and FY 1994.

Meanwhile, the controversy over the actual distribution formula grew more complex and heated, with governors still unable to agree. At issue were questions of what year to use for a baseline, the minimum federal match, minimum and maximum growth rates, and—above all—what to include and how to weight such factors as tax base, population growth, poverty ratios, health care costs, and case load severity. Especially on this last issue, various states and regions had their own perceived needs, theories, and numbers. The hours spent negotiating were endless and the computer runs countless. The NGA appointed a special task force of seventeen governors, which also failed to agree, with only days to go before the Commerce Committee markup.[93] No consensus was ever reached.

The eventual resolution was what policy people call "satisficing," or "good enough" and rational in critical respects (cf. Simon 1955:99–118). The formula that was worked out by the Commerce Committee staff was responsive to state needs and met committee majority constraints. It was based on number of poor, case-load severity, and a health care cost index for the particular state. It guaranteed a minimum growth rate as well as setting an upper limit. These limits would ratchet down in succeeding years, but would do so less for states with historically lower Medicaid spending. To this formula, the NGA agreed not to disagree. And the bill passed, after a sweetener was added, largely to benefit rural states, that would raise minimum payments for HMOs over a period of three years.[94]

One question that arises is, Why did it take so long to reach a sensible outcome? One reason, of course, is that, politically, the Republican leadership had to work though the National Governors Association and, at a minimum, get the assent of the Republican governors. In the best of circumstances, that process was likely to be difficult and time consuming. However, another important factor was the overblown rhetoric and dubious purpose of the Republican leadership in the beginning: setting a goal of a block grant and a 5 percent cap on growth and using a minority of enthusiasts to lead their campaign in the Republican Governors Association. This simplistic formula was handy for developing the initial budget resolution and had the merit of rallying partisans for the achievement of a single objective, but it raised expectations in one quarter and fears in another. Cooling out the first group and providing assurances for the second took time; and reaching a certain level of weariness seems to have been necessary before more sensible compromise solutions became possible.

An important provision of the House bill was to continue the longstanding requirement of a state plan setting forth eligibility, benefit packages, and administrative guidelines. States were to seek the approval of the secretary of DHHS, though no provision was made for what to do should the secretary not approve. Also, states did not have to guarantee that those meeting the criteria would necessarily receive the specified benefits—so that Medicaid would cease to be an individual entitlement, so far as states were concerned, even though set-asides and other forms of earmarking would remain.

Several state mandates were continued. These included provision of emergency treatment for illegal aliens, though not other medical assistance; payment for immunization for poor children covered by Medicaid; and creation of fraud units.

Various protections for Medicaid recipients were either terminated or considerably attenuated. The federal nursing home standards, established in 1987, were eliminated—though states were required to develop their own standards and describe them in their MediGrant state plan. The Boren Amendment was repealed with a further measure virtually denying any suit in a federal court against a state for its compliance or noncompliance with the federal legislation or its own MediGrant plan. The legislation also dropped an earlier Medicaid provision designed to protect the spouse of a nursing home resident from becoming impoverished by "spend down" requirements.

Assuming that the objectives were to take substantial savings from Medicaid but also fix the funding formula, give the states discretion to manage their own Medicaid programs as they saw fit and still provide essential protections to Medicaid recipients, the House bill substantially met those criteria. It also provided a template for further modification by the Senate. Many observers of this legislative episode commented on the remarkable discipline with which the Republican majority pushed through a bill.

Yet the bill that passed the House was considerably modified from its original and rather simplistic conception of a block grant with a 5 percent cap. One important factor working toward this modification was the governors' associations and the "formula fight." It also seems pretty clear that advocacy group efforts, the administration's rhetoric, and committee infighting affected some details of the legislation but not the major principles. An important intangible influence, though, was the education of the majority itself—including governors, committee members, and individual representatives, especially freshmen, to a greater understanding of Medicaid and what is prudent, conscionable, and politically safe to do about it. This kind of education was a work in which many participated, often across party lines, including Commerce Committee staffs, individual representatives, and wiser heads among advocacy groups. Had the environment been less combative, more of this education and more bipartisan collaboration might have taken place.[95] Yet when purposes are wrong-headed, it is also hard to educate.

In broad outline, the Senate Medicaid package closely resembled that passed by the House both in savings and program revisions. But in the Senate, the notion that Medicaid needed reforming was less widely shared, block granting more suspect, and the quest for beneficiary protections more salient. To an extent, this would be the normal posture for the Senate in the reconciliation process: in large measure following the lead of the House, but with a "show me" attitude and a concern to ease the pinch where justified. In this situation, though, there were special circumstances—in particular, the history of this specific reconciliation, Senator Chafee and the makeup of the Finance Committee, and the role of individual senators, both Republican and Democratic.

With respect to the reconciliation process, the Senate Republicans did not start from the same position as their House colleagues. They did not share the speaker's "transformational" goals; nor had they experienced "one hundred days" passing the Contract with America. As noted, the Senate Republicans came eventually to accept the budget-balancing objectives of the House and deficit reduction numbers that were nearly as high. But $182 billion seemed like a reach at the time for Senate Republicans. Moreover, there was no Newt

Gingrich in the Senate, no collective mobilization similar to the Contract with America, and no intense lobbying and pressuring of the authorizing committees as there had been in the House. In short, there was some agreement about where to go, but lack of a revolutionary mood or an enthusiasm for "transforming" institutions such as Medicare or Medicaid.

In any event, no Senate leadership was likely to be notably successful in pressuring the Senate Finance Committee of 1995 on reconciliation issues. Sometimes referred to as a "Democratic" committee by Republicans, Senate Finance was often liberal on health issues. The majority was thin, eleven Republicans and nine Democrats. The Democrats, moreover, were moderate to liberal with several senators, such as Rockefeller (W.Va), Graham (Fla.), and Moynihan (NY), both deeply concerned and knowledgeable about health affairs. On the Republican side there were some staunch conservatives but also John Chafee (RI), a health liberal, and various others, such as Bob Packwood, chairman until September 7, Orrin Hatch (Utah), Charles Grassley (Ia.), and Alfonse d'Amato (NY), who would sometimes vote with Democrats on specific health issues. Particularly when Medicare or Medicaid were concerned 11–9 "liberal" majorities or 10–10 ties were common.

Senator Chafee should be mentioned separately. A long-time senator from Rhode Island despite its overwhelming majority of registered Democrats, Chafee came from a patrician family and had a strong sense of responsibility for the poor or handicapped. He was a tireless negotiator, could work effectively across party lines, and was a skillful leader of a small group of moderate Republicans, mostly from New England and sometimes referred to as "Snow Birds." The group included at that time William Cohen (Me.) and Olympia Snowe (Me.), Arlen Specter (Pa.), and James Jeffords (Vt.). Chafee, who was chairman of the Senate Finance Medicaid subcommittee,[96] was knowledgeable, persuasive, deeply committed to the Medicaid program, and especially protective of children and the handicapped. Given the balance in Senate Finance, his views would often prevail there. And with the small 54–46 Republican majority in the Senate, he and his allies could sometimes tip the balance of a floor vote. He was, in few words, committed, powerful, and a critical factor in many of the decisions about Medicaid.

Even though the Senate followed the House in adopting a modified block grant, there was less enthusiasm for the concept and more concern about vulnerable populations. Senator Chafee, along with almost all Democrats, opposed block grants outright. An alternative strongly supported at one point was block grants only for the AFDC population, leaving the rest of Medicaid as it was. Senator Nancy Kassebaum, Chairwoman of Labor and Human Resources, proposed a "swap," similar to the one recommended by the Reagan administration in the 1980s, which would let the states deal with welfare and Medicaid for the AFDC population and make health care for the elderly poor and the disabled a straight federal program. Strong support for a block grant came from the leadership, from the Budget Committee, from more conservative Republicans and from Senator Packwood, then chairman of the Finance Committee. But this support was qualified by emphatic statements that block grants would come with "strings" and protections for vulnerable populations.[97]

Unlike the House, the Senate Finance Committee did not get into a formula fight over Medicaid. For an item, they were already engaged in one over welfare. Also, the House had started earlier on Medicaid and was better equipped with staff and other resources. In hearings, though, the Finance Committee heard from governors and other senators about their preferred alternatives, including several not reviewed by the House. Per capita caps were given careful consideration, including testimony by outside experts on their technical feasibility. Ultimately, Finance followed the House approach, ending the entitlement, but with set-asides.

Details of the Finance Committee's Medicaid proposals were released on September 22, with the markup to begin on September 26. The major provisions included a state plan, a matching requirement, a block grant (or capped entitlement) with a modified formula, set-asides, and some additional "strings," but much greater freedom for states to manage on their own. Like the House, the Senate version called for $182 billion in savings. Some important differences from the House bill were the use of 1985 for a baseline rather than 1984 and revision of the Medicaid DSH formula rather than termination of payments.[98] In broad outlines, the chairman's draft tracked the House bill; but that was before the markup and Senator Chafee's contribution.

Senator Chafee, who was deeply opposed to block granting or ending the entitlement, used his committee leverage and personal influence in the markup and beyond to fight the block grant and, through amendments, to protect vulnerable populations. One of his first proposals was to require states to provide a minimum benefit package, which would have largely vitiated the block grant. This failed to pass on a 10–10 vote, all Democrats voting with Chafee.[99] A follow-up to protect low-income mothers, children, and the uninsured was defeated 10–10. Also lost, 9–11, was an attempt to delete a ban on the use of federal funds for abortions except in case of rape, incest, or danger to the mother's life.

Committee Republicans knew that no bill would get out of committee without Chafee's vote and agreed, in return for his support, to back a number of his amendments.[100] Most important for these amendments, also supported by Senator Rockefeller, was a requirement that states provide benefits for poor pregnant women, children under twelve, and the disabled. The level of support was up to the states, but an earlier amendment, sponsored by Chafee, provided that the set-aside for mandatory populations had to equal not just 85 percent of historic expenditures on mandatory populations, but 85 percent of total spending—for some states, a much larger sum. Another Chafee amendment, passed 15–5, mandated that federal funds be used to cover prepregnancy family planning.

Individual senators, some of whom were close to Chafee on health issues, offered successful amendments during the markup, protecting Medicaid recipients or imposing other limitations or mandates. A Hatch amendment required a 1 percent set-aside for local health centers. A Graham amendment prohibited states from excluding any beneficiary because of a preexisting health condition. Amendments by Mosely-Braun and Hatch required states to specify goals and standards for children with special needs. A pair of amendments restored the spousal protection against spend-down requirements and prohibited any lien against a home or a family farm of moderate value. And another Graham amendment barred states from shifting the costs of matching to local governments without their written consent.[101] Only two of the amendments significantly lightened the burden on states. One was a change in the formula to reduce the minimum a state would have to contribute to qualify for federal funds. And the other, backed by Senator D'Amato, lowered the minimum match from 50 to 40 percent, so that no state would receive less than 60 percent federal dollars.

For Chafee and his allies there were two major losses. One was the proposal by David Pryor (D., Ark.) to restore the nursing home standards or, in the alternative, permit federal review and approval of state laws. This failed twice on a 10–10 vote. The second was the Chafee-Rockefeller amendments to guarantee protection of the disabled. This was a matter about which Chafee cared deeply. But because of the enormous expense, especially for long-term institutional care, governors strenuously resisted a mandate. During the markup, the committee had approved a Chafee amendment including the disabled along with poor pregnant women and children under twelve. As the committee was finishing its work, a group of twenty-four Republican governors wrote to Dole complaining about this mandate as well as the restoring of spousal protections. With Dole's intervention, and after sharp floor debate, the Finance Committee agreed on October 17 that states—even though they had to protect the disabled—could decide who qualified as "disabled."[102]

The Senate had yet to pass the reconciliation bill, for which the support of Chafee and his "Snow Birds" was essential. Augmented by several other moderates, including Nancy Kassebaum (Kan.), Mark Hatfield (Ore.), and Ben Campbell (Colo.), this group negotiated individually and collectively with Dole for additional modifications.[103] A chairman's (Roth) amendment reinstated most of the nursing home standards, also adding $10 billion to compensate states hardest hit by the Medicaid DSH cuts. The Senate adopted (60–39) a Chafee amendment that would require states to use the Federal Social Security Income (SSI) definition of "disabled." It deleted language that would have barred use of federal funds to pay for abortions except in cases of rape, incest, or danger to the mother's life. One motion that would have recommitted the bill with instructions to restore the Medicaid entitlement was defeated by a vote of 51–48, and another to restore existing Medicaid eligibility for women and children was defeated by a vote of 50–49.

The conference report added some further adjustments, mostly sweeteners. Conferees agreed to a reduced $163 billion savings target for seven years, by now almost $20 billion less than the number in the original budget resolutions. It added $3.5 billion to help those states with the largest health care expenses for illegal aliens. And states could choose whichever funding formula—House or Senate—that provided them with the most money. The Conference Report[104] also mandated coverage for pregnant women and children under age thirteen and agreed to retain the nursing home standards, but rejected the Chafee floor amendment, and allowed states to define "disabled," rather than using the federal SSI definition.

On November 17, the House passed the conference report by a vote of 237–189. The same day, the Senate passed the bill, with a vote of 53–47. By then, President Clinton had vowed to veto the bill, and the first shutdown of the federal government had begun.

NOTES

[1] Federalist, No. 10.

[2] Gingrich (1995). Note the use of "renew." Like many leaders, Gingrich knew the importance of invoking past ideals to move into the future.

[3] An interesting historic comparison would be Henry Clay (1777–1852). Six times speaker of the House, Clay also sought to use the office to dominate national government.

[4] He was, for instance, skillful at adapting traditional institutions, with a few deft strokes, to radically new purposes, leaving observers wondering what had happened.

[5] Gingrich took charge of the legislative agenda and was involved in negotiations and much of the detail, even though he had never had extensive experience on a major committee.

[6] As one admirer said, "I know he's deeply flawed, but when he's on he's a genius."

[7] GOPAC was founded in 1979 to aid Republican candidates for state legislative offices. Gingrich took over GOPAC in 1986 and used it to support Republican candidates for Congress and other party activities.

[8] An amendment that seeks to add extraneous material to a bill under debate, especially to "must pass" legislation such as an appropriations bill.

[9] Vin Weber as quoted by Drew (1996:27).

[10] The Clinton budget reconciliation of 1993 not only cut expenditures $353 billion over five years, it included a substantial tax increase.

[11] Though a historic precedent was the Reagan budget reconciliation act of 1981, especially as conceived by David Stockman, then director of OMB.

[12] Congressional Quarterly Almanac (1995), pp. 2–3.

[13] Many expected the party to lose seats in the election, but still hoped to retain control of the House.

[14] Jack Ebeler of the RWJ Foundation, formerly deputy assistant secretary for planning and evaluation, DHHS. Interview, January 6, 1999.

[15] Passing the provisions in the Contract with America was labor-intensive activity requiring 487 hours in session—compared with one-fourth as many in the same number of legislature days in 1993. There were 278 roll call votes with a total of 111 bills passed. During this same period, in the preceding Congress, only five public law bills were passed by the House, so that the Contract, whatever its merits as a unifying and mobilizing tactic, exacted a high price in time and energy. *Congressional Quarterly,* April 8, 1995, p. 990.

[16] *Congressional Quarterly,* April 1, 1995, p. 919.

[17] Additional revenues or savings that would "offset" expenditures that exceed a discretionary spending cap or (for entitlements) would add to the federal deficit. See Collender (1995:33ff.).

[18] *Congressional Quarterly,* February 18, 1995, p. 509.

[19] Cuts in funds already authorized—in this instance for the current fiscal year.

[20] *Congressional Quarterly,* March 18, 1995, p. 794.

[21] Ibid., p. 797.

[22] Drew (1996:264). According to one Democratic staffer, when the Democrats saw this "big, fat pitch" coming their way, they couldn't believe their good fortune. Needless to say, they did not waste the opportunity. J. Ridgway Multop, Democratic Policy Committee. Interview, December 18, 1998. Thereafter, Republicans spoke warily about being "school-lunched" again.

[23] Though Elizabeth Drew compares the rescissions episode to the Spanish Civil War, often considered the preliminary to World War II (1996:183).

[24] As to why the specific year 2002, Gingrich said there was no special reason, except that he thought seven years would be needed to reach a balance (Drew 1996:128).

[25] *Congressional Quarterly,* January 21, 1995, p. 205.

[26] Ibid., p. 205.

[27] *Congressional Quarterly,* April 8, 1995, pp. 1012–13.

[28] Howard Cohen of Greenberg Traurig, formerly Commerce Committee staff. The prospects for "stealing a march" were considerably improved by the low morale and disorganization of the House Democrats; also by the reduction of minority committee staffs.

[29] *Health Care Policy Report,* December 5, 1994, p. 1987.

[30] Ray Sheppach, executive director of the NGA, believes it was "given the nod" at the same time. Interview, June 16, 1999.

[31] *Health Care Policy Report,* January 23, 1995, p. 107.

[32] Ibid., February 2, 1995, p. 190.

[33] The governors were Jim Edgar (Ill., chairman), George Allen (Va.), Arne H. Carlson (Minn.), John Engler (Mich.), Gary E. Johnson (N.M.), George E. Pataki (N.Y.), Tom Ridge (Pa.), Tommy Thompson (Wisc.), George V. Voinovich (Ohio), and Pete Wilson (Cal.). Congressional leaders included Pete Dominici (N.M., chairman of the Senate Budget Committee), Bob Packwood (Ore., chairman of Senate Finance Committee), Thomas Bliley (Va., chairman of House Commerce Committee), and John Kasich (Ohio, chairman of House Budget Committee).

[34] Certainly the issue that generated the highest volume protests. Mandates for women and children alone were estimated to account for 12.8 percent of program

expenditures between 1986 and 1990. Other important mandates were ESPDT, premiums and cost-sharing for low-income Medicare beneficiaries, asset and income protections, nursing home regulations, and coverage for legal aliens. Cf. Holahan, Coughlin, Ku, Heslam, and Winterbottom (1993:28ff.).

[35] *Congressional Quarterly,* March 25, 1995, p. 872.

[36] *Health Care Policy Report,* February 20, 1995, pp. 269–70.

[37] For an example of the format and instructions, see Collender (1996:Appendix A).

[38] Drew has a good account (1996:Ch. 16).

[39] James Capretta, Senior Policy Analyst, Senate Budget Committee. Interview, October 7, 1998.

[40] HconRes67.

[41] Interview, August 19, 1998.

[42] Interview, June 16, 1999.

[43] *Congressional Quarterly,* January 7, 1995, p. 34.

[44] Mark Hatfield (R., Ore.), who was a hold-out, even offered to resign—an offer rejected by Robert Dole, the 16 minority leader (Drew 1996:163).

[45] *Health Care Policy Report,* March 6, 1995, pp. 347–48.

[46] *Congressional Quarterly*, February 11, 1995, p. 403.

[47] Ibid., p. 403.

[48] *Health Care Policy Report,* March 6, 1995, p. 346.

[49] *Congressional Quarterly,* April 8, 1995, p. 1012.

[50] Sheila Burke, Kennedy School of Government, Harvard University; then chief of staff for Sen. Robert Dole. Interview, January 5, 1999.

[51] *Congressional Quarterly,* May 6, 1230.

[52] For instance, Judith Feder, then deputy assistant secretary for planning and evaluation, and Andy Schneider, until 1995 a member of the Democratic Commerce Committee staff.

[53] James D. Bentley, senior vice-president, American Hospital Association, interview, November 18, 1998.

[54] Howard Cohen. Interview, May 19, 1999.

[55] Ray Sheppach, executive director, National Governors Association. Interview, June 16, 1999.

[56] Mary McGrane, senior director of government affairs, Rhone-Poulenc-Rohrer; then Commerce Committee staff. Interview, December 2, 1998.

[57] The process used by Congress to enforce a budget resolution when also making changes in mandatory spending and revenues.

[58] Director of health legislation for the NGA. *Health Care Policy Report,* March 13, 1995, p. 412.

[59] Ibid., April 17, 1995, p. 626; also Howard Cohen, interview, May 19, 1999.

[60] Ibid., p. 627.

[61] Ibid., May 29, 1995, p. 868.

[62] Formula fights occur over the formulas used to distribute among the states grant money that funds activities and programs such as highway construction, water pollution control, welfare programs, and, of course, Medicaid. They are common and often protracted and hard fought. The size of the stakes and the complexity of the issues made Medicaid special.

[63] Interview, June 16, 1999.

[64] Howard Cohen, for instance, thought Medicare policy was technical and prosaic compared with the variety, drama, and pathos of Medicaid.

[65] Since the payment formula involved distribution to the states, the Senate might have been more prominent. According to Howard Cohen, the House Commerce Committee had more staff and "we had Ed Grossman" (the legislative counsel). Interview, May 19, 1999.

[66] Ibid.

[67] *Health Care Policy Report,* September 18, 1995, p. 1438.

[68] Andy Schneider, Health Policy Group, formerly Democratic staff, Commerce Committee. Interview, June 15, 1999.

[69] Jack Ebeler. Interview, January 6, 1999.

[70] Burney substituted in part for an actuary, though the group also sought information from the HCFA actuary. One major problem was the lack of hospital data and projections. Judith Feder, dean of Policy Studies, Georgetown University, then deputy assistant secretary for planning and evaluation. Interview, April 7, 1999; and Jeanne Lambrew, then a special assistant to Jack Ebeler.

[71] Especially Karen Nelson and Bridgett Taylor.

[72] Bridgett Taylor, Commerce Committee, Democratic Staff. Interview June 2, 1999.

[73] Howard Cohen. Interview, January 13, 1999.

[74] Ray Sheppach. Interview, June 16, 1999.

[75] Andy Schneider. Interview, June 15, 1999.

[76] Judith Feder. Interview, April 7, 1999. An anecdote recounted by Bridgett Taylor illustrates this theme. Henry Waxman and John Dingell had an amendment on nursing home standards that they wished to have considered. Taylor, aware that repeal of the Boren amendments was coming up next, alerted Dingell, the ranking member. With some old-fashioned oratory about the Boren amendments and the shame of earlier days when patients were tied to their beds or kicked out, Dingell got the repeal defeated in subcommittee. But Republicans besieged the White House with such dire threats about how this vote might prejudice other good causes that Chris Jennings (health policy adviser to the president) called back, imploring Dingell to negotiate a compromise through Howard Cohen. Repeal of the Boren amendment went back, but it was agreed that the Dingell-Waxman quality amendment would not be opposed on a later voice vote. According to Taylor, the Democrats later got even more in the Senate.

[77] Including Feder, Nelson, and Taylor.

[78] The "double M, double E" or "Medicare/Medicaid, Environment and Education" was a developing strategy, but firmly in place by August. Jack Ebeler, interview, January 6, 1999.

[79] Karen Nelson. Interview, August 19, 1998.

[80] On one occasion, in the midst of the block grant controversy, President Clinton was to attend a governors' meeting in Nevada. Worried about the president's tendency to "schmooze" with his former colleagues over Medicaid and that he might unintentionally "give away the store," one of Dingell's staff called Chris Jennings in the White House. Together, they agreed to orchestrate a full-fledged demonstration at the meeting site in Nevada to remind Clinton of the other and "human" side of the argument. Bridgett Taylor. Interview, June 2, 1999.

[81] Judith Feder, then in DHHS, said that she did not trust Clinton or think he was

"solid" on Medicaid and that only when advocates for the program began to be successful did he think he could defend Medicaid. Interview, April 7, 1999.

[82] In 1994, the AARP was keeping a low profile in part because of member reaction to the association's involvement in health care reform and the Medicare Catastrophic Coverage Act. According to Ray Sheppach, the AARP leadership was also aware that the Republican Medicaid proposal was not likely to succeed.

[83] James Bentley, senior vice-president, American Hospital Association. Interview, November 18, 1998.

[84] Herb Kuhn, vice-president for federal relations, AHA. Interview, January 13, 1999.

[85] *National Journal,* June 10, 1995, p. 1399.

[86] Herb Kuhn. Interview, January 13, 1999.

[87] *National Journal,* June 10, 1995, p. 1399.

[88] James Bentley. Interview, November 18, 1998.

[89] Per capita caps had been proposed in the Reagan administration, at which time Clinton opposed it. The proposal came from Jack Lew, of OMB, via the task force.

[90] *Health Care Policy Report,* June 26, 1995, pp. 1002–4.

[91] Most who were associated with this initiative seemed to think so, but one staff person said PCCs were "a great defense play" that "threw a spanner in the works."

[92] Ray Sheppach, interview, June 16, 1999.

[93] *Health Care Policy Report,* September 26, 1995.

[94] *Congressional Quarterly Almanac,* 1995, pp. 7–20. This addition was also of interest because the push for it was led by Gregg Ganske (R., Ia.) one of several physicians turned legislator in the House.

[95] Howard Cohen, interview, June 6, 2000; Eric Berger, professional staff, Commerce Committee. Interview, November 12, 1998.

[96] Medicaid and Health Care for Low Income Families; also chairman of Public Works and Environment.

[97] For instance, from Pete Domenici, Bob Packwood, and Bill Frist (R. Tenn.), a physician.

[98] *Congressional Quarterly,* September 28, 1995, p. 2898.

[99] *Congressional Quarterly Almanac,* 1995, p. 7–21.

[100] Ibid.

[101] Ibid.

[102] Ibid.

[103] Ibid., p. 7–23.

[104] H.Rept. 104–350.

4

Medicare—1995

"If we solve Medicare, I think we will govern for a generation." This statement, by Newt Gingrich in a June 28 interview with the *Atlanta Constitution,* could be dismissed as an example of the speaker's robust and often inflated rhetoric.[1] But it should not be, since he meant what he said. It raises a question of why he and other members of the House Republican leadership attributed such importance to Medicare and to "solving" it.

At an obvious level, large Medicare savings would be needed to balance the budget, especially with Social Security and defense off the table. Not all Republicans accepted the first premise of a need to balance the budget or, as Pete Domenici said, to make more than a "down payment" on the deficit. Even so, with savings of $900 billion projected over seven years, few believed[2] that amount could be achieved without substantial Medicare reductions. Moreover, leadership Republicans—John Kasich, Richard Armey, and Pete Domenici—recognized that savings of that magnitude would require structural changes in the Medicare program, which would be a major undertaking.

Among the savvier participants in Newt Gingrich's House revolution, the budget process and, especially, budget reconciliation were valued as engines for transforming government as well as for reducing budget outlays because they could be used to restructure programs or curtail activities without requiring the time-consuming and uncertain processes of ordinary legislation. Since much of their agenda was to shrink government and to deregulate, devolve, or privatize rather than to initiate new programs, budget reconciliation could serve well as a primary vehicle.

In taking this path, the House Republicans were following a lead of President Reagan in the drastic budget and program reductions enacted by the Omnibus Budget Reconciliation Act of 1981.[3] Of course, in 1994, Republicans controlled the Congress rather than the presidency, but Democrats had shown, especially under the Reagan administration, what could be accomplished under divided government when one party controlled the budget and appropriations process and how the reconciliation process could be used to expand or to amend entitlements such as Medicare and Medicaid. So there were precedents. What the House Republicans did was to take maximum advantage of their legislative powers over the budget, appropriations, and taxation.

Newt Gingrich often spoke of reforming Medicare, not just of reducing outlays or ending the entitlement as such. He knew that savings from Medicare would be needed. He was also aware of the sacrosanct status of Medicare, the political power of the provider and beneficiary constituencies, and the daunting complexity of the program. When he spoke of "solving" Medicare, he meant that—along with ending the entitlement—the program had to be substantially improved and modernized. More than budgetary reductions, he was interested in "successor" institutions—those that could take the places of the ones we have today.[4] The largest entitlement after Social Security, Medicare was popular, well defended, and highly visible. It was also a tangled thicket of problems, having gone for thirty years without a major overhaul. It would be a challenge. But the speaker's expansive statement expressed a hope, shared by many who worked on the Medicare Preservation Act, that it could be a showcase demonstration of the soundness and fairness with which Republican ideas such as personal responsibility, consumer choice, and competition could be applied to this historic (and antiquated) program. One premise, not unreasonable, is that Medicare could be made more competitive through added choice and that competition would save money both for the government and for beneficiaries. Another was that by shifting much of the risk from the government to private insurers—for instance, as done by the Federal Employees' Health Benefits Program (FEHBP)—greater efficiency and adaptability could be achieved even as government intrusiveness and micromanagement were reduced.

At the same time, the budget reconciliation process—especially when associated with a campaign style of legislating—creates a tension between the objective of reform or restructuring and that of deficit reduction. The strategic objectives of the party leadership and the budget committee chairmen tend to encroach upon the substantive policies of the authorizing committees. Deficit reduction and reconciliation emphasize "scoreable"[5] savings over more experimental options that might receive wider, bipartisan support. Motives become suspect as to whether, for instance, Medicare is being preserved or only more money taken from the program. And, combining major reform or restructuring with deep budget cuts raises the political stakes very high, leading to partisan mobilization on both sides of the aisle. Partisanship sows distrust, invites demagoguery, and hardens positions, all of which work against compromise on substantive policy.

People studying the Medicare Preservation Act in 1995 were often surprised to discover how sensible it was, especially considering the opprobrium heaped upon it. Not only was much of it well crafted but it seemed for the most part driven by policy rather than politics, as though the principals and their staff were earnestly seeking a "successor" institution to traditional Medicare. Much of what it sought to achieve was later incorporated into the Medicare+Choice legislation, adopted in 1997 with overwhelming bipartisan support. But the rhetoric and tactics that accompanied the reconciliation process in 1995 as well as some of the proposals advanced for Medicare seemed aimed at its destruction rather than its preservation. With little opportunity for compromise or reassurance as to the majority's intentions, the situation lent itself to assuming the worst, to judging the Medicare Preservation Act by the company it kept and the rhetoric it inspired, and to countering this assault with "Mediscare" demagoguery. One side won a major political victory; but useful reforms were delayed and a pestilent partisanship still infects efforts to restructure or reform Medicare.

I. PREPARING THE WAY

In the new Congress, there was a broadly shared consensus that 1995 would be a big reconciliation year, with much of the initiative coming from the leadership and the Budget Committee. Balancing the budget was a campaign pledge; and a Balanced Budget Amendment was the first item in the Contract with America. In the House, the budget process got off to a running start, not waiting for the president's budget to appear in February. Within the first week, John Kasich, chairman of the Budget Committee, announced hearings to revise the budget for the existing fiscal year, and Robert Livingston—whom Gingrich had picked to chair the Appropriations Committee—began hearings on February 1 for a rescissions[6] bill that might amount to as much as $20 billion. Their presumption, widely shared, was that balancing the budget, with Newt Gingrich overseeing the process, would be a top priority in 1995.[7]

Along with more comprehensive schemes, health care reform of an incremental variety was another salient objective. One reason was public expectation. Despite the Clinton health care reform debacle, Republicans did not wish to be seen as purely negative. Some thought that a modest incremental package, successfully passed, might make their efforts look good in contrast to the Democrats' more extreme behavior.[8] Moreover, Republican members of the committees of jurisdiction—Ways and Means, Commerce, and Economic and Educational Opportunities—had ideas of their own and cherished projects that had long been bottled up by a Democratic majority. Strong interest was expressed both in the House and Senate for an incremental bill, or bills, that would include such items as limited insurance reform, medical malpractice reform, tax deductions for health insurance, and medical savings accounts.[9] There were also discussions about budget reductions for Medicare and Medicaid, but no ambitious projects for structural change.

Medicare (and Medicaid) were not included in the Contract with America in part because debate over health care reform was still continuing while the contract was being drafted in 1994. The House Republican leadership, especially Newt Gingrich, also thought that Medicare and Medicaid merited independent consideration, needed more time for preparation, and might derail the contract. As previously noted (see pp. 33–34), the contract helped encourage a campaign mode of legislation and give impetus to the budget-balancing effort. But only one item on product liability dealt even remotely with health care.

Midway through January, Speaker Gingrich called upon House Republicans to set up task forces to study possible reforms in Medicare and Medicaid along with budget reductions. These task forces would be led by the chairmen and subcommittee chairmen of the relevant committees and were charged with writing the legislation that would ultimately be sent to the committees of jurisdiction for their approval. The task force on Medicaid was to be formed immediately; that on Medicare could wait until spring. In this particular initiative, Gingrich associated reform and budget reductions, though not emphasizing Medicare.[10]

The use of task forces to develop legislative proposals had been a standard House Republican practice when they were in the minority, used especially for initiatives that involved two or more committees. It saved time, pooled staff resources, and promoted collaboration. Since it shifted much of the activity from the committee or subcommittee to the chairmen and their staffs, it cut down on time spent in committee hearings and sharing information with the opposition and listening to their views. Such task forces could also be an effective way to bring the leadership closer together and increase its influence over the committee's ultimate decisions.[11]

On January 30, Newt Gingrich and Bill Thomas, chairman of the Ways and Means Health Subcommittee, addressed an annual meeting of the American Hospital Association (AHA). Both spoke of the need for a fundamental reexamination of Medicare, but added that reform came before reductions in the program. Gingrich said that savings would be minor, probably less than those for Medicaid. Responding in part to President Clinton's State of the Union message, they added that Medicare savings would not be used to pay for the tax cuts promised in the Contract with America.[12]

In February, as the budget process moved forward, House Republican leaders with an interest in health formed an advisory panel or "steering committee" to advise the speaker on health reform, Medicare, and Medicaid. This group included the chairmen and health subcommittee chairmen of Ways and Means, Commerce, and Economic and Educational Opportunities. In this and subsequent meetings they discussed among themselves and with the House leadership such issues as overall strategy, whether to focus on a number of incremental bills or one omnibus reconciliation, and what role bipartisan collaboration should play.

On February 17, the same day that the advisory panel convened, John Kasich announced a leadership agreement with unusually tight spending targets. He warned at the time that members would have to be "creative" in coming up with structural changes needed to reach a balanced budget. Speaker Gingrich, who had been gradually taking a larger part in the budget process, said that he would be the "final arbiter" in any disputes with the budget committee—a statement that acknowledged both the role anticipated for him and the priority assigned to budget reconciliation.[13]

Early in March, the rescissions bill, which sought to eliminate or "rescind" $17 billion in existing appropriations, cleared the appropriations committee and was being debated on the floor of the House. Meanwhile, the Budget Committee was busy with a $190 billion package of budget reductions for the coming year, intended to pay for the tax cut promised in the Contract with America. One hundred billion dollars of these proposed reductions would be achieved by lowering caps on discretionary spending, but $90 billion of the savings was parceled out among entitlement programs including Medicare. Coming off that, John Kasich signaled on March 22—a month in advance of the committee's April report—that Medicare cuts might top $300 billion over seven years. He also introduced a new Republican theme, adding that he would move more quickly than the administration because of the impending insolvency of the Medicare hospital insurance trust fund.[14]

A speech to the AMA's National Leadership Conference on March 28 revealed some of the speaker's thinking at that time. He stressed in particular that part of the agenda would be incremental reforms such as increasing the health care tax deduction for the self-employed, establishing medical savings accounts, and extending ERISA protections to the small group market. But he added that the most important challenge would be "transforming Medicare" to provide more choices for seniors and to make the program more responsive to competitive market forces.[15] With characteristic flair, he urged the AMA members to share their views with their representatives in Congress about how best to change Medicare.

Early in April, immediately after passage of the Contract with America, Gingrich announced that he would be directly involved in the drafting of a Republican health care reform plan and the passage of an incremental package.[16] He then merged the earlier Medicare and Medicaid task forces and appointed himself chairman of the joint task force. These moves assured a dominant leadership role in developing the legislation, which would, initially, be drafted by the speaker's task force and only then submitted to Ways and Means and Commerce for their approval.

This evolution helped to mark out the agenda as well as to provide a method of pursuing it. There would be either an aggregated package or separate incremental bills, ultimate role and content to be determined. There would be a budget reconciliation with savings from Medicare on the order of $300 billion over seven years. Savings of this magnitude would both require and facilitate a transformation of Medicare, which would receive the attention of a special task force as well as the independent scrutiny and approval of the committees of jurisdiction. Leadership concerns within the task force would be protected by the chairman (Gingrich) and the added presence of John Kasich, the Budget Committee chairman.[17]

In a little over three months, the health care agenda had moved from one in which incremental reform had top priority to one in which deficit reduction was primary, restructuring of Medicare next, and incremental reform subsidiary. Given the shared understandings about the leadership role, and the importance of balancing the budget and of transforming institutions, this change in emphasis is not surprising, though the speed and effectiveness with which it was brought about were remarkable. As a way of achieving fundamental reform, the underlying strategy could be a good one, for it made use of the urgency and mobilizing energy of the reconciliation process but provided for the time, expertise, and policy input needed to draft a competent piece of legislation. The political danger of associating comprehensive reform and budget reconciliation was still considerable, because of the high stakes, the confounding of motives, and conflicting rhetoric about "saving Medicare" while getting rid of entitlements

Of particular note was the task force appointed by Speaker Gingrich to develop the Medicare draft. Like other Gingrich innovations, it was an adaptation of familiar institutions. Yet participants said that it was unlike any task force they had worked on, before or since, in the scope of its assignment, the time and resources committed, and the intensity of the work.

Members of the "task force," as it was generally called,[18] were the speaker; Archer and Thomas from Ways and Means; Bliley and Bilirakis from Commerce; at times, Fawell from Economic and Educational Opportunities; Hastert, the chief deputy whip, and John Kasich. Particularly notable about this list is the bringing together of committee chairs and leadership representatives.

The task force met regularly, though not according to a set schedule, in the speaker's Policy Office. This office was also known as the "Dinosaur Room," because of a huge Tyrannosaurus Rex skull that the speaker—a genuine dinosaur buff—had gotten on extended loan from the Smithsonian Institution. Gingrich acted as chair, but in his absence was represented by a spokesperson, Ed Kutler—a method he used to protect both his time and policy interests.[19] Members sat around a long table, with staff often behind them on chairs. The staff also worked there, especially on joint problems. The meetings were long and frequent and went on steadily until the budget negotiations finally collapsed, well into the next year. One staff aide recalled looking through a window at the trees, during occasional quiet moments, and watching the leaves change as the seasons completed a full cycle.

Staffing this task force presented a special problem for two reasons. One was that the House Republicans had been in the minority for forty years and were short of experienced committee staff to deal with legislation of this scope and complexity. Instead of hiring against this need, the new Republican majority cut committee staffs by one-third, leaving the Democrats with skeleton staffs and themselves with shortages of experienced junior staff. Also important was the mood of partisan hostility and the limits put upon communication or collaboration with Democratic counterparts or the Clinton administration. As one result, whatever limited benefits might have been obtained from the minority or from HCFA and DHHS were sharply limited.

This shortage of staff and expertise was dealt with in several ways. One was the task force itself, which pooled staff resources and economized on the number of member briefings. The Commerce Committee had two highly professional senior staff: Howard Cohen and Mary McGrane. Ways and Means hired two experienced staff people from outside. One was Chip Kahn, a staff veteran with many years of experience, that had included putting together major statutes. As a second to Bill Gradison at the Health Insurance Association of America (HIAA), he had orchestrated the "Harry and Louise" campaign that was so effective against the Clinton administration's health care reform. He had also been a manager in two of Newt Gingrich's campaigns. The other was Kathy Means, an economist, with experience both in HCFA and with the Senate Finance staff. The task force drew, variously, upon congressional staff agencies, including the Congressional Budget Office, the Congressional Research Service, and the General Accounting Office.

The two commissions, ProPAC and PPRC, were especially valuable as sources of institutional memory and politically neutral policy expertise. Each of the commissions had a history of working with Congress and especially the relevant committees of jurisdiction. Their reports provided a rich policy history for any number of cost-saving recommendations. Their chairmen were available to testify. And the commissions, through their directors, could provide data, simulations, and the results of computer runs.[20] Many participants commented on the value of these commissions, and on their "neutral competence" although working in a politically charged environment.[21] It is worth noting in this context, that ProPAC was created largely because Congress had been unable to get facts and figures from the Reagan administration and that PPRC was initially established so that Congress would have a source of information and policy options available to help it design a fee schedule for Medicare.

Another important staff aid was the House Office of Legislative Counsel, and especially Ed Grossman—whose institutional memory, capacity to express complex thought in written text, and grasp the parts and the whole of a huge bill may be unique in the annals of legislation. He was present at all task force sessions in which legislation was being written. In a special drafting room, he had a computerized projection system that could be used to project text and amendments on a screen, radically reducing the time needed for drafting, as sentences were quickly altered and paragraphs transposed for comment. Always mentioned with both awe and affection, he was regarded as a major resource. A senior staff person, explaining why the House often did better in conference on Medicare issues than the Senate said: "We had more staff than the Senate—and we had Ed Grossman."[22]

The special task force was one indication of the political and strategic importance that Speaker Gingrich attributed to Medicare. Another was the preparations he made to co-opt or reassure some of the potential opposition, especially the big advocacy groups for providers and for beneficiaries.

A salient characteristic of legislation dealing with Medicare, as opposed to Medicaid, is the importance of large, national advocacy groups. For Medicaid, there are few powerful champions of the poor, except occasionally the DSH hospitals or the National Governors' Association. For Medicare, by contrast, there are powerful, well-heeled, and savvy national organizations such as the American Association of Retired Persons, the AHA, the AMA, the American Association of Health Plans (AAHP), and a large number of smaller, specialized groups that follow their lead or lobby on related, niche issues. In addition to these, there are a number of business associations, such as the Health Insurance Association of America or the American Trial Lawyer's Association, that have a stake in issues related to Medicare such as medical savings accounts or malpractice reform. Almost any one of these groups, given the right issue and good timing, could threaten or defeat major legislation, as the famous "Harry and Louise" campaign of the HIAA had demonstrated in 1993.

Newt Gingrich was well aware of the power of these national advocacy groups and their importance for Medicare policy. Earlier, he had expressed some misgivings about taking on Medicare, thinking it might be a political "third rail"[23] like Social Security. By any sort of calculation, this particular problem was a major challenge, which the speaker dealt with in characteristic fashion—adapting familiar institutions with his own personal flair.

One practice that had grown up in the 1980s, though beginning with the Carter administration, was legislating by inducing industry or advocacy groups to "come to the table" with responsive alternative proposals of their own. For hospitals, especially, this practice began with a growing awareness of their common interest and the need to negotiate at the peak with committee or subcommittee chairmen. On the congressional side, the approach was to initiate a proposal designed to soften up the providers and "bring them to the table" with an alternative. It also helped if lead associations such as the AHA would represent the industry as a whole and do some of the work of sorting out differences. The presumption was that a reasonable offering brought to the table would be recognized, not with a quid pro quo, but where possible and appropriate with some kind of accommodation. This kind of approach—helpful in making unpleasant redistributive decisions—often characterized tax legislation. It was also generally employed in the budget reconciliation acts of the 1980s and beyond.[24]

Beginning early and continuing through the legislative cycle, Gingrich was assiduous in his cultivation of important advocacy groups, including the AARP, the AHA, the AMA, the AAHP, and other smaller and more specialized ones. His particular adaptation of inviting people to the "table" was to be positive and expansive—reaching out first; seeking to persuade, cajole or intimidate; and working to develop ententes of mutual interest.[25] People who participated in the process commented especially on the openness with which the speaker solicited their views, the persuasiveness with which he explained his own policies, and his eagerness to find common ground. As with tax legislation, people shared the pain, but got enough to prevent open opposition. More positively, Gingrich sought to co-opt or get people to share in his vision of a creative transformation. He also gave individual attention to each of the advocacy groups and its leaders, varying his approach as appropriate.

One group especially sought out was the AARP, a giant advocacy group with a membership of thirty-three million senior citizens, enormous lobbying resources, and a long history of successful campaigns. Even before 1995, when still the minority whip, Gingrich had begun overtures to the AARP. With Medicare on the agenda, he actively courted this group, going to their headquarters in Washington, and speaking to their board and top executives. He was described as "very pragmatic, quiet, a realist—all the way through" and his message was, "I can't get done what I want to do without you; you can't get what you want without me."[26] What Gingrich wanted was for the AARP to lay off—not oppose him. For his part, he intended to make additional burdens on beneficiaries as light as possible, to retain the traditional FFS program as one of the options, and to put some limits on medical savings accounts. Chastened by membership reaction to earlier support of health care reform and mindful that they were not likely to do better in the House, the AARP leadership concentrated its efforts on the Senate.[27]

The AMA already shared much of the philosophy and objectives being pursued by Gingrich and the House Republicans, so that accommodating them presented little difficulty. The AMA had long supported the idea of a defined contribution and of private sector medical savings accounts.[28] Medical malpractice reform and modifications to the antitrust laws were agenda items for them as for the House Republicans. Especially important for the AMA was legislation facilitating provider-sponsored networks (PSNs), which would have given physicians a larger role in managing care and strengthened them in relation to HMOs and insurance companies. This innovation, which also expanded choice for beneficiaries, was supported by Gingrich as one way the physicians as well as the hospitals could be accommodated.[29] Other than that, the AMA was concerned that physicians not be singled out for big hits, and that implementation of the resource-based practice expense payment schedule be delayed.[30]

The health plans had much to gain and much to lose. On the loss side would be subsidies for medical education, which they shared with FFS Medicare, and their comfortable payment formula, based on average payment rates for FFS Medicare patients. They, along with the insurance companies such as Aetna and Blue Cross/Blue Shield, had a major stake in the certification requirements and insurance standards for the PSNs or provider-sponsored organizations (PSOs). There was much either to lose or to gain in the new payment formulas and updates. And there was an enormous amount to be gained, or so it seemed at the time, from access on favorable terms to the anticipated flow of Medicare patients into managed care entities.[31]

For the health plans, the situation was one that counseled staying engaged, and bargaining and maneuvering so as to reap future benefits. Moreover, Gingrich was reassuring, encouraging the AAHP and individual health plans to develop proposals of their own, explaining the schemes for "modernization" that he and other Republican leaders had in mind, and inviting the health plans to participate in a better future.[32] Like the AARP, the AAHP largely reserved their objections for the Senate.

The AHA was especially favored with outreach, though more to neutralize the association than to win it over.[33] For the most part their relations with Gingrich and the Republican majority were those of an ongoing, sporadic dialog, punctuated by periods of open hostility.[34] Like the AMA, the AHA had an interest in medical malpractice and antitrust policy. The AHA also supported PSOs, its own version of PSNs, and it shared with the AMA and the Republican House a desire to "modernize" the system and to move toward a successor to the contemporary hospital. But it differed with the Congress over a matter of money—specifically the size of the cuts the hospitals would be expected to absorb.

In a year of deficit reduction, the AHA leadership was well aware that they could expect substantial cuts in payments. They hoped for something in the neighborhood of $80 billion as a total figure for Medicare, with an opportunity to get specific reductions "well placed" so as to cause the least harm. According to one AHA representative, they might even "give them [Congress] a road map" to $180 billion.[35] But the Congress wanted $260 billion and over that number and the Medicaid DSH cuts (see pp. 58–59). The AHA parted company with Gingrich in early May[36] and launched a major newspaper, TV, and grass-roots campaign. They renewed the dialog later, but intermittently and warily.

On the whole, Newt Gingrich's strategy for winning over or neutralizing the opposition was successful. Only one major group opposed him on Medicare and that not very effectively. One way of looking at this process would be to say these stakeholders were "bought off" or induced by various "sweeteners" to go along.[37] But people who witnessed or participated in the process resisted the notion that "deal making" or specific inducements were important. In general, it seemed like the usual "coming to the table" and the kind of implicit trades typically associated with the reconciliation process—but with more outreach on the speaker's part and a greater effort to co-opt or to associate the participants with the "transformative" process. Although described as dazzling, Gingrich's approach probably made few converts. But it did achieve two other purposes, aside from muting the criticism. One was to make the Republican leadership "bulletproof" by giving the advocacy groups a stake in the process.[38] Another was to provide some "cover" for the representatives, who, along with the budget cuts and obvious pain, could point to important benefits received by their constituents.

Early in April, the House Republicans—conscious of their rising disapproval ratings—were developing the message that they would use to justify the deep cuts in Medicare (Drew 1996:185). Gingrich and other Republican leaders had for some weeks been insisting that language such as "cutting" or "slashing"—appropriate enough for taxes—not be applied to Medicare, and that more soothing phrases such as "slowing the rate of increase" be used instead. Gingrich stressed modernizing Medicare and offering more choice, and pollsters, who had been testing various themes, recommended "protect, improve, and strengthen Medicare" as a phrase that resonated well with the electorate.[39]

On April 3, the Medicare trustees reported, as they had nine times since 1970, that the Hospital Trust Fund would soon be "bankrupt"—this time, in seven years. The coincidence seemed almost providential. Indeed, Haley Barbour, the Republican national chairman, proclaimed this news "manna from heaven." The message that developed—of slowing the growth of Medicare expenditures in order to save the Trust Fund and improve Medicare for future generations—was one that Republicans used with remarkable effectiveness throughout the summer of 1995. This message cast Republicans as preserving an entitlement, not destroying it, and as concerned about a future generation—an issue that Democrats had so far chosen largely to ignore. This revised Republican theme not only avoided blame, it shifted it (Weaver 1987).

In early May, the House Republicans held a two-day retreat in Leesburg, Virginia, to discuss the budget. At this meeting, they were lectured by pollsters on the approved message and the way to refer to the impending cuts in Medicare (Drew 1996:206). The next week, on May 11, the House Budget Committee reported out its resolution. One week later, the House approved spending reductions of $282 billion for Medicare and $184 billion for Medicaid. On May 25, the Senate followed with $256 billion for Medicare and $175 billion for Medicaid.

II. THE DEMOCRATS COUNTER

On February 6, President Clinton sent Congress his fiscal year 1996 budget. This budget was a "placeholder," making the gesture but conceding little and nicely masking the administration's substantive intentions.[40] It contained something for everyone: incremental program increases, a middle-class tax cut, modest deficit reduction, and $178 billion for Medicare, an 11 percent increase. Especially lacking were serious budget cuts that would give Republicans precedent or guidance for their own deficit reduction efforts. President Clinton invited the Republicans to go first, challenging them to provide "specific and real details" of how they would set about reducing the deficit. Leading Republicans deplored this "abdication" of the president. Pete Domenici, Senate budget chairman, said that without a more substantive budget from the president, "I don't know where we are going," and John Kasich called it a "tragedy," saying that the president was setting "a trap for people who are serious about deficit reduction."[41] Some of the background for this episode is instructive.

Deficit reduction and tax cuts were the centerpiece of the House Republicans' agenda. Among their campaign pledges were a tax cut of $200 billion over five years, a balanced budget amendment to the Constitution, and ending the deficit by the year 2002. Some House Republicans arrived in January proposing to put together their own budget and make the president's budget irrelevant.[42] But more moderate counsel prevailed, with arguments that the president's budget could guide them, force the president to share the pain, and provide cover for the Republicans. They were disappointed, even disconcerted, by the president's budget, since it forced them to go it alone. There was talk of trying to seek a budget summit—like that between President Bush and a Democratic Congress in 1990—but the prospects seemed poor and, besides, that particular precedent was not encouraging.[43]

From the president's perspective, the choice was not obvious, since he shared some objectives with the Republicans, such as deficit reduction and tax cuts. Some weighty members of his own party and administration were deficit "hawks" and thought that he should go farther in this direction. Among Democrats, though, there were memories of 1993 when not a single Republican had voted for the Democratic deficit reduction effort. Understandably, they thought the Republicans ought to have a turn of their own. Furthermore, as one former Budget Committee staffer observed at the time, Congress would pass whatever it saw fit, and "if your [Democratic] proposals are not going to be enacted, why take the heat."[44] The president made no moves to encourage a summit or even to engage in serious consultations with the Congress. He waited for their budget.

At this juncture, the administration and congressional Democrats were busy with skirmishes over the Contract with America, welfare reform, and the rescissions bill. They were also struggling to reposition themselves politically and develop a new message with appropriate strategies. In large measure, the House Republican majority, with its zeal and inexperience, made the Democrats' initial strategic choice for them. That choice was generally described as "counterpunching"—waiting for Republican initiatives and then coming to the defense of popular programs or principles when the Republican majority overstepped. An early case in point was the school lunch program, where the Democrats could accuse Republicans of taking food from poor children to provide tax cuts for the rich (see pp. 44–45). The veto was also considered, including likely occasions for its use, such as cuts in loans for higher education or attempts to weaken or repeal the Safe Water Drinking Act of 1974. Medicare was specifically mentioned.[45]

This defensive strategy had a number of advantages, some of them not obvious. Most immediately, the Democrats avoided making a stand prematurely and gained time to take stock and regroup. At a stage when the administration desperately needed a new message—something that resonated more deeply than the "New Covenant"—this approach, especially the veto part, prompted thought about priorities and principles that had to be defended.[46] Moreover, as the battle over rescissions demonstrated, this strategy let Republicans do much of the work of mobilizing Democrats.

While not apparent at the time, these maneuvers also put the House Republicans at a strategic disadvantage. Congress, the naturally pluralistic and more responsive branch, would propose the budget, while the administration, with its advantages of unity and capacity to develop agendas and frame debate, would be in a position to wait, find the points of weakness, and counterattack. In Congress, Republicans would be challenging seasoned congressional Democrats on familiar home ground: entitlements they had watched over and worked with for many years. Moreover, the Republicans had themselves associated Medicare and Medicaid in their budget strategy, which helped strengthen the defense of each of these entitlements.[47]

Much of early Democratic tactics, both in Congress and the administration, amounted to attacking Republicans for "excessive" cuts and trying "to put a human face on the numbers."[48] In doing so, they were disadvantaged by a lack of detail to go with the Republican numbers being proposed and by not having a counterbudget of their own.[49] In this respect, they were aided by the informal task force that had developed within the executive branch (see pp. 56–57) and, within Congress, by the cumulative political experience and policy expertise of the members and their staffs and their well-established ties with health care advocacy groups. Indeed, one of the most important achievements of Democrats during this period was to hold together and help mobilize these resources—another reason why a period for regrouping was so important.

Despite advantages, the defensive strategy was inadequate by itself, in large measure because the counterpunching lacked much punch: Republicans were not listening.[50] and the public was little moved by data on the impact of the budget cuts or Medicare structural issues and arcane problems of risk selection.[51] They began to get "traction" only when they associated the Medicare reductions with tax cuts for the rich, a theme used at the time of the rescissions controversy, especially on the school lunch issue. It worked well for both the administration and the congressional Democrats, even though Democrats disliked taking such a negative posture.

According to standard texts, with a defensive strategy should go a consideration of whether, when, and how to go on the offensive. At the White House these issues were being debated largely in terms of whether the president should do his own version of a balanced budget. Some within the administration shared the view of many House Democrats that they should continue with their present strategy and let the Republicans hang themselves.[52] People who were strong on program, like Gene Sperling and George Stephanopoulos, were loath to abandon cherished campaign pledges, especially "investments in people," and opposed budget cuts (Stephanopoulos 1999:343). Taking the other side, Dick Morris was urging "triangulation," i.e., a compromise budget (Drew 1996:217–18).[53] Democratic deficit "hawks" were arguing that the president ought not to concede all of this issue to the Republicans, and still others said that the president needed a serious budget to bolster House moderates who might defect to the Blue Dog coalition.[54] The debate was intense, but consensus among the White House staff was elusive.

During much of this debate, Clinton was concerned about timing: whether to seek a balance in seven years or ten, and what priorities came first. But he was more pushing than being pushed on whether there should be such a budget. One reason, according to George Stephanopoulos (1999:345), was that he was by nature positive and optimistic and did not like playing defense. Chris Jennings, health adviser to the president, shared this view, saying that Clinton believed, "If you don't play, you don't win," that it was not enough merely "to hold off the enemy." He added that doing a serious budget—as opposed to merely positioning himself—helped Clinton decide what he stood for.[55] Clinton himself—as reported by Stephanopoulos (1999:343)—provides an additional insight from a conversation with his advisers: "You guys want me to go out and criticize the Republicans, and when they say, 'Where's your plan?' you want me to say, 'Well, who am I? I'm just the President of the United States. I don't have a plan.'"

Taken in context, his statement reflected a view that the president must provide leadership and not merely object to what Congress was doing. At the

same time, the observation would also be much to the point if he were contemplating a veto.

These discussions were taking place in May, only days before the president's
proposed budget to reach a balance in ten years was made public. Such decisions are not often made without carefully thought out options and some plausible numbers to consider. In other words, there had to be an earlier decision
to develop a proposal with realistic expenditure and revenue projections, baseline numbers, credible savings, and acceptable substantive proposals. That
decision came early in April, after both the House and Senate Republicans had
clearly signaled that the budget resolution would contain drastic reductions,
with the heaviest weight to be borne by Medicare and Medicaid. President
Clinton, explaining that he needed something with which to respond and had
to have alternatives, asked his staff to develop a budget that would reach a balance and to have it ready for June.[56]

Medicare and Medicaid would, of course, be part of a larger proposal that
involved other entitlements and mandatory spending, discretionary spending,
tax cuts or increases, revenue projections, and many other variables. Medicare
and Medicaid reductions together were actually less than the total cuts in discretionary spending. But Medicare, along with Medicaid and welfare, had
been targeted. not only for deficit reduction but for structural changes that
would end the entitlement status of the program and fundamentally change
its operation. As the largest entitlement with the most political support,[57]
Medicare was also the easiest to defend. And winning on Medicare could help
protect Medicaid as well. Because of considerations like these, Medicare
acquired great strategic and symbolic importance for both Democrats and
Republicans.

The particular challenge for the Medicare part of the budget proposal was
not unlike that faced on a larger scale for health care reform in 1993–94:
developing a complicated structural design that would plausibly work; satisfying, or not alienating, key constituencies; hitting a budget target for which
the component parts were moving and interacting; developing a compelling
message and mantra[58] for the whole package; and doing it in a matter of
weeks and under great stress.

The informal task force (see pp. 56–57) already working on responses to the
Republican Medicaid and Medicare initiatives was well suited for this kind of
effort. The key members of this group were almost all veterans of health care
reform, experienced in this kind of activity, well-acquainted with each other
and with established channels of communication in the administration. They
had developed proposals for Ira Magaziner during health care reform and
began working together again after the electoral defeat of November 1994 on
such issues as what to do about a budget or a cap on Medicaid expenditures.[59]
Early in 1995, they resumed functioning as an irregular staff agency, supplying the administration with numbers, policy options, and talking points, and

helping to coordinate quick responses to Republican initiatives. Several members of this group said that they welcomed the challenge of a budget proposal, as a specific task and as a way of moving beyond a defensive posture.

This group met, mostly on call, about once a week in Room 211 of the Old Executive Office Building. As work progressed, the DHHS members met on a daily basis, at 8:00 in the morning. Members were frequently in touch via memos and conference calls. They kept their own superiors informed and "in the loop." But the important line of communication upward was through Chris Jennings to Gene Sperling, a political appointee to the National Economic Council with a strong interest in health policy and a regular in the daily meetings of the White House budget group. In a word, the task force had a ready channel of communication all the way to the president.

In the division of labor that developed, all of the principals brought as resources their own considerable knowledge of policy and politics as well as the staff resources of their administrative divisions. Bruce Vladeck, as the administrator of HCFA, was responsible for program substance, especially the Medicare Choices option and postacute and subacute care. He drew upon the policy expertise and data capabilities of HCFA. Nancy-Ann Min, an associate director of OMB with a staff of fifty on call, was a critical source of timely and authoritative estimates and of a budget perspective. Judith Feder (later Jack Ebeler), as a deputy in Assistant Secretary for Planning and Evaluation [ASPE], worked with her staff to add numbers, do impact analysis, assemble the elements, and negotiate within the department. Chris Jennings coordinated the task force's efforts with high-level policy—communicating to the group the needs and views of his superiors and working to integrate the task force's product into the larger strategic objectives and budget requirements of the White House.

In developing a budget proposal, the task force had some materials with which to begin, such as the president's February budget and OMB option papers, projections, and other supporting information. HCFA could be mined for any number of demonstrations and policy options with which to improve Medicare. There were also OMB and CBO suggestions of where to cut, along with years of accumulated recommendations from ProPAC and PPRC. Another source of guidance was whatever was known of Republican proposals, which could be used to distinguish the administration's position and present it in the most favorable light.

The career civil servants detailed to this group brought specialized expertise and institutional memory that helped develop the specifics of the budget proposal. Ira Burney, knowledgeable about the particulars of the Medicare FFS program, was a source of quick and fairly accurate estimates of expenditure increases and the impact of budget cuts. Peter Hickman, from HCFA's Office of Legislation, could advise about what would seem plausible and play well in Congress, and how best to present it. Mark Miller, from OMB, could add the big numbers about the economy and the deficit and the "scoring" or expected savings of their proposal, as well as guide the task force in using OMB's formidable resources. The HCFA actuary was another resource, not formally incorporated into their group, but frequently consulted and indispensable for reaching their final estimates.[60]

Before leaving the department, the task force's work was fully vetted in the ASPE office, with care taken to keep the secretary and other key staff people informed. Above that level, Chris Jennings was the key coordinator within the Executive Office of the president. Others frequently involved at that level were Gene Sperling of the National Economic Council and Jack Lew, associate director for legislative affairs at OMB. They and their superiors—Laura Tyson and Alice Rivlin—helped articulate the Medicare and Medicaid proposals with the overall economic numbers, political strategy, and presidential message.

On May 23, President Clinton announced that he would have his own plan to offer—after Congress approved its budget resolution in June—which would balance the budget in "eight to ten years." The plan he announced on June 13 would achieve a balance in ten years with proposed reductions of $127 billion for Medicare and of $55 billion for Medicaid.[61] Of the total amount, $156 billion would go for deficit reduction, with $26 billion earmarked for various reform initiatives, such as premium subsidies for the uninsured. This compared to projected House savings of $288 billion for Medicare and $184 billion for Medicaid; and in the Senate, $256 billion for Medicare and $175 billion for Medicaid.

One reason for the ten-year timetable, as opposed to the seven-year period for the House and Senate, was to have more money to spend for the president's other priorities, especially environmental protection and education.[62] As the budget proposal had been developing, the Clinton administration had also been coming to closure on its fundamental priorities for domestic policy—the familiar "Medicare, Medicaid, Education, and the Environment"—which figured prominently in the campaign for a second term.[63]

As expected, the Medicare proposals were friendly to beneficiaries and, for providers, built incrementally on existing administration and HCFA approaches. The Part B premium contribution was permanently set at 25 percent of program costs. Deductibles, copays, and balance billing protections for FFS Medicare stayed essentially as they were. For managed care, the proposal added point-of-service and preferred-provider options and some beneficiary rights but largely adapted existing law with the addition of some pieces from HCFA's "Choices" demonstrations. Postacute and subacute proposals were what HCFA had ready to go or in prospect. Other features, for the most part growing out of HCFA demonstrations, aimed at "modernizing" Medicare, such as competitive bidding, "centers of excellence," and modifications enabling HCFA to act as a "prudent purchaser" of health care.

Initial reactions to President Clinton's deficit reduction proposals were mixed, with a fair amount of favorable comment from Republicans and a considerable amount of grumbling from Democrats. Republicans welcomed Clinton's joining the cause of budget balancing. John Kasich said that the president deserved credit for proposing a "serious budget."[64] Pete Domenici pointed out that Medicare savings using a CBO baseline would be $192 billion, much higher than Clinton's own figures, so that the two sides were closer than might appear. Other Republicans challenged Clinton's projections, saying that his proposal would not come near to balancing the budget within ten years.[65] Moderate Democrats generally applauded Clinton's initiative, one saying that it would make a case for his reelection.[66] Others, especially liberal House Democrats, were angry at the size of the cuts and for, as they saw it, rescuing Republicans from their self-made predicament.

Democrats in Congress

The situation of the House Democrats in 1995 was not a happy one. Many were both physically and emotionally exhausted by the demoralizing health care reform disaster. They had lost the House for the first time in forty years. Minority committee staffs were all but eliminated. Disorganized and without an overall strategy, they saw little but the relatively passive option of objecting to whatever the Republicans proposed. And the Republican majority seemed unstoppable in its resolve to remake the House and repeal much of what Democrats had achieved from the New Deal to the present.

Relations with their own president varied from strained to downright hostile. A number of House Democrats saw Clinton as the man who had lost the House for them. During this period, Clinton worked more with the Senate than the House, in part because of his access, through John Hilley,[67] to Tom Daschle, the Senate minority leader. It was a time, moreover, when Clinton was "triangulating" and following Dick Morris's counsel to distance himself from liberal House Democrats (Drew 1996:65). For their part, these Democrats understandably felt unsure of Clinton, and of whether they could count upon him to stand up when needed or to follow through on his veto promises. Liberal Democrats, including the leadership and a number of ranking committee members, felt strongly that the Republicans should be allowed to "walk off a cliff" if they wished—and that the president ought not to intervene in that process with some "triangulating" compromise budget of his own.

House Democrats were further disadvantaged by shortage of staff and lack of access to information. One of the first acts of the new Republican majority was to reduce committee staffs by one-third, which devastated minority staffs, especially at the subcommittee level, where legislation for Medicare and Medicaid would normally get most intense consideration. Developing legislation through the speaker's task force tended especially to keep minority committee members and staff in the dark. Both Ways and Means and Commerce held hearings, but they were on general issues, not on specific legislative proposals, and the Republican leadership directed that the Balanced Budget Act be closely held and details not disclosed to the minority or the administration until immediately before committee markups.[68] Despite such strictures, majority and minority staff often collaborated;[69] and information, of course, leaked out. But the constraints hampered a more effective political response by Democrats.

Under these circumstances, Democrats in the Commerce and Ways and Means Committees did what they could. They spoke out, in committee or on the floor, against "excessive" cuts or "harmful" program modifications. They and their staff worked with advocacy groups to stir the grass roots and support beneficiary and provider representatives in the hearings.[70] They developed both substantive and "message" amendments for the committee markups. And for Commerce and Ways and Means, the minority developed proposals of their own, which were presented and rejected in the markups. At midnight, during the one day allowed for the Ways and Means Health subcommittee markup, the minority submitted a complete substitute bill that would, they claimed, hold the beneficiaries harmless, get equivalent savings, and extend Medicare Trust Fund solvency as many years as the Republican majority proposal.[71] It was a feat appreciated by insiders, but unnoticed by the larger public.

The Democratic leadership in the House never developed a budget proposal of its own. One reason was that Richard Gephardt, the minority leader, preferred to fight it out with Republicans over their Medicare proposals and did not want a budget that would inevitably communicate a message of concession and going part of the way. Many Democrats shared that view. Even their own Budget Committee members lacked enthusiasm for doing a budget, because they had little to offer and doubted they would get much cooperation from the authorizing committees in developing the numbers. Martin Sabo, the ranking member of the Budget Committee, believed that the Democrats needed a more credible alternative than the president's February budget, with "deficits of $200 billion as far as the eye could see." But for that, Sabo had to join with the Blue Dog coalition.

The Blue Dogs[72] were initially a group of twenty-two or twenty-three conservative Democrats, mostly from the South and West, who felt at odds with the policies of the liberal wing of the party. Some of them supported much of the Contract with America, voting more frequently with Republicans than with Democrats. They came together in mid-February and started working on a budget—a budget that could have decisive importance because of the twenty to forty other Democrats from marginal districts who might desert their party in a critical vote. For this reason, they were assiduously wooed by

Republicans and watched nervously by Democrats and the president. They remained a significant and incalculable factor throughout 1995 and 1996, and are still active today.

Their budget proposal was about midway between the Republicans' and the president's. It called for a $174 billion cut in Medicare and block-granting Medicaid with a 5 percent cap on increases. It included the Democratic version of welfare reform and more money for education. It would balance the budget in seven years, but would allow no tax cut until the budget was in balance. This proposal was one of several voted down—with none of its provisions incorporated—as the House passed its budget resolution on May 18;[73] but it was a plausible alternative and helped rally the Democrats during a bleak season.

The House Democratic leadership largely stood aside from the budget debate in its early stages and offered perfunctory and lukewarm support to President Clinton's alternative. Many of them, including Richard Gephardt, thought that the Republican budget effort would fail to achieve what it promised and might even implode.[74] Some also believed that Medicare would be their ticket back to power and, after the school lunch and rescissions debates, were spoiling for a fight. The leadership saw the Blue Dogs and Clinton as dividing the caucus and diluting their efforts. In Gephardt's view, they should fight for Medicare and attack and rally votes against any proposal with Medicare or Medicaid budget reductions of the size being currently discussed. Their other strategy was to hold enough Democrats so that the minority leadership could count on somewhere between 140 and 190 or 200 votes, depending on the issue.[75] The 140 would sustain a veto; and 200 would enable them to bargain to advantage with the majority.

For the Senate, the most important development during the budget resolution phase was the movement of Democrats from a mode of cautious bipartisanship into one of partisan mobilization. This transformation was largely brought about by the Senate Republicans themselves, following too closely the priorities of the House Republicans and their radical budget strategy.

As noted (see pp. 51ff), the Senate began working toward a budget resolution in its traditional fashion, waiting for House initiative and hoping, at least, for a large measure of bipartisan collaboration in their own efforts. Pete Domenici, chairman of the Senate Budget Committee, was himself a pragmatic moderate who never fully accepted a tax cut, wanted initially only a "down payment" on the deficit, and thought mostly in terms of achieving Trust Fund solvency for Medicare. Both the Budget Committee and the Finance Committee, which was the relevant authorizing committee, had among their members deficit hawks and moderates who, in fact, did support bipartisan collaboration for some weeks.

But Domenici and Senate Republicans were frustrated by the absence of counterproposals from Democrats and were carried along by party loyalty and the budget-balancing enthusiasm generated in the House. Late in March, Domenici and most Senate Republicans had accepted the goal of reaching a balance in seven years. Outlines of the Senate Budget Committee plan, made public by Domenici in the first week of April, called for over $1 trillion in budget reductions over seven years. Medicare would be reduced by $250 billion and Medicaid by $160 billion—figures almost as high as those being developed in the House. A tax cut was not included at the time, though Senator Dole said in an NBC "Meet the Press" program that room would be provided for one. It was added, later, in the form of a $170 "contingency fund" that could be gotten from lower interest rates and increased revenues, assuming the deficit reduction was successful.[76]

Absent an effective basis for negotiation, partisan debate and maneuvering were shaping the issues and helping establish the policy positions that would be important in the future confrontations over Medicare. The Senate was involved in a nasty fight over the rescissions bill that mobilized both parties and sharpened partisan opposition. About this time, congressional Republicans were also going on the offensive with their public relations themes of "save the Trust Fund" and "preserve, protect, and strengthen" Medicare. Since the Senate Democrats had no budget proposal of their own, their primary strategy in countering the Republicans was to attack "excessive" cuts in popular programs, either to win concessions from Republicans or to inflict maximum political damage on them. They also began to feature the theme that Medicare was being sacrificed to pay for tax cuts for the rich. Unfortunately, both the Democratic and the Republican mantras proved effective, so the incentives to resort to demagogic rhetoric mounted on both sides.

At the time, Dole, Gingrich, and Bill Archer, chairman of Ways and Means, were sending out signals that they would like almost any kind of counteroffer from the Democrats. Yet neither side was in a good position to compromise. Senate Democrats had no budget of their own, so were poorly situated to bargain. For the Republicans, any easing of the budget reductions would require offsets taken from other programs and risk a loss of collective will or defections from their tenuous majority. In fact, the Republicans badly needed actionable counteroffers. Yet Democrats feared they would lose even more by making them. In a time of partisan mobilization and rhetorical escalation, there was little to encourage collaboration.

One source of counteroffers and bargaining points could have been the administration. Under the circumstances, the administration's response was interesting. Leon Panetta, writing for the White House on May 1, declined the invitation, saying that the Republicans would have to pass a budget resolution first. He also censured Republicans for seeking "the largest Medicare cut in history to pay for tax cuts for the well off."[77] There was, of course the president's closely held June budget, which the Republicans did not know about. It was released after budget resolutions were passed in both houses.

On April 27, Domenici announced plans for over $1 trillion in budget reductions, which would achieve a balanced budget by 2002. The proposed resolution included cuts of $250 billion for Medicare and $160 billion for Medicaid. During the Senate Budget Committee markup and the floor debate that followed, partisan opposition sharpened dramatically. Four days of markup produced little give and take as the bill passed 12–10, strictly along party lines.[78] The floor debate generated mostly partisan bombast, with the Democrats emphasizing the Republicans' "heartless cuts" in Medicare to provide tax relief for the rich, and "Mediscare" themes about the impact upon the program and the beneficiaries.[79] Subsequent appeals by Republicans for bipartisan collaboration were distrusted and discounted, so that passage of the budget resolution marked not just another stage in the process but a shift in mode of conduct as well.

In all of this, one is led to wonder about the propriety of the games our highest leaders play and about the way in which the game itself becomes dominant—which, like war, can lead to outcomes that serve neither the public nor the participants.

III. THE MEDICARE PRESERVATION ACT

Toward the end of March, as the House concluded work on the Contract with America, the speaker's task force began meetings to develop its Medicare proposal. This date was about six weeks before the House Budget Committee approved its reconciliation instructions, directing that the authorizing committees report back by July 14 on policies to meet the new spending targets. At the time, two additional months were allowed for Medicare, a recognition of the importance of this entitlement and the policy and political issues that would confront the task force.

The Medicare Preservation Act of 1995 was the catchy title given to the House Medicare bill, echoing the Republican theme of preserving and strengthening Medicare.[80] Despite the cosmetic wrappings, the Medicare bill had substance. It was a technical feat of impressive magnitude, setting forth in closely articulated text the comprehensive design and the specific details to transform one of the most complex programs in American history. Of course, little that happens in government is entirely new; and most of the elements of this proposed statute had been around in one form or another, from earlier legislative hearings, CBO options books, HCFA demonstrations, and so forth. But few of these possibilities and options had ever been really "done"—shaped into politically acceptable proposals, put into legislative language, scored by CBO, marked up in committee, and passed.[81] Making a workable and politically viable whole from the parts was another major challenge. Complex parts and a complex whole interacted dynamically. Powerful and vocal groups had a stake in each part and would be quick to make the most of any inconsistencies, technical flaws, or injustices. The Republicans also labored under a self-imposed constraint to reform or "strengthen" Medicare, not just to save money.[82]

In rough outline, the Medicare Preservation Act can be divided into four major parts. (1) The most ambitious and far-reaching was MedicarePlus, which offered a number of private plans, ranging from standard HMOs to provider-sponsored networks, private FFS plans, and medical savings accounts. (2) Associated with this restructuring were measures that would both save money and put traditional FFS Medicare and the private plans on a more competitive footing: by " delinking" managed care plans from FFS Medicare and by ending or reconstituting a number of the subsidies or bonuses built into payment systems. (3) A third rubric was money savers—including the familiar hospital and physician reductions and a variety of strategies for extracting savings from outpatient and skilled nursing facilities, home health agencies, durable medical equipment, etc. (4) The last major category was various initiatives that had been part of the "incremental" reforms currently being considered by the authorizing committees, such as medical malpractice, antitrust amendments, and fraud and abuse.

MedicarePlus

The two concepts underlying MedicarePlus were increased choice for Medicare beneficiaries and competition between the health plans. The latter was especially important, since competition was expected to lead to efficiency and efficiency to savings. One notion popular then and now, especially among Republicans in Congress, was "competitive bidding"—the idea that plans would submit premium bids and then the government would decide what contribution it would make. One example of competitive bidding much discussed at the time was the Federal Employees Health Benefit Plan (FEHBP), which provided for a contribution to the subscribers' premium and allowed plans to compete both on price and by varying the benefit package. Another model derived from Senator Durenberger's proposed reform of Medicare, advanced in 1994 in the course of debates over the Health Security Act. This approach followed closely the Ellwood-Enthoven[83] "managed competition" model, which required a "defined" or standard benefit package and then structured and monitored competition over price.

The first approach developed by the task force staff, and ready in draft form by June, was a competitive bidding model that followed the earlier Durenberger proposal.[84] Circulated among the staff, it was sharply criticized both on technical and policy grounds. Kathy Means, the leading Medicare expert in the group, recalls getting the draft from Chip Kahn and reading it over the weekend. In her view, as she said to Kahn, the infrastructure was not there, the government lacked the expertise to do competitive bidding, there was not enough time for the decisions that had to be made, and there were serious issues of public policy.[85] Her appraisal seems to have been persuasive. The forty-page draft was buried, and the task force turned in a different direction.

For a time, according to Means, the staff talked about FEBHP as a model, but ran into difficulty working out an acceptable method for setting the government contribution. Ultimately, along with Julie James, another Medicare expert, she developed the administrative structure and regulatory principles working from Section 1876 of the Social Security Act; the TEFRA amendment governing most current Medicare HMOs; and from a HCFA "Choices" demonstration that tested choice and competition among a number of managed care plans. This incremental approach had the advantages of familiarity and political acceptability. At the same time, it tilted in the direction of choice versus competition, and raised an issue of how much of a factor competition between managed care plans was likely to be in containing costs.

One important step toward a more competitive system was to "delink" managed care payment from the FFS program. As provided in TEFRA[86] HMO payments were based on 95 percent of the adjusted average per capita cost (AAPCC) for a Medicare FFS beneficiary in a particular county. Over time, this led to enormous variation in payments throughout the country, for example, $313 per month for the one hundred lowest counties and over $760 per month for the highest.[87] Moreover, HMOs that could deliver care for less were allowed to add benefits, but could not keep the surplus nor return it as cash payments to the beneficiaries. This was a wasteful form of competition that, because of the favorable selection HMOs enjoyed, probably resulted in the government losing money on a supposedly competitive system that, in principle, should have saved a substantial amount.

Almost everyone who looked at this system, with the exception of high-end managed care plans, agreed that it needed fixing. But doing so was a complicated matter. The easiest step was to delink managed care payments from the county-based AAPCC. An important proviso was that the plan benefits had to be at least equivalent to the standard FFS Medicare package. Beyond that, the scheme devised by the task force would phase in payment changes as done with other administered pricing systems, such as the Prospective Payment System or the Medicare Fee Schedule. Capitation payments would be calculated annually by "the Secretary" with separate rates for the aged, the disabled, and end-state renal dialysis enrollees. Payments would be further adjusted using both the familiar AAPCC risk factors of age, gender, welfare eligibility, and institutional status, as well as "other factors as the Secretary determines to be appropriate" to insure "actuarial equivalence."[88] A next step was to begin equalizing payment rates across the nation by assigning health plans to classes according to their "utilization of services," i.e., expensiveness. Each year, low utilization plans would be raised and high ones lowered: for instance, in year one, the lowest class would be assigned a growth rate of 9 percent and the highest a rate of 4 percent—but no plan would receive less than $300 a month per member. In subsequent years, plans would receive a percentage increment, according to class, ranging from 187 percent of the national average to 75 percent—no plan to receive less than $320 per month for each enrollee. Meanwhile, quite a lot of money was to be taken out of the system, by capping annual growth beginning in 1996 at variable percentages ranging from 3.8 to 5.6 percent to reach a steady state of 5 percent by 2002. A rough calculation indicates that, assuming a then current growth rate of 8 percent, the cuts would amount to about 40 percent of a seven-year projected growth.

Various complexities and uncertainties made this scheme even more difficult than it might seem. One was the split among health plans, especially as between lean, high-efficiency ones such as those in Minneapolis/St. Paul and Southern California, with rates so low that there was no fat to spare; those in Florida and the Northeast, with historically high AAPCCs and attractive pharmaceutical and preventive care benefits they could pass along to beneficiaries; and rural HMOs, many of them struggling to exist. There were also major uncertainties about how much of the variation was surplus and how much represented different levels of severity, practice patterns, or beneficiary attitudes, say, as between rural areas and urban ones. In any event, the impact upon the health plans would be painful and, in some cases, might be devastating. Another major problem with all of this was lack of adequate impact data.

For the task force staff, the process was similar to the formula fight over Medicaid block grants, except that the American Association of Health Plans and the managed care constituency lacked the political clout of the governors and, in 1995, did not have good impact numbers that would enable them to press their case effectively.[89] It was "very political, very difficult,"[90] with everyone working on the managed care rates, scrounging data from CBO and PPRC, pressed for time, and trying to get the formula right.[91]

Several points about this effort are worth mentioning. It provides an indication that, despite Speaker Gingrich's various "inducements," the House was hard on some providers. The requirement that health plans provide actuarially equivalent benefits for the health plan enrollees was seen as a way of promoting competition; but it also showed a concern for the plan members and is one way in which the House proposal went beyond a bare "defined contribution" scheme.[92] From a policy perspective, it is interesting that the AAHP did not protest more and more effectively. One reason is that the health plans did make important gains, though of a nonobvious sort. They wanted the freedom a defined contribution proposal would give them and they pretty much got that. Health plans also hoped to make money from the "bonanza" of Medicare patients who were expected to enroll in the new managed care options. In addition, opposition to MedicarePlus was divided or ineffective.

The equalization features were a wedge issue for them, putting their own constituency on different sides. Also, AAHP lacked good impact numbers in 1995 that would have enabled them to make a better case for distributive justice. Much that the House Republicans were proposing needed doing and they had better numbers to support their proposal.

Decoupling FFS Medicare from the Medicare managed care plans was one way of moving toward more competitive choices. Another step, and a money-saver, was to reduce the provider subsidies that had long been charged to the program, largely on the ground that such subsidies should be paid for directly. While there were a good many of these, particularly for special categories of hospitals, the largest were the Medicare disproportionate share (DSH) payments and the teaching allowances.

The Medicare DSH, a counterpart to the Medicaid DSH that was abolished in the Medicaid Transformation Act, provided extra payments for hospitals serving a disproportionate share of low-income patients. The payments were made on the theory that these patients were more expensive to treat, though also at times because a category of hospital was in financial distress and needed help. The subsidy was especially important for urban and public hospitals that typically had large numbers of poor patients, both Medicare and Medicaid. Much smaller than the Medicaid DSH, the Medicare payments had also been less abused. At the same time, they were criticized as double payment for services already adequately compensated and as providing a general benefit to the hospitals that was paid for solely by the Medicare Part A Hospital Trust Fund.

The medical education allowances helped cover the extra expenses of teaching hospitals. The general medical education (GME) payment (often referred to as direct medical education or DME) covered salaries for residents and faculty and some related educational expenses for patient care attributable to Medicare. Indirect medical education (IME) covered a number of additional expenses or effort attributable to patient care in teaching hospitals, such as extra demands on staff, additional tests and procedures associated with teaching students, and the costs of treating larger numbers of severely ill patients.[93]

Generally, legislators took pride in their local hospitals, especially if they were prestigious teaching institutions; and the teaching subsidies were popular. Still, like many such subventions, they had grown incrementally over the years, often adapting to new purposes and, in the view of some, increasing the supply and specialization of doctors. For many years there had been pleas from the medical schools and within the policy community to put these subsidies on some more publicly avowed and broadly shared footing.

The approach taken for Medicare DSH was almost as simple and drastic as that chosen for the Medicaid DSH: a reduction by 25 percent a year for the next seven years. That would have reduced the allowance 87 percent by the year 2002.[94] Medicare DSH was not a big issue, amounting to about $5 billion, as compared to Medicaid DSH, which was $19 billion that year. However, the AHA protested the aggregate of hospital cuts and, as Congress moved from global to more specific figures, began mobilizing their member hospitals by sending them data from computer runs showing how DSH, DME, and IME cuts would affect them.[95] One bit of soothing balm for the health plans in the House version was the omission of a "carve out" provision removing DSH payments from the AAPCC. That was added by the Senate.

A dramatic and far-reaching proposal in the House bill was to establish a new Graduate Medical Education and Teaching Hospital Trust Fund for the annual payments in support of Medicare direct and indirect teaching expenses. This new trust fund would be funded by carving out existing payments from the Prospective Payment System and from managed care. The proposal would broaden the sources of support and make them more visible. Distributions could be made to "qualified consortia" as well as to medical schools. At the same time, restrictions and payment reductions would be imposed. For general medical education, the number of residents would be frozen, support for the individual resident limited to five years, and that for alien residents phased out by the end of 1998. The IME payment would also be limited by reducing the adjustment made for future increases in the resident-per-bed ratio, which was the established proxy for teaching intensity. Recognizing the issues likely to be stirred up by these changes, the House bill created a new commission to study and report on financing issues relating to medical education.

Basically, the medical schools made out well. A cap was put on GME support for residents; but residents largely paid for themselves. Though IME payments were to be cut, it would be from a 1984 PPS base that was almost twice what it should have been.[96] AAMC initial fears of steep reductions[97] were allayed by the eventual formula. The proposal itself was put together, late at night by Representative Thomas, chairman of the health subcommittee, Chip Kahn, chief of staff for the task force, and Donald Young and Lauren LeRoy, executive directors of ProPAC and PPRC, respectively. A representative from AAMC said that they claimed no credit for the result, but that it was pretty much what they hoped for, at least for the short term.[98] A larger issue, of course, is that this move would get the federal government more explicitly into the complexities of health manpower—a venture for which the precedents were not reassuring. A subtle point was raised by some of the theory accompanying this proposal, to wit, whether medical education should be considered a public good or not. For some Republicans, this concept provided both a justification for support as well as a criterion for limiting public funding.[99] AAMC representatives feared that "public good" might be too confining, limiting funding that was desirable but hard to justify theoretically: for instance, support of alien residents who staff inner-city hospitals and clinics for the poor.[100]

One major objective of Medicare "restructuring" was to disengage the MedicarePlus plans from traditional FFS Medicare and make the plans more competitive. A second was to offer a number of competing plans, relying mainly on HMOs, but including other options, such as point of service, provider-sponsored networks, private FFS plans, "Taft-Hartley" and "association" plans, and medical savings accounts. The two prime reasons for these additions were to increase choice and to foster competition. Some were pushed by providers, such as the provider-sponsored networks and private FFS plans and others by insurance companies, such as the MSAs. Traditional FFS Medicare would be retained; but these plans would add a second part that was closer in motivation and behavior to the private market, more attuned to personal choice, and more competitive.

One important step was to give the health plans a margin of increased freedom to vary price and product. For the first time, plans could increase premiums if additions to the Medicare core package were made or they could rebate the difference (in tax-free dollars) if their premiums were below the Medicare Adjusted Community Rate.[101] Copays, though not deductibles, were allowed for core benefits. And deductibles, copays, and balance billing would all be allowed for additional benefits, though not beyond the limit of out-of-pocket expenditures under the traditional FFS plan. For private FFS plans or out-of-plan point of service, no such limits applied. In short, the amendments protected the core benefit package and kept the beneficiary as well off as under FFS Medicare while allowing the market to work more freely in the supply and demand for alternatives.

Two of the additional plan offerings were of relatively minor significance and occasioned little discussion. These were the private FFS option and the limited enrollment ("Taft-Hartley" and "association") plans.

The private FFS option was for plans that reimbursed their providers with privately determined fee schedules or on some "other basis." Subject to review by the secretary, they would be licensed and regulated by the states and have separate solvency standards. They would not be subject to Medicare balance billing limits—one reason that they were supported by the AMA. They also appealed to sectarians—such as antiabortion groups or Mennonites—because they could be limited to practitioners who shared the faith. From a policy perspective, it was an option that increased choice, would not be much used, won some support, and would do little harm.

A more important option was plans for trade unions and other "qualified associations," which could include fraternal and professional organizations, such as AARP, the Masons or Shriners, American Bar Association, the National Federation of Independent Business, or even the Farm Bureau.[102] A major restriction was that such plans could be offered only to the association members and spouses. Most of the likely candidates were already regulated either under the Taft-Hartley law, other federal authority, or by the states. But these would be risk-bearing associations spending Medicare dollars, so there was some federal responsibility to see to standards that would protect beneficiaries and providers. The formula devised combined both federal-state and public-private elements. Association plans already regulated by the states would continue as before. Those that were not would be subject to standards devised by the secretary, working from proposals submitted by the National Association of Insurance Commissioners. Union and Taft-Hartley standards would also be developed by the secretary, consulting with the Secretary of Labor.

A high-profile issue that occasioned a great deal of controversy was the provider-sponsored networks (PSNs) or provider-sponsored organizations (PSOs) as they were eventually termed. These touched upon important and sensitive interests and raised major issues of policy and ideology as well. A top priority for the AMA and strongly supported by the AHA, they had been pretty much promised by Newt Gingrich. They were just as strongly opposed by major health insurers, such as Blue Cross/Blue Shield, and by the health plans. In conception, they were one of the few new plan offerings that might have made more than an incremental difference, which makes their fate of some interest. Major changes in Medicare are rare, and so it was a time of opportunity and decision and the big providers and insurers weighed in on this one.[103]

As the term itself indicates, doctors, hospitals, or other providers would be the sponsors. The motives varied, ranging from high-minded professionalism to crass materialism. Some physicians and hospitals wanted to practice better medicine[104] or to bring health care to poor or underserved areas. Others saw it as countervailing power against the HMOs. Still others wanted to cut out the insurance companies and gain access to the Medicare beneficiaries expected to move to managed care. From a larger perspective, whatever their personal interest, many health professionals saw this as an opportunity to take back health care from the insurance companies, the HMOs, and the accountants and MBAs.

Insurance companies, health plans, and even hospitals resisted especially the PSNs, the AMA-sponsored version, which would have allowed physicians to get into the market with comparatively small and specialized groups. In the view of other provider groups, PSNs were too likely to be in it for quick profits. As one observer put it, "They spook the pool, don't know how to compete, go broke, and leave the patients in the lurch."[105] Given the fresh fields of new Medicare beneficiaries, they would also be in an excellent position to engage in favorable selection, make a lot of money on the healthier ones, and leave the sicker cohort for the established plans. When the controls began to bite, they could still get out with a bundle. Clearly, some kind of admission criteria for providers were desirable.

One important criterion was the proportion of health care for which a PSN would be responsible. If no standard were specified, then almost any group would be eligible, including narrowly specialized preferred-provider organizations. At the opposite extreme, for instance, responsibility for a majority of care for the enrollees, only hospital-based PSOs could qualify. This issue was intensely lobbied in both the House and Senate, with the AMA and physician groups trying to keep the stated proportion as low as possible and hospitals, health plans, and insurance companies pushing for a majority standard or even higher. The House, reluctant to shut out the physicians, specified that a "substantial proportion" would have to be provided, either directly through the provider or by an affiliated group, but that the secretary would define "substantial proportion" considering the need to assure "financial stability and other factors." Practically, this approach left either the Senate or the secretary to make the hard choice.

Especially important for PSNs was the treatment of solvency standards. Since health plans are at risk, reserves are an important requirement, just as they would be for an insurance company. Precisely this point was argued strenuously by large health care insurers such as Aetna and Blue Cross/Blue Shield. If these were low, so their argument went, all sorts of plans could easily enter the market, and lacking the usual reserve requirements would compete at an advantage meanwhile leaving their enrollees unprotected. On the other hand, meeting insurers' solvency requirements is difficult—legally complex, time consuming, and conditioned upon large cash and capital reserves. These conditions would be too stringent for all but a few physician groups and quite difficult even for hospitals. The AHA argued strongly for "going-concern" value and "sweat equity" to count as reserves; but the insurance companies opposed that. The physicians wanted special plans with partial risk. And the hospitals opposed that.

For the most part, the task force was open on the topic of PSNs or PSOs, but also aware that the issues were difficult and that resolving them would be like stepping into the middle of a marital dispute—somebody, and maybe everybody, was likely to be angry with the mediator. They surveyed state practices in this area, but found little support for special treatment on the reserve requirements. According to Chip Kahn, their own language was carefully drafted so as to provide some slack—for instance, recognizing going-concern value, but not conceding much on the issue of solvency. For this, they resorted to an ingenious but little-used device—negotiated regulation.[106] With this scheme, representatives (typically, attorneys or accountants) from interested or expert groups such as the AHA, AMA, BC/BS, and the NAIC would convene with a presiding magistrate and a government representative to negotiate within limits set by legislation. Their product would then become the basis for an administrative rule. This was a convenient device that survived in the 1997 legislation and, when implemented, worked quite well (see p. 261ff).

Among the MedicarePlus plans, the one most driven by ideology and yet with the least support on policy grounds was "Medisave," otherwise referred to as a "high-deductible" plan or as a "medical saving account." In general outlines, Medisave combined features of a major medical or high-deductible policy with those of an individual retirement account. The basic idea was that the federal government would contribute a set percentage of a premium amount and the beneficiary would enroll in a qualified high-deductible plan. The difference between the government contribution and the plan premium would be deposited in a designated medical saving account, which could accumulate and be drawn on for qualified medical expenses or, with a penalty similar to that for IRAs, be used for nonmedical purposes. Another important feature was an upper limit of $10,000 on beneficiary liability, so that the MSA insured against catastrophic expense.

Some of the support for this proposal was rooted in a Republican view that people should spend their own money as they pleased, without the intervention of regulations or bureaucrats. MSAs were also seen as a useful experiment in a high-deductible policy[107] and a way to make the market more competitive by sharpening consumer self-interest. The AMA supported them in part because of a belief that they would encourage patients to take more responsibility for their own health care, one of the association's long-term strategies. Another appealing feature for physicians was that Medicare balance billing limits would not apply. MSAs were fairly well established in the commercial market, were offered by some of the major plans, and provided a way for isolated individuals or small groups—for instance, farmers or artisans—to get some coverage, though at relatively high prices. Very much to the point, MSAs were popular in Texas. John Goodman, head of the Center for Policy Analysis in Texas, a conservative think-tank, was a leading theoretical supporter of MSAs (Goodman and Musgrave 1992). The Golden Rule Insurance Company, the leading purveyor of this product, and Patrick Rooney, its colorful president, were a presence in Texas, and made large campaign contributions to Republicans. Both Dick Armey, the House Budget Committee chairman and Bill Archer, chairman of Ways and Means, were from Texas and strongly supported MSAs.

Interest groups such as Blue Cross/Blue Shield or the AARP did not weigh in heavily on this issue, in part because of doubts that Medicare MSAs were likely to happen. But there was strong opposition from the AARP, the administration, most Democrats, and some Republicans in Congress over the issue of risk selection. The fear was that MSAs would especially appeal to the healthier beneficiaries and skim them off from the insurance pool, adversely affecting both FFS Medicare and other risk plans. There was further concern about victimization of individual beneficiaries by get-rich-quick artists, flashy and misleading advertising, and plans with loss ratios (paid out benefits) as low as 50 percent. Even Bill Thomas, the Health Subcommittee chairman, who faithfully supported his own committee chairman, was skeptical of the proposal. A personal aide to Gingrich said, however, that the organized interests were "quite strong," and that they "had to tell them there would be an option."[108] But most of the staff people seemed not unhappy with the thought that MSAs would almost certainly be "stripped"[109] in the Senate or radically reduced in number.

A fundamental premise of MedicarePlus—the new Part C—was that plans would be marketed fairly and the enrollees or "consumers" well informed. Accordingly, the provisions for marketing and election of plans by enrollees were carefully specified and prominently positioned at the beginning of the House bill. The specifics were developed from the existing Section 1876 of the Medicare statute, from the HCFA "Choices" demonstration, and from other lesser parts lying around in the legislative bone yard[110] The centerpiece was an annual "Health Fair" to be held each October, at which time enrollees would make their "elections," i.e., choose their plans. Preceding this choice would be a regulated national "campaign," during which plan literature and materials prepared by "the Secretary" would be disseminated.

A large role was assigned to the secretary to promote an "active, informed selection" and to regulate and monitor the election process. Each year the secretary was to conduct the Health Fair, which would include a nationally coordinated education and publicity campaign. Also mandated was an information booklet in standardized format that would set forth in "plain English"[111] benefits and premiums; comparative data on quality indices including consumer satisfaction and beneficiary rights and responsibilities; and a toll-free "hot-line" for inquiries about the MedicarePlus program. The secretary was authorized to establish procedures and conditions under which eligible Part C plans could market their wares. No brochures, application forms, or "other promotional or informational material" could be distributed without the review and approval by the secretary.

A number of protections for enrollees were carried over from existing statutes and others were added. The House bill came down heavily on disclosure, especially of items likely to get omitted in advertising brochures or buried in fine print—such as coverage exclusions, prior authorization requirements, and enrollee satisfaction data. Other protections were fair-marketing standards, guaranteed issue, nondiscrimination because of health status or medical history, and limits on disenrollment. Patients were guaranteed timely and reasonable access to services, protection of confidentiality of records, grievance and appeal rights, and emergency care without prior authorization. The bill also carried over and added to the array of "intermediate sanctions" that gave the secretary authority to impose civil monetary penalties (CMPs) and suspensions as alternatives to the clumsy and seldom used remedy of contract termination.

The marketing provisions were especially notable both for the attention given to them as well as for the large amount of authority and discretion assigned to the secretary. Much was spelled out in terms such as disclosure requirements; but the secretary would have wide discretion to set up the program, administer it, promulgate standards of fair advertising, conduct the Health Fair, and prescribe materials that would contribute to an "active and informed" selection. The delegation of authority and discretion was deliberate and calculated for it was widely assumed that marketing the MedicarePlus plans would require experimentation, including borrowing state-of-the-art information technology from the private sector.

At the same time, the House (and Senate) took precautions to unburden the secretary and HCFA in some ways as well as to change the organizational culture. The House bill provided, for example, that the secretary could contract with the Social Security Administration—which had local offices throughout the country—to administer the enrollment and disenrollment in Medicare-Plus plans. With respect to beneficiary information and promoting an informed choice, the secretary was enjoined to contract with appropriate outside public and private agencies to carry out these activities. Most important, the secretary was directed to create a separate agency within DHHS, separate from HCFA, to administer MedicarePlus and Medicare Section 1876 managed care plans.

These provisions were motivated at least in part by a practical consideration that neither DHHS nor HCFA was, at the time, well organized to conduct such an information campaign and by a further belief that the marketing of managed care plans and, more generally, educating consumers were highly sophisticated enterprises. Even as this matter was being considered in Congress, the Institute of Medicine was completing a draft report that made these same points and suggested delegating the activity to a private sector entity (Institute of Medicine 1996:esp. vol. 1, 105ff.). There was also a widespread belief, among Republicans in Congress and managed care providers in the private sector, that HCFA had a fixed antipathy to HMOs and could not be trusted to administer fairly a program like MedicarePlus.

Leaving aside the merits or motivation of these provisions, they were being discussed, along with the IOM study, at a time when champions of the traditional Medicare program were on the offensive and looking for good points of attack. To them, the marketing provisions seemed tainted by a Republican aim to devolve and privatize wherever possible. And the "two HCFA's" directive to the secretary, whatever its justifications, looked like one more nail in the coffin that was being built by people hostile to Medicare.

Saving Money

Creating the design and devising the legislative language for the new MedicarePlus option with all of its moving parts answered one major priority of the House Republicans, which was to restructure Medicare. A second, closely related cluster of objectives was to reduce expenditures, save enough for Part A Trust Fund solvency, balance the budget by 2002, and provide for a tax cut.

In some ways this task was more straightforward and familiar, but it also involved difficulty. It was a test of whether the Republicans could deliver—both save money and "preserve, protect, and strengthen" Medicare.

On June 29, after several weeks of intraparty negotiation over a tax cut, the House and Senate passed the 1995 budget resolution that, inter alia, called for $270 billion in Medicare expenditure reductions and set a reporting deadline for the authorizing committees of September 22. On September 21, one day short of that deadline, Speaker Gingrich outlined the Republican plan for reform of Medicare and for savings over seven years. CBO scored the plan at $270.2 billion in Medicare savings but also noted a payout to the Graduate Education Trust Fund of $15.8 billion, which would reduce the net savings to $254.4 billion.[112]

In the package that was ultimately presented, a notable feature was the extent to which the savings were back-loaded, that is, concentrated toward the end rather than the beginning of the seven years. Roughly speaking, about one-eighth of the savings would occur in the first two years and about half in the last two. A solid policy ground for such an approach would be to allow a period for start-up and to evaluate impact and continuing need over time. Cynics point out that such adjustments usually put serious pain safely beyond the next election. Of course, Democrats do it as well as Republicans, but it is important to realize that in deficit reduction as elsewhere, the fanfare and regalia may be more impressive than the bodily presence.

Hospitals and Physicians.   One part of budget reduction that was relatively easy was extracting savings from the traditional Part A (hospitals) and Part B (physicians) FFS program. It was easy because Congress had been doing this for years, as part of the budget process, and had ready for help the formidable expertise of ProPAC and PPRC as well as the Congressional Budget Office, the General Accounting Office, and the Congressional Research Service. All of these agencies were accustomed to working with both parties and providing a comparatively neutral technical expertise. ProPAC and PPRC had been purposely built for just such a task.

The savings—$59.7 billion from the physicians and $67.6 billion from hospitals—were achieved mostly using two basic approaches. One was to be systematic and ruthless in going after the "usual suspects," known to ProPAC, PPRC, and CBO—those providers with inflated payments, subsidies, pass-throughs, or other cozy arrangements—and postpone updates, cap subsidies or freeze payments, prescribe a fee schedule or prospective payment system, and even, in some cases, "zero them out." In all, roughly $50 billion of projected expenditures were eliminated through this method, with a minimum of complaint from the producers.

A second, wholesale method was simply to reduce the updates for the Prospective Payment System and the Medicare Fee Schedule globally. These updates, which took account of a number of variables, increased or decreased most of the individual payments by a flat percentage amount, much like a cost-of-living adjustment. For PPS hospitals, the update was set at "market basket"[113] minus 2.5 percent for FY 1996 and minus 2.0 percent annually through FY 2002. As for the Medicare Fee Schedule, following a recommendation of PPRC, a "sustainable growth rate" was adopted that, through a complex formula, would set a rate of increase equal approximately to the real growth in GDP plus 2 percent, with limited bonuses or penalties depending on performance. According to CBO, changes in the PPS update should save $29 billion and the MFS changes another $26 billion for a total of $55 billion.[114]

The size of these reductions, along with the Medicaid DSH issue led the AHA and several other hospital groups that especially served the poor to mount a brief but intense campaign opposing the House proposal. As for the physicians, and especially the AMA, they were more interested in some of the structural changes and regulatory relief and had relatively little to say about Part B cuts. The AMA did express serious concern about the penalty provision of the new update and the single conversion factor—which projected possible dollar reductions in the CF of more than 20 percent by 2002.[115] As a general observation, though, the volume of complaint seemed about normal for a reconciliation year, with the exception of the controversy over Medicaid DSH. The task force was, of course, working throughout with both ProPAC and PPRC to advise them on tolerable limits and placement for specific reductions. Even Democratic staffers acknowledged that the cuts were not excessive. According to one, "Pete Stark always said that you could take a lot of money out of Medicare."[116] Another said that $270 billion was not unreasonable—that, in fact, the Republicans could have taken more. He added, though, that the cuts were too front-loaded, especially for providers serving the poor.[117]

Several apparently minor provisions had large consequences politically, for deficit reduction, or for both. One of these was the Medicare Part B premium. Historically, the Part B premium was set to cover 50 percent of program costs. Congress in 1974 limited dollar increases in the premium to the same percentage as the cost of living adjustment (COLA) for Social Security, but when that proved too small the contribution was set at 25 percent. For 1995, because of an estimating error, the premium was set at $46.10 per month, which represented 31.5 percent of Part B program costs. H.R. 2485 proposed making that 31.5 percent permanent rather than reverting to the scheduled 25 percent—a change that would have netted about $12 billion dollars by year 2002.[118] Compounded over the seven years it would double beneficiary premiums, though actually raising them only $27 dollars above the figure they would have reached anyway. In addition, the Part B premium was income related so that well-to-do beneficiaries would pay more. Beginning at incomes of $75,000 for individuals and $125,000 for couples, beneficiaries would pay steadily higher premiums until, at $150,000 and $175,000, their contributions covered 100 percent of their Part B costs. This feature was calculated by the CBO to produce an additional $2 billion in savings, for a total of $14 billion. These provisions were among the very few that explicitly imposed higher burdens on the beneficiaries; but they were to cause the House Republicans much grief (see pp. 180, 229).

A change with no significant budget impact but large political consequences was the "Part A–Part B switch." This provision set a per episode limit for home health care of 165 days and shifted payments beyond that limit from Part A to Part B. In a protective gesture toward the beneficiaries, the bill further provided that these Part B billings not be counted in calculating the Part B premium. Probably, the underlying concept of separating the longer term care made sense, at least in recognizing that home health services were increasingly being substituted for nursing homes, not acute inpatient hospital care. Also some money might be saved since home health care that is not hospital related is usually less expensive. Much more important, though, was the political effect. The Part A Trust Fund would gain an estimated $54 billion over seven years, considerably easing the solvency problem,[119] achieved not by additional savings taken from providers but by a transfer of the ledger account. It was one of those steps that seemed good at the time, but eventually benefited most the Clinton administration.

Outpatient, Post-Acute, and Long-Term Care.   Included under this rubric is an assortment of services and procedures that have in common that they are not covered by the Prospective Payment System or the Medicare Fee Schedule and that they are not delivered in the typical acute inpatient hospital setting or the doctor's office. The most important for the House bill were outpatient services, skilled nursing facilities (SNFs), home health care, and the non-PPS or "exempt" hospitals (psychiatric, rehabilitative, cancer, children's and long-term care). Collectively, they were an unkempt and forbidding tangle of problems because of the variety of settings and patients involved and the different ways in which the service modalities and payment systems evolved. They had tended to receive less attention because less money was involved, because they had historically been ignored, and because of a lack of expertise needed to reform them. As for the payment systems, they may not have been "broken," but they needed some fixing. Given the state of the art, the task force did what it could. And it deserves credit for recognizing the limits imposed by circumstance and their resources.

Hospital outpatient services was a situation that badly needed fixing but one where the task force temporized. Outpatient services and procedures had been growing rapidly—about 14 percent a year in dollar volume—since 1983. Much of this growth was driven by a payment methodology that mixed costs and charges, invited site shifting, drastically increased copays for Medicare beneficiaries. and cost the federal government about $1.7 billion a year in "formula-driven overpayments." In its March 1995 report, ProPAC had strongly urged Congress to provide immediate relief to the beneficiaries, remedy the formula-driven overpayments, and support the development of a prospective payment system. But ProPAC also indicated that rescuing the beneficiaries would cost money and would be tricky to implement and that the outpatient PPS method currently under study needed an effective volume control.[120] Given that situation, the task force opted for a minimalist solution: it extended some cost limits and remedied the formula driven overpayments by providing that coinsurance amounts would be deducted later in the payment cycle. The savings were considerable: CBO scored the provision at $16 billion for seven years. This left the beneficiaries without relief, except that some of the incentives for ratcheting up on copays were removed. A prospective payment system was subsequently mandated in 1997, and the sequel to that is dealt with later (see p. 279ff).

The cost of skilled nursing facilities (SNFs), while not a huge item in absolute amount, had been rising 35 percent a year since 1986, reaching $11.7 billion in 1996. From 1 percent of Part A expenditures in 1986, SNFs had grown to 9 percent by 1996 (Medicare Payment Advisory Commission 1998:95). Several inflationary factors were driving this remarkable rate of increase, among them a repeal (temporary) of the three-day hospital stay requirement, earlier discharge from hospitals, and a payment system based on traditional per diem and ancillary cost reimbursement. As with hospitals earlier, the biggest problem was controlling the "nonroutine" costs, which for the SNFs meant especially labor-intensive therapy and rehabilitation. By 1995, costs were growing five times as rapidly as the number of patients, showing the importance of increased intensity (ibid.).

Devising a remedy depended in this instance on the state of the art. Congress liked prospective payment systems, and Stuart Altman, then chairman of ProPAC, urged a system similar to the hospital DRG-based PPS.[121] However desirable, this prescription seemed an instance in which the ideal was an enemy of the good. In the view of Donald Young, executive director of ProPAC, that approach required the development of an adequate case-mix adjuster that could discriminate reliably between routine and high-intensity stays. And that, in turn, depended on work being done in HCFA on resource utilization groups (RUGs) and other case-mix adjusters—work that was "moving along" but not there.[122] Under the circumstance, the House proposal prudently went with the state of the art: requiring the secretary to extend routine cost limits to most ancillary services but to exempt a selective list of high-intensity nonroutine services for future consideration.

Home health care was another high-growth area, with a 32 percent annual increase in expenditures from 1988 to 1992 and a 16 percent increase in visits per beneficiary from 1989 through 1995. In 1995, Medicare home health expenditures were $17 billion a year, having risen from a mere $2 billion in 1988. The $17 billion amounted to almost 10 percent of the total Medicare budget. The reasons for this explosive growth illustrate the political dynamics of a widely shared and much needed benefit. The Social Security Amendments of 1972 eliminated the 20 percent copay for home health visits. OBRA 1980 removed the limits on number of visits and opened the program to for-profit providers. By 1995, half of all certified agencies were for-profit. Then, in 1989, in settling Duggan v. Bowen,[123] HCFA modified the "part-time or intermittent" eligibility criterion, a major constraint on volume of use. In addition to rapid growth, one consequence of these changes was to transform the program increasingly into a substitute for long-term care or nursing homes. Another was to make it a mainstay for the infirm, elderly, and poor, and increasingly popular with the electorate. Congress was of two minds, deploring the runaway costs, but not disposed to be the bad guys.

For home health care, both Congress and the industry would have preferred a prospective payment system with an adequate case-mix adjuster. That option was being developed as a part of Phase II of an ongoing HCFA demonstration, but the results had yet to be evaluated. Nevertheless, the task force went ahead with what was available, adopting the HCFA Phase II methodology with minor amendments. The payment system had three basic elements. (1) It set per visit limits at 112 percent of a national average for the major categories of home health service covered by Medicare (such as skilled nursing, physical therapy, and speech pathology). (2) Beside the per visit limits, home health agencies would have aggregate limits based on 120 days per episode of care. Within a given region, aggregate costs for 18 different categories of service would be calculated for the prescribed 120-day period. These would then be used to develop a case-adjusted target figure for the individual agency. (3) As a final step, total payments to a specific agency would be compared to the target figure. From 120 to 165 days the agency would be at risk. If below 120 days, it would receive 50 percent of the savings. If above 120, the agency would be penalized according to a formula to be devised by the secretary. Beyond 165 days, the agency could apply to have the cases treated as outliers and reimbursed on a cost basis.

The home health proposal had several additional cost adjusters commonly used for prospective payment systems, such as a wage index, a market basket with updates, and periodic rebasing for both per visit and per episode limits. An additional cost-saver provided that future payments would be based on "current payment levels," i.e., there would be no "catch up" for FY 1994 and FY 1995 inflation, which had been disregarded under current law. The CBO score for the home health savings was $17.3 million over seven years, noting primarily the limit in growth of visits per user and that Medicare would reduce payments for visits on days 121–165—representing about 7 percent of all visits.[124]

In putting forward this proposal, a summary report of September 21 acknowledged that this Phase II scheme was a "substitute for a true case-mix adjustment not yet available."[125] In this connection, one remarkable feature of the House bill was the "marching orders" given to the secretary, directing her to carry out specific provisions, monitor quality, abnormally short episodes, and "code creep," and to be watchful for various provider scams and gaming strategies. In addition, the new Medicare Review Commission—to be created by a merger of ProPAC and PPRC—was directed to report annually for three years on the new payment system and rather comprehensively on whether some better alternative might be feasible.

Managed Care. As for budget savings, probably the most disappointing experience for House Republicans was MedicarePlus and managed care generally. This disappointment resulted, in part, from the high expectations for this showcase program: the numbers that would enroll, the force of market competition, and the savings that cost containment could generate. The other source of bad news was CBO, which refused to score managed care savings without a credible way to assure those savings and, even when fail-safe and look back provisions were added, remained very conservative in its scoring. The result was a difference of $50 to $65 billion between some of the early estimates in the House and the CBO final scoring—a serious matter.

The central point at issue was the amount of savings that could be credited to increased enrollment in MedicarePlus managed care plans and to the competition that would be stimulated among these plans by their bidding for enrollees and by the comparison shopping of these same enrollees. For Republicans, this expectation had long been bolstered by policy advocacy and think-tank studies, and was a strong talking point for managed care. Moreover, much of the argument for restructuring Medicare rested upon the supposition that competition and market-oriented practices would generate big savings. At the same time, this supposition had tended to become an article of faith or an inspirational myth, supported by scant evidence that what may or may not be true of the private sector or the FEHBP would hold true for Medicare.

For CBO scoring, the whole point is calculable, enforceable savings based upon an explicit mandate or credible mechanism that would produce the savings. Accordingly, CBO accepted the scheduled reductions in the capitation payments and scored these at $33.6 billion. But the agency had a number of objections with respect to the projected savings through competition. The major point made was that FFS Medicare was also being reduced, so that additional savings through managed care, even with the delinked AAPCC, were likely to be "relatively small."[126] They also assumed that some of the putative savings should be offset since they would result from favorable selection by the managed care plans. Even accepting a favorable 9 percent estimate of increased enrollees, CBO concluded that the savings for seven years would be only $5 billion.

Awareness that CBO would not score increased managed care enrollments as a saving was one factor that prompted Republicans in both House and Senate to consider a fail-safe or sequester mechanism that would impose automatic reductions if program expenditures exceeded the spending targets.[127] Aside from meeting CBO constraints, this device could also serve to make midcourse corrections and maintain a rough parity between FFS and managed care, in a way similar to the fail-safe proposed for the graduate medical education trust fund.[128] Some believed—and more hoped—that the fail-safe would never be needed; but some such device had to be in place for CBO to score BBA as reaching a balance by 2002.

The fail-safe methodology was roughly similar to that in use for the Medicare Fee Schedule, with both prospective and retrospective adjustments. It applied only to the FFS part because managed care limits were specifically set elsewhere. The scheme was based on projected and actual expenditures in each of nine FFS sectors, such as inpatient hospital services, physician services, diagnostic tests, and durable medical equipment and supplies. Each year, beginning with FY 1998, the secretary would determine whether the estimated expenditures for a particular sector matched the baseline amount set in the statute, and reduce payment rates for projections in excess of the baseline as well as reallocate proportionally any amounts by which the baseline exceeded the projected expenditures. There was also a retrospective or "lookback" feature. Beginning in 1999, the secretary was to estimate the actual spending for the second preceding fiscal year and compare that to the adjusted budget limits. Any spending amount above the budget amount would be subtracted from that sector's next fiscal year allotment. CBO scored the fail-safe provision for $33.4 billion in savings.

The fail-safe mechanism in the House bill eventually occasioned sharp, partisan controversy and on that account merits comment. On its face, it seemed a reasonable attempt both to assure scorable savings and to monitor implementation.[129] Still, applying it only to the FFS program might seem unfair, even though heavy exactions were imposed upon managed care.[130] Several provisions were especially hard on providers. CBO pointed out that because sector growth rates were based on 1995 rates, rather than those likely to occur after implementation began, projection errors would be frequent and accurate corrections difficult to make. The penalty reductions would be 133 percent of the amount by which spending limits were exceeded because of the CBO behavioral offset of 25 percent.[131] Moreover, in contrast to treatment under the Medicare Fee Schedule, providers got no rewards to offset the penalties, except that they would not be worse off than the scheduled reductions. Some critics thought the scheme unworkable since it relied upon sanctions applied to groups of providers two years after the event, sanctions that were expected to induce restraint among individual providers whose unit prices were being squeezed in present time.[132] CBO concluded that the large reductions and uncertainty of the rates "would probably increase the incentive" for providers to move from fee-for-service to MedicarePlus.[133] And if large numbers of providers were to leave FFS Medicare, beneficiaries would, too—so that to partisan eyes the fail-safe could be seen as a squeezing device, aimed at driving both providers and beneficiaries out of the FFS program.

Most other cost savers were relatively minor, notable only for the thoroughness with which ProPAC, PPRC, and the task force scoured for savings among the various Medicare subsidies and payment systems. These included such expedients as reducing rates of capital reimbursement, payments for hospital bad debt, and updates on clinical laboratories; rebasing payment systems for long-term hospitals; and freezing payment rates for clinical laboratories and ambulatory surgical centers. Also notable were the small savings attributed in some instances to big changes. For example, an elaborate statutory scheme to control fraud and abuse was scored at $2.8 billion in savings, despite estimates that as much as 20 percent of program costs could be attributed to this source. Medical malpractice reform was estimated to save only $200 million over seven years. On the other hand, regulatory relief would probably cost about $640 million and the Medical Savings Accounts another $4 billion.

As this account may suggest, CBO scoring is stringent and can seriously affect substantive policy and political outcomes. Several congressional staffers have noted that CBO emphasis upon calculable and enforceable scoring works against experiment and corrigible approaches that might still be the best option. The same emphasis may also tend to peak and sharpen controversy over the formula itself—losing sight of broader concerns. And it can tempt party leaders to go far out on a comparatively weak limb. Still, all of this may be preferable to letting politicians get away with technically unsound budget proposals and reliance on smoke and mirrors to create the illusion of savings.[134]

Fraud and Abuse, Regulatory Relief, and Malpractice Liability

Three chapters of the House bill related to fraud and abuse, to regulatory relief, and to medical malpractice liability. They were much more the work of the regular committees—not the task force—and less relevant to the reconciliation process as such. Malpractice liability was stripped from the Senate bill under the Byrd Rule as "nongermane."[135] CBO thought that the regulatory reforms would cost money rather than saving it. These chapters tended to favor providers, though not uniformly. They also embodied a philosophy more inclined toward private sector approaches than regulation. They were there because they seemed like needed reforms, to gain support within Congress, and to address some long-standing grievances of providers. Only fraud and abuse had bipartisan support.

Malpractice liability was one of those issues that had traditionally belonged to the states, along with auto accidents and ordinary breach of contract. However, it had been an issue in the health care reform debates of 1994 and had figured, along with product liability, in the Contract with America. In fact, an opening gambit, early in 1995, was the successful effort by the Health Care Liability Alliance—a coalition of two dozen trade associations and malpractice insurers—to add three medical malpractice provisions to H.R. 10, the "Common Sense Legal Reform Act," which was moving through the House Judiciary Committee as part of the Contract with America. The amendments were attached to the product liability bill because of a widely shared conviction, especially in the House, that malpractice reform had little chance of survival as a stand-alone bill facing a presidential veto.[136]

The amended bill, the Common Sense Product Liability and Legal Reform Act (H.R. 956) passed the House on March 10 by a vote of 265 to 161. In the course of passage the medical malpractice provisions had both changed and grown beyond the original conception. One change was to focus more specifically on medical malpractice, providing for a $250,000 cap on noneconomic damages (such as pain and suffering) in all health liability suits.[137] This amendment, offered by Representative Cox (R., Calif.) drew upon California experience with the Medical Injury Compensation Reform Act (MICRA), a 1976 statute widely cited for its effectiveness in reducing medical malpractice judgments. A second Cox-sponsored amendment was to eliminate "joint and several responsibility," which encouraged going for "deep pockets" rather than the most responsible party. A collateral source rule for determining damages was considered but did not pass. By a voice vote, the House added the so-called "FDA defense," which would protect manufacturers from punitive damages if their products had been approved by the FDA. Intensely debated, these amendments were defended especially as a way to contain health care costs, by reducing incentives to practice defensive medicine. On the other side, they were attacked as taking remedies from poor working people. Little was said about any relevance to Medicare.

How the medical malpractice provisions of H.R. 956 became part of the Medicare Preservation Act can be briefly recounted. In the Senate, the Judiciary Committee was considering a broad product liability bill, the Civil Justice Fairness Act sponsored by Senator Hatch, which included several malpractice provisions. Meanwhile, the Labor and Human Resources Committee was working on a more comprehensive medical malpractice bill (S 484) but the principal sponsors, senators McConnell (R., Ky.), Kassebaum (R., Kans.) and Lieberman, (D., Conn.), had little hope that it would pass. The Hatch bill was reported out of committee and seemed assured of passage when Senator McConnell moved to attach the H.R. 956 provisions to the Hatch bill—a way to provide a legislative vehicle. The McConnell amendment was carried by a close vote: 52–47. But the result rankled and the Republican majority lacked the votes to end the protracted floor debate that followed and were unable to bring the amended bill to a vote.[138] On May 10 the Hatch bill passed but only after all the medical malpractice provisions had been stripped.[139] The provisions of H.R. 956 were subsequently included in the House Medicare bill, with several additional measures. Eventually, that part of the Medicare Preservation Act met the same fate in the Senate—it too was stripped.

As an ironic comment, most of the senators wanted malpractice reform—but not the bill that ultimately developed. For that matter, so did most members of the House: H.R. 956 passed with a healthy majority of 100 votes. Yet their bill wound up as part of the Medicare Preservation Act where it did not belong, where it was a political liability, and where it would add a paltry $200 million in savings.

Subtitle C of the House bill dealt with regulatory relief and "self-referral." These were particularly troublesome because they involved activities where business and medicine came together and where individual providers often wanted to venture but feared to do so, especially without a good attorney. Judging from the volume and intensity of complaints in popular medical journals,[140] this was one area in which regulatory relief or clarification would be welcome, as a gentle rain falling upon a parched land. It was also an area in which providers, and especially physicians, could be rewarded for their political support at a relatively low cost.

The whole field was both vast and dauntingly complex, but the provisions in the House bill fell into a small list of categories: (1) self referral, and especially the Stark I and Stark II limits; (2) antikickback rules and safe harbors; (3) level of intent required for imposition of sanctions; and (4) an antitrust exception for medical self-regulatory entities.

The Stark laws—named after Rep. Fortney H. (Pete) Stark, former chairman of the Ways and Means Health Subcommittee—had been crafted over the years to deal with physician self-referral. Self-referral, in this context, occurs when a physician refers Medicare patients to an outside entity in which he/she or a member of the family has a compensation arrangement or an ownership or investment interest: for example, a referral to a clinical laboratory, an MRI center, or a medical supply company. Stark I applied to clinical laboratories, but Stark II reached out to include various "designated services," such as radiology, physical and occupational therapy, and durable medical equipment and supplies. There were exceptions, especially for in-office, group practices, or directly supervised services—but these tended to be like IRS exceptions—subject to all sorts of requirements that often seemed to physicians to be ignoring the realities of medical practice, keeping them out of a legitimate line of business, or presuming that they were crooks.

For good or ill, the Health Subcommittee, which dealt with Stark issues, went in the direction of greater market freedom: drastically reducing the list of designated services; repealing the "compensation arrangement" as a ban; eliminating restrictions on site of service; modifying the definition of prepaid health plans to accommodate new entities such as PPOs and PSNs; and declaring a moratorium on Stark II implementation until final rules on Stark I physician referral were published.

Delay in publication of these rules had long been a sore point. Stark I goes back to OBRA of 1989. Six years later the final regulation on physician referral had not been published—a testimony to the complexity and difficulty of rule-making in this area. Stark II was perhaps biting off too much; and Representative Stark acknowledged that he, too, would like to have seen the law simplified. For Representative Thomas there was a genuine concern about freedom for provider entities to develop new methods of treatment. He also protested that Stark II would "get into the detailed workings of physician group practices, hospitals, medical schools, and entities that employ or contract with practicing physicians" adding that the law may already "be overreaching, too complex, and intrusive."[141] Viewed from this perspective, the task force treatment of the amendments seems like a reasonable effort to move toward a less regulatory emphasis.

At the same time, the House amendments may themselves have gone too far—for instance, in preempting thirty states that had their own self-referral laws. The BBA provisions would unsettle a large body of common law, and they would open up new loopholes, for example, exempting compensation arrangements, which could in practice cover many forms of "interest" other than direct financial ones such as rent or consulting arrangements; or allowing "general supervision" instead of "direct," which, combined with repealing the "site of service" requirements, could allow for almost any kind of joint venture.[142]

The Senate did not deal with the Stark laws, possibly out of courtesy to another house as well as the complexity of the subject. That may have been wise, since the reconciliation process is a blunt instrument, not ideal for fixing complex arrangements. Yet the example also illustrates a dilemma: between caution and moving when opportunity offers. For seldom in our system of government do we get the chance to deal comprehensively with some of these rank overgrowths produced by the tendency of Congress and other institutions to increment, micromanage, and overregulate.

Antikickback provisions were of a more venerable origin, dating back originally to the Social Security Amendments of 1972. Section 1877(b), as amended, prohibits "knowingly and willingly" offering or paying any remuneration directly or indirectly to induce referrals or the purchase, lease, or ordering of goods or services. Steep penalties are prescribed for anyone convicted of a violation. As with the Stark laws, however, there were questions of interpretation and many exceptions, including a provision whereby the secretary (in practice, the DHHS inspector general) could establish a "safe harbor" for any payment practice. Not surprisingly, especially in view of the money involved and the penalties for kickbacks, providers sought additional safe harbors, especially as managed care and new kinds of provider activities and organizations developed.

For the most part, the Thomas bill left antikickback legislation as it had been. One important addition, though, was an exception for HMOs and managed care that would allow reductions in cost sharing or increases in benefits. The DHHS inspector general was also required to solicit proposals for new safe harbors and, as appropriate, modify or promulgate them. This step was seen as important in keeping regulations responsive and abreast of industry developments, although a representative for OIG testified before the subcommittee that encouraging such applications could "open the floodgates" and become "all encompassing."[143]

Potentially the most far-reaching of all these amendments were the changes made in the specific behavior and requirements of proof for various offenses. These cut across the whole field of Stark I and II, antikickback, fraud and abuse, and antitrust violations. For civil monetary penalties (CMPs) under the False Claims Act, the "should know" in establishing an offense was changed to acting with "deliberate ignorance" or "reckless disregard" of the truth or falsity of a claim—just short of criminal intent. For antikickback penalties, seeking to "induce" referrals was changed to "significant purpose" of inducing. In proposals for a safe harbor, the secretary would not be allowed to look behind the proposal for its underlying intent. Medical self-regulation entities (such as PROs) were exempted from antitrust suits, and PSNs or PSOs would be judged under the "rule of reason" standard and could not be charged with per se violations.

Together these statutory changes would have two effects. One would be to legitimate some activities previously regarded as illegal or questionable. They would also make law enforcement more difficult. The Department of Justice, the Federal Trade Commission, and the Department of Health and Human Services all testified that these changes would sanction objectionable behavior and make the work of policing offenders more difficult, costly, and time consuming.[144] At the same time, other parts of the Safeguarding Medicare Integrity Act (H.R. 2389) came down hard on objectionable behavior, especially that which seriously affected costs or program integrity. A clearer separation between the legitimate and the criminal or legally actionable, where it can be done, is usually seen as a good thing. Reasonable persons disagree about where that line should be drawn.

Medicare fraud and abuse were part of the Safeguarding Medicare Integrity Act and eventually incorporated into the Medicare Preservation Act as Subtitle C. Activities of this nature had been a concern since the Medicare and Medicaid programs began. Fraud and abuse legislation also received a considerable amount of bipartisan support during health care reform with bills sponsored by Senator Mitchell (for the Mainstream Coalition), Senator Dole, and Repre-setative Gephardt, the House majority leader. Despite the collapse of health care reform, fraud and abuse was seen as a topic that should receive attention in the coming year. In January, 1995, Sen. William Cohen (R., Me.) then chairman of the Senate Aging Committee, introduced a health care fraud pre-vention bill (S 245), which, though it covered all payers, had many of the same principles and provisions included in the later House bill. Various factors had stimulated an increased interest in fraud and abuse, and the bill had bipartisan support. Moreover, one consideration important to House Republicans and to their constituents was that deep cuts for Medicare would be hard to defend unless strenuous efforts were made, at the same time, to reduce Medicare fraud and abuse.

A theme strongly developed in the fraud and abuse provisions of H.R. 2389 was education and prevention. One way these objectives would be pursued was by educating beneficiaries: explaining their benefits; informing them about fraud and abuse problems in their areas; and publishing fraud alerts in the Federal Register and through other means. Education of providers was also included, with emphasis upon payment integrity. A program to encourage voluntary disclosure allowed the secretary to reduce or mitigate penalties (which were mandatory under current law) for individuals who would come forward and admit to violations or omissions—premised on the belief that many providers would like to do the right thing but did not know how and feared prosecution despite good-faith efforts. The act would further authorize an Anti-Fraud and Abuse Trust Fund, which could draw upon moneys generated by fines to support preventive activities of the Medicare Integrity Program.[145] Along with this provision went increased authority for the secretary to negotiate with carriers and intermediaries.

Effective enforcement received special attention. One expression of this emphasis was authority for DHHS to provide rewards for information on fraudulent or abusive practices. Other measures increased the civil monetary penalties for various offenses and provided new intermediate sanctions, such as stopping enrollments for a term or temporary exclusions from the Medicare program. To help coordinate fraud and abuse prosecution, the bill ordered the establishment, within 120 days after enactment of the statute, of a nationwide Health Care Fraud and Abuse Task Force. This task force would combine the efforts of the Department of Justice, the inspector general of DHSS, and the attorneys general of the states and coordinate their efforts both nationally and locally. The legislation also authorized use of "strike forces" similar to those under the RICO statute.[146] Extending this RICO approach, the bill created a new category of Federal Health Care Offenses—some applying to any health plan—with enforcement powers that included wire-tap authority and procedures for establishing a pattern of racketeering activity under RICO, all of this, no doubt, terrors to the unrighteous, but often to the righteous as well.

The Safeguarding Medicare Integrity Act involved much work and contained a number of useful provisions. At the same time, it could have used a dose of cautious incrementalism and the benefit of thoughtful criticism. That goes especially for amendments changing standards of illegal conduct and shifting around burdens of proof and for the symbolically imposing but seemingly thoughtless addition of an array of Federal Health Care Offenses with its *ad terrorem* enforcement mechanism. But caution was not the mood of the Republican majority; and the minority had little effective voice.

Passage in the House

Passage of the Medicare Preservation Act was another striking example of party discipline and organization. In a word, the Democrats had no visible effect on the legislation. Hearings were held, but only on general issues, not on legislation. The work of the task force was not made public nor shared with Democrats. Legislative drafts were given to the minority immediately before markups in the Ways and Means and Commerce Committees. No subcommittee markups were held. Medicare markups in full committee were constrained to one day. Floor debate was limited to five hours, with one hour for a Democratic substitute. The seven-hundred-page bill was passed on October 19 with only six Republicans breaking ranks. At no point in the entire history of this legislation did the minority prevail on a significant amendment.

Under the circumstances, much of the Democrats' activity amounted to theatre or efforts to build their own morale. To protest the lack of legislative hearings, House Democrats staged a "hearing" of their own on September 22, in the rain, outside the Capitol.[147] Commerce Democrats stalled the markup by demanding roll-call votes on petty procedural motions and then walking out.[148] During the markup, they made speeches and offered "message" amendments, covered by C-Span, for the benefit of "those who are watching." In the Commerce Committee, one small victory for the Democrats was an amendment prohibiting HMOs from excluding doctors solely because they were not board certified. In Ways and Means, Democrats were able to introduce a last-minute substitute, scored by CBO, assuring equivalent trust fund solvency. It was voted down, but figured in subsequent debate. Both committees reported out their bills, with no significant Democratic amendments, on straight party-line votes. Democrats were "outraged" and, surely, this is not the best way to legislate, though staffers who had been around for some time said that when they were in the majority Democrats had been equally hard on Republicans.[149]

Along with rules for the floor debate, the Rules Committee included, as customary, a number of amendments, mostly sponsored by the leadership, to gratify some constituency or to add or delete minor or controversial items. Many such amendments were relatively insignificant; but some were important. Among the latter was a guarantee to all Medicare/Plus providers of a minimum payment per patient of $300 per month for FY 1996 and $320 for FY 1997. This was a critical item, since a number of Republicans from rural states, led by Gregg Ganske (Iowa), threatened to join with Democrats to defeat the bill without such a provision. The rule front-loaded payments for teaching hospitals. It also added the list of Federal Health Care Offenses along with fines and prison terms for each. And it made good on one of Newt Gingrich's promises with a small formula change that increased physician payments by $300 million for FY 1996.

The floor debate produced nothing of significance. One hour was allotted to debate on the rule, three hours for the majority proposal, and an hour for the Democratic substitute. Democrats complained about these limits, with the venerable Sam Gibbons, ranking member of Ways and Means, remarking, "Yesterday the Republicans spent four hours on shrimp [fishing and shrimping regulation]. Today we are spending three hours on 40 million people's benefits and 270 billion dollars."[150] After passage, the Medicare Preservation Act along with the Medicaid Transformation Act was included in H.R. 2491, the reconciliation bill, to be sent to the Senate.

Senate Action

In general, the Senate produced a shorter and less exhaustive bill that tracked the House version with respect to its most important provisions. In many areas, S 1357 had no provision, adopted the House version, or modified it only slightly. Only with respect to beneficiary obligations did the Senate bill differ notably in content or philosophy. In general, it was more moderate and showed the benefits of a second iteration. It was also a less partisan product, though more because of senatorial individualism than a genuine spirit of bipartisanship. The most important moderating influence, aside from individualism, would seem to have been the Senate's own institutions, such as committee structure and membership and the Byrd Rule against nongermane provisions in a reconciliation bill.

It is important to remember that the Senate experienced no "revolution" in 1995 and was, at most, going along with the House and not seeking to lead. Though eventually committed to trust fund solvency and balancing the budget, even Republican senators had second thoughts. And despite a liking for managed care options, restructuring Medicare or seeking "successor" institutions was not a high priority for them.

Policy in the Senate is seldom "leadership driven." Both the rules and the temperament of the Senate make disciplined, majoritarian efforts well nigh impossible. Even if that were not so, the existing leadership had little interest in such an effort. Senator Dole liked to delegate, not actively manage; and he was most interested, in 1995, in a run for the presidency. Pete Domenici, the

Budget Committee chairman, was a cautious negotiator, not a militant of the John Kasich species. Two additional antimajoritarian institutions were the Senate Finance Committee and the Senate tradition of unlimited debate: the filibuster.

The membership and some of the institutions of the Finance Committee were important influences in the passage of S 1357. Finance had eleven majority and nine minority members—a close balance that needed only one defector to produce a deadlock. Furthermore, in 1995, several of the Republicans, such as Chafee, Dole, Grassley, Hatch, and Packwood, were sometimes on the liberal side of health care issues while most of the Democrats were moderately to strongly liberal. The staff, which traditionally was very good, worked for the whole committee and with senators of the opposing party. Finance would often meet or hold hearings in full committee and did not have subcommittee staff or markups. All of these factors worked toward moderation and against one-sided or strongly partisan legislation.

Several Republicans on the committee had individual interests that moderated their views on comprehensive reform or led them on occasion to press for specific concessions. William Roth, who succeeded Packwood as chairman, was mainly interested in taxes, not Medicare. John Chafee, a liberal on health issues, was chairman of the Medicaid subcommittee and weighed in mostly on those issues. Charles Grassley was especially concerned with access to health care in rural areas and with managed care payment issues rather than restructuring Medicare. Alfonse D'Amato was facing a tough reelection contest and disposed to defend beneficiaries and New York medical schools. They and other Republicans on the committee worked on their own version of the budget numbers and pushed for particular amendments. They shared a desire to support the party and go along with the House, but no one had a compelling, comprehensive vision for Medicare.

Putting together a bill was hectic though relatively uncontroversial for the Senate Republicans, in part because of earlier experience with developing managed care options while in the minority and during the debates over health care reform. Largely because of this experience, the Finance Committee staff was able to develop a "Choices" draft by early June that worked from existing HMO legislation, remnants in their own "bone yard," and some pro-competition elements of the FEHBP.[151] Like the House, the Senate Republicans had a long-standing health care task force that could advise the leadership and committees working on health care issues. This task force had a proposal, developed legislatively by Senator Gregg and his staff, that closely tracked the FEHBP but would have kept traditional FFS Medicare as a separate entity.[152] This initiative was sufficiently developed to be scored by CBO but did not figure significantly in the final legislation. The Finance staff finished drafting the chairman's mark by the end of August. A week thereafter, on September 7, Senator Packwood resigned following a lengthy scandal and adverse report of the Senate Ethics Committee. The final markup was delayed for several weeks to brief the new chairman, Senator Roth, on the whole reconciliation bill, but no significant changes were made in the Medicare provisions.[153]

The committee's three-day markup produced little of additional significance. Senators Moynihan and Rockefeller offered a Democratic substitute that was voted down. It would have saved $106 billion over five years and called for a bipartisan commission to consider long-term problems of Medicare structure and financing.[154] The committee amended slightly a proposal for income-relating the Part B premium, but voted down a series of other amendments. The bill was reported out on September 30.

As for Part A and Part B savings, the Senate and House bills were similar, which is not surprising since the potential money savers were generally known and both House and Senate were advised by ProPAC and PPRC. The Senate was more generous on hospital updates, rural hospitals, and Medicare DSH payments and about the same as the House, both in payment and methodology, on hospital outpatient overpayments, physician payment updates, skilled nursing facilities, and home health care. The Senate did not capture as many small savings. On the other hand, it went farther than the House by taking twice as much from the PPS-exempt hospitals. Although the Finance Committee had two New York senators, the Senate bill was not especially considerate of medical schools or hospitals, cutting almost as much from the IME as the House did and making no provision for a trust fund.

An important difference was the Senate's less favorable treatment of beneficiaries. One reason was that the Senate, unlike the House, made no particular point of protecting the beneficiaries. The Senate had been more impressed by some of the statements and alternative proposals coming from the Bipartisan Commission on Entitlement and Tax Reform that had reported late in 1994. This commission, much concerned with intergenerational equity and the fiscal impact of future retirees ("baby-boomers"), had recommended postponing eligibility and shifting more of the burden of health care to the beneficiaries. Senators John Breaux (D., La.) and Alan Simpson (R., Wyo.), members of the Finance Committee, had served on the commission. John Chafee (R., R.I.), a consistent liberal on health issues, felt that more attention needed to be paid to children and the poor and less to the elderly.[155] It was also sound policy to look ahead and plan for future demand.

With that said, the Senate's onslaught on the beneficiaries was more bark than bite. Like the House, the Senate would return to a premium level of 31.5 percent of Part B program costs. But the Senate eased the pinch by scheduling the increase over seven years. On more affluent beneficiaries, the Senate was a bit tougher than the House, phasing out premium support at $100,000 for individuals and $150,000 for couples. The Part B deductible was increased from $100 to $150, with $10 increments in succeeding years. Beneficiaries would also be liable for premium costs over the Medicare payment rate and for balance billing by health plans.[156] And the Senate bill would raise Medicare eligibility from the current sixty-five to sixty-seven years of age; but, like Social Security, with a transition period of twenty-four years that would not begin until year 2003. The burden may have been shifted, but it was relatively light and most of it would not be felt soon.

The managed care options were similar to those in the House bill, except for use of the term "Medicare Choice" rather than "MedicarePlus." One major difference was the absence, in the Senate bill, of any specific provision for provider-sponsored organizations (PSOs). In principle, other provisions were almost identical but the Senate bill did not spell out in detail the enrollment and marketing procedures and the protections for beneficiaries and providers. The only other major difference was with respect to payment for managed care plans.

The Senate version of managed care payments went several steps beyond the House bill, both in severing links with the traditional AAPCC and in adopting a powerful technique for equalizing payments across the nation. Pushed especially by Senator Grassley (R., Iowa) this plan would primarily capture more overall savings and help make HMOs feasible in rural areas. In essence, it involved a partial nationalization of rates linked, eventually, to growth in the gross domestic product. The payment area would be either Metropolitan Statistical Areas (MSAs) or rural non-MSA areas. For these a rate would be calculated based on the historic AAPCCs and the mix of services provided in the area. A health plan would be paid at this rate averaged with an increasing percentage of the national per capita rate until a 50–50 balance was reached—in effect raising low-payment plans and reducing high ones. At that point, the link with the traditional AAPCC would be severed and new updates based on the percentage increase in the gross domestic product—a much lower figure than typical health care market-baskets or the Medicare Economic Index. In the first two years, the indirect teaching allowance, the direct medical teaching payments, and the Medicare DSH would be drastically reduced: 50 percent each year. Taken as a whole, the scheme was both a powerful equalizer and a potent money saver. CBO scored this part at $43.7 billion dollars over seven years, roughly $10 billion more than the House plan.[157]

With respect to fraud and abuse and much of the regulatory field, the Senate did less and also built more on existing approaches. It left Stark I and Stark II to the House. On fraud and abuse, the Senate went along with the House on intermediate sanctions and the new criminal offenses but, in general, put more emphasis on data collection and strengthening in-house capabilities rather than beneficiary mobilization. It allowed fines and other penalties to go into an enforcement fund—which was an important precedent. Medical malpractice and most of the antitrust amendments were stripped under the Byrd Rule as not germane to reconciliation, and the Senate, thanks largely to Senator Chafee's efforts, restored the nursing home standards.

Several significant items were added in the course of floor debate. A chairman's amendment by Senator Roth restored $13 billion in health care spending, most of it for Medicaid, but $2 billion targeted for teaching hospitals[158] The amendment also retained most of the nursing home standards. Two anti-HMO amendments were adopted: one by Sen. Jesse Helms (R., N.C.) that required HMOs to offer a point-of-service plan and another by Sen. Bob Graham (D., Fla.) that assured access to emergency care despite HMO rules. Several items were struck under the Byrd Rule: Medicare savings accounts; the increase of the eligibility age from sixty-five to sixty-seven; and the Senate version of a fail-safe (Budget Expenditure Limiting Tool, or BELT)—because CBO refused to score it as saving any money.

After conference negotiations that lasted over two weeks—mostly to deal with tax provisions—both houses passed the final reconciliation bill on November 17. On most items, the report followed the House bill, and important differences were few.[159] The beneficiary deductible was kept at $100 instead increasing it to $150 with $10 annual increments; but beneficiaries were made liable to health plan charges under some circumstances. Medicare-Plus plans were guaranteed a monthly minimum of $300, rising to $350 in 1997, with a minimum 2 percent annual increase thereafter. A compromise on PSOs was reached which called for state licensing and separate solvency standards for doctors and hospitals. Medical savings accounts were restored; but antitrust provisions were removed on procedural grounds.

IV. DENOUEMENT

According to the dictionary, "denouement" is "the outcome of a complex series of events." It is a descriptive heading for the final episodes in the 1995 reconciliation process. Another possibility would be "end game," alluding to the calculated moves and countermoves that were involved, though many of the activities seemed less like chess and more like some cosmic game of poker with high stakes, secrecy, and bluffing. Another term then current was "Kabuki," suggesting that much of the activity, like theatre, was stylized and primarily for the audience. Most commonly, though, people spoke about an impending "train wreck," aware of the serious consequences for both sides. These are all good characterizations of the mobilization politics and campaign-style legislation that was going on. It had much in common, at different times, with a political campaign, aimed at the voter; a diplomatic campaign, seeking to bargain with the opposition; and a military campaign, inflicting damage with the aim of subduing an enemy.

Like most situations that lead to war, there was an early recognition on both sides that the political stakes in this process were high and that a major confrontation or "showdown"[160] was likely. Recall Speaker Gingrich's comment in June, just after final agreement on the budget resolution, that Republicans could "govern for a generation" if they would "solve Medicare." According to report, he believed that winning on Medicare was essential to retain control of the House. At the same time, Democrats, especially in the House, were thinking that Republicans had dangerously overreached and that Medicare might be the Democrats' ticket back to majority status. For that matter, the House Democratic leadership was operating on a primary strategy of holding enough loyalists to sustain a presidential veto.[161] The Republicans were planning to go them one better, with a debt ceiling "hammer" that would preclude the Treasury from borrowing to keep the government running if President Clinton vetoed the reconciliation bill or whatever continuing resolution Congress offered.[162]

Over the long summer, from June through September, the Republicans were pushing a message that Gingrich and their pollsters had urged: that Medicare was going bankrupt in seven years, that they were restructuring the program to save it now and for a future generation, and that they were reducing the rate of increase, not actually cutting the program itself. According to observers, they stayed "on message" with remarkable consistency and were making up much of the approval ratings they had earlier lost. Meanwhile, Republicans were demanding details of the president's June budget, denouncing it as based on phony numbers, accusing the Democrats of resorting to "Mediscare," tactics and condemning them for refusing to confront the long-term problem of baby boomers.

Republicans in both House and Senate continued to work actively with interest groups on specific formulas and numbers as well as putting out several brush fires. At one point, the AARP, which had gotten restive over the budget cuts, was checked by a timely "shot across the bow." This shot took the form of a Finance subcommittee investigation into AARP's nonprofit status by Sen. Alan Simpson The message was quite clear and was perfectly understood: lay off or expect trouble.[163] When the AHA went public with its opposition to the Medicare and Medicaid DSH cuts, it got a harsh warning from the Republican Conference chairman, John Boehner, about "mimicking of the Democrat line" and "running a paid fear campaign in the media." At one point, even the AMA was threatened with a lack of cooperation, but was also mollified with a "correction" in a technical payment formula worth $900 million in FY 1996.[164]

The Democrats sharpened their message: hammering on excesses; and arguing that the Republican scheme was not motivated by a desire to save Medicare but would destroy the program as it was then known; that beneficiaries would be forced into managed care plans; and that the real purpose was not to make the plan "solvent" or save the trust fund, but to end entitlements and give a tax break to the well-to-do. At times the message was more sophisticated—pointing out, for instance, dangers of adverse selection with the

MedicarePlus scheme—but as one staffer acknowledged, few understood that argument, so they had to "demagogue it" with the cruder messages.[165]

Despite their denunciations, Democrats in both House and Senate worked on their own versions of a budget. In the House, the Democratic leadership never produced a budget—for tactical reasons, from a principled opposition to balancing the budget with Medicare and Medicaid reductions, and because of divisions among themselves. However, the Blue Dog–coalition did submit an alternative budget resolution in May (which was rejected) that closely resembled the Senate Republican bill. This bill and the Blue Dog coalition continued to play a role in the reconciliation process, but primarily as forces moving Democrats more toward the Republican position, not in mounting a Democratic opposition.

In the Senate, after the passage of a Republican budget resolution, a small task force of seven senators, representing a spectrum of Democratic opinion (Kennedy, Rockefeller, Harkin, Graham, Daschle, Breaux, Lieberman) began working, together and with their staffs, on a proposal that was to become the Senate Democratic budget. Usually referred to as the "Daschle budget," because Tom Daschle—the minority leader—chaired the task force, this budget aimed at scorable savings from Medicare that would preserve solvency until 2006. It included a Democratic version of structural changes, emphasizing the concept of HCFA as a "prudent purchaser" of quality health care.[166] The projected savings were much below the Republican budget. In part, this level represented an amount that the task force thought Senate Democrats would tolerate. It was also in accord with their avowed policy that Medicare savings should not be used to balance the budget.

The president's June budget, although it remained in outline the president's proposal, was not a finished product, relied on OMB numbers and not the more conservative CBO scoring, and would reach a balance in ten years rather than seven. Republicans welcomed the president's change of position, especially as giving them some cover, but quickly condemned the budget proposal itself as little more than an outline (totaling twenty-nine pages), and as too little, too late. Robert Reischauer, former director of CBO, observed at the time that by using OMB numbers Clinton had "lowered the bar" so much that he could figuratively "step over it," adding that he would be nowhere near a balance by the end.[167] Over the summer, the administration task force continued to work on this budget, to improve its scoring, recalculate savings as deficit and baseline figures changed, develop alternative scenarios or fall-back positions, brief administration officials and congressional representatives and supply them with talking points.[168] But neither then nor later did Clinton move more than incrementally from his June proposal.

The secrecy surrounding the budget and reconciliation proceedings is worthy of note. As one consequence, neither friend nor foe knew what the president had in mind. Democrats in the Senate, for instance, were not aware until

December either of the total Medicare reduction in the president's budget or the accompanying details.[169] A number of House Democrats saw his budget as a sign that he was moving away from a veto strategy and would "cut a deal," going even farther toward the Republican position.[170] Republicans saw the president's budget as making their task easier, especially by helping to win votes and bolster morale. At just about that time, the president vetoed the rescissions bill. According to administration insiders, the president was, by then, settling on his priorities, articulating his "double M–Double E" message, and preparing to go on the offensive.[171]

The timing of Clinton's budget was important. It came shortly after the passage of budget resolutions in House and Senate and could have been a window for negotiations. Once the conference report was accepted, with its instructions and deadlines for the authorizing committees, it tended to lock in the reconciliation process and work against compromise. That factor seems to have been important. For the Republicans, budget reconciliation was bloody work: costly in time and effort, in political resources, and in public good will. They were losing support among their own members and in the country. Over the summer, Democrats were out-polling them on favorable Medicare ratings by as much as two to one. Yet compromise, even if the votes were there to do it, risked an appearance of weakness as well as loss of their political base. So a compelling logic for the Republicans was to push harder, see the reconciliation through to victory, and then negotiate from a position of strength.

For the Democrats there were also reasons not to compromise. A number within the administration thought that the reconciliation would stall or fail, and that would increase the president's leverage. Even though Democrats were losing the fight in Congress, they were beginning to reap a harvest in the opinion polls. Further concessions would make the Republicans seem more reasonable and give them cover, might cut Democratic gains in the polls, and could risk losing still more of their own base.[172]

If there were any window of opportunity for compromise, little effort was made to hold it open. Both parties were mainly pursuing tactical advantage— short-term gains and positioning for a future showdown. In mid-July, at a White House meeting with leaders of both parties, Clinton said that he hoped to avoid a "train wreck" and urged the Republicans to speed up the legislative process. This would provide earlier details on the reconciliation, which the president would like to have, but he shared nothing with the opposition. Newt Gingrich emphatically ruled out a budget "summit," considered a bad word in Republican company, especially because of President Bush's summit agreement to raise taxes in 1990 (Drew 1996:302). Neither side pushed negotiation. Meanwhile, Republicans hired consultants to advise them on post-veto strategies and Robert Rubin, secretary of the Treasury, planned how to keep the government running if Republicans used their debt ceiling "hammer." By August, many in leadership positions in Washington assumed there would be a veto. In a National Public Radio address on August 7, President Clinton said, "No, I am not going to blink" (ibid.:303–34). Speaker Gingrich, in one of their frequent informal talks, pointed out to Clinton that a veto might be good for both sides as a way to maintain legitimacy with their base constituencies and still gain some bargaining leverage.[173]

When the Congress reconvened after the August recess, only three weeks remained until October 1, which would terminate the authorizations for that fiscal year. The Republican majority faced an impossible schedule. Because of time spent on the Contract with America, they were far behind on appropriations, with half of the thirteen bills—including the most controversial ones— not expected to meet the deadline.[174] September 14 was the original date for the reconciliation bill to be assembled, scored by CBO, passed in both houses, negotiated and agreed upon in conference, and finally adopted. At that point, not even one of the committees had reported—though House Ways and Means had released a detailed outline. Senator Packwood resigned on September 7 just before the Finance Committee markup, another occasion for delay. The deadline slipped to September 22 and then to September 29, but even that date was unrealistic. Meanwhile, any expectation that the appropriations bills would be ready had been abandoned. Eventually, the reconciliation bill was passed, but that was not until November 20, after the first week-long shutdown of the government and two months past the original deadline.

With a budget not completed by October 1, the usual procedure is to pass a continuing resolution (CR) temporarily extending spending authority, typically with some reduction in the level of funding and the addition of various riders. One problem with such a measure is that a first CR can lead to another, and another—extending the budget process or budget reconciliation well into the next year. Several reconciliation bills—in 1983, 1985, and 1987—came unglued after a series of CRs and fell apart. So delay can be costly. With this consideration in mind and to gain additional leverage for a final push, Speaker Gingrich signaled his intentions in a September 21 speech to a securities group, saying that he would block a debt limit increase unless Clinton agreed to the Republican reconciliation bill.[175] He was strongly supported in this initiative by Pete Domenici, who added that leaving the debt limit where it was for forty or fifty days might be worth doing if it could get a budget agreement from Clinton.[176]

The opening move of this hammer strategy was not auspicious. As predicted, the stock market was jittery. Congress and the president, concerned about who would be blamed for repercussions, moved slowly and cautiously, without significant concessions. Meanwhile, the appropriations bills and the reconciliation were falling farther behind. Only Finance had completed its part of the reconciliation by September 29. Ways and Means was trying to get its scoring to work and did not expect to vote until October 9. Commerce would not report before that. Dissension among Republicans over the interior and defense appropriations made further delay almost imperative.[177] With a respite attractive to both sides, a temporizing agreement was negotiated in which the Republicans stripped out those appropriations riders most objectionable to the White House and the administration agreed to a reduced level of spending for the term of the CR. The CR would run until November 13. At this stage, no mention was made of accepting the Republicans' reconciliation bill or their formula of a balance in seven years with CBO scoring. The hammer was held in reserve to see what progress could be made through negotiation. November 13 was calculated as the date the administration would run out of various discretionary funds needed to keep the government running.

Meanwhile, quite a bit of positioning and implicit bargaining did take place once the details of the reconciliation bill were known. On October 19, the day the House bill passed, Clinton announced that he would veto the reconciliation bill if it cut Medicare as deeply as projected. But he added that he would seek to reach a balance in nine years and was open to a plan for seven. He suggested ways in which the White House and Republicans could meet halfway. And he made some specific concessions: agreeing to means testing for the Medicare premium and to a capital gains and a middle-class family tax cut.[178] Informal lines of communication at critical levels were also open: Clinton and Gingrich; Pete Domenici and Leon Panetta; and Gingrich's staff and counterparts at the White House (Drew 1996:310). Republicans were willing to yield some ground on the size of the family tax cut, on Medicaid DSH, possibly even on the earned income tax credit.[179] They also initiated, at Senator Dole's prompting, a meeting with the president on November 1 that led to two hours of "constructive discussions" at the White House.[180]

There was positioning and talking but no serious bargaining or concessions. Here, several factors worked against quiet deal-making. One was the publicity and rhetoric attending almost any shift of position or conciliatory gesture. In this high-stakes diplomacy, "open covenants" tended to mean "no covenants." As with a military confrontation, both sides were highly mobilized, struggling to hold their forces together, and captive in some measure of their own partisan ideology and militants. Seldom mentioned, but perhaps most decisive was that neither side could give what the other had to have. The administration never developed a budget that reached a balance in seven years with CBO scoring, and, given the deficit and baselines at that time, it is doubtful that they could without cuts in Medicare and Medicaid that would be unacceptable for them.[181] From the Republican side, any sizable reduction in the reconciliation cuts would require an arduous restructuring, slow the momentum, and pose a grave threat to the coalition. House Republicans were especially impatient, suspicious of the old "go halfway" approach to negotiation and, as John Kasich put it, loath to lose the "crusade" spirit of the reconciliation effort that had inspired the struggle and made the pain seem worthwhile.

Not unlike cooling-off periods in strike negotiations, the rhetoric during the six-week period of the first CR grew more intense and attitudes seemed to harden. Democrats tweaked up their "Mediscare" tactics and, with the reconciliation package before them, could point out, for example, how the fail-safe device could be used to force Medicare beneficiaries into HMOs. Republicans continued with their message of saving Medicare, attacked the Clinton budget as phony, and increasingly demanded he get serious with a budget that CBO would score as reaching a balance in seven years.

October 24 for the Republicans was one of those star-crossed days—two leaders stumbling at the same time. Making the point that Medicare had flaws, Senator Dole told a gathering of the American Conservative Union about his early opposition to Medicare, saying, "I was there, fighting the fight, voting against Medicare—1 of 12—because we knew it wouldn't work in 1965."[182] On the same day, before the Blue Cross/Blue Shield Association, Newt Gingrich made his famous and ambiguous "wither on the vine" speech, long debated as to whether it was HCFA or Medicare that was to "wither."[183] Bill McInturf, a pollster for the Republicans, upon hearing of these statements, said, "There goes the election." Senate Democrats blew up the quotes and carried them to the Senate floor on poster boards; the Democratic National Committee ran television clips from the speeches; and Mike McCurry, the president's press secretary, commented to reporters that Republicans would probably like to see senior citizens wither away too.[184] In the political turbulence, these events soon got lost. But this kind of attack from Democrats along with the restive opposition of conservative House Republicans to discussions that seemed to go nowhere were factors that induced Gingrich to break off the talks and move toward a more punishing CR for the next round.

The next resolutions, passed on November 13 a few hours before the earlier debt limit extension was scheduled to end, led to the first shutdown. One of these, a CR, continued until December 1 the funding for the agencies that fell under the unfinished appropriations bills. The second extended the debt limit until December 12 but contained provisions aimed at forcing the president to agree to a budget deal or veto the debt extension and face the prospect of a default. There were a number of "poison pills" in the bill, including several regulatory measures, but most important was a requirement that the president agree to enact a seven-year balanced-budget plan using CBO scoring. There was a "snap-back" scheme that would raise the debt limit through December 12 and then lower it. And the secretary of the Treasury was forbidden to borrow from trust funds to keep the government running. In other words, agree on our terms or throw the government into default.[185] That same day, Clinton vetoed the bill. On November 14 the federal government "furloughed" 800,000 workers and shut down a large number of "nonessential" activities. The first shutdown had begun.

This kind of doomsday strategy was not without precedent. For instance, the government had several times shut down for a few hours during the Reagan administration and for three days in 1985, during a confrontation over the Gramm-Rudman-Hollings deficit control legislation. The threat of a Gramm-Rudman sequester forced George Bush in 1990, most reluctantly, to agree to a budget "summit" that led him to renege on his famous "no new taxes" pledge. And the March 1995 fight with President Clinton over the rescissions bill was seen by some Republicans as a likely precedent for what might happen with the reconciliation bill. The president would veto, but make a realistic assessment of the disposition of forces and "cut a deal" with Congress. Both sides would talk tough for a while, give on some of their priorities, and go home claiming victory. This strategy, though heavy-handed, would seem a reasonable gamble, given past precedents and the current situation.

Whatever the ultimate strategy, this opening move by the Republicans was premature. The reconciliation bill was still unfinished and less than half of the appropriations bills had passed Congress. One consequence of an early shutdown was to divert attention from larger issues of policy, such as deficit reduction and the substantive measures contained in the reconciliation bill to the highly dramatic confrontation over a shutdown. Moreover, the Republicans seemed almost spoiling for a fight—indeed, trying to start one before the public knew what the argument was about. This perception was not helped by Newt Gingrich's statement that he had forced the shutdown in part because of his resentment over having to leave Air Force One through the rear door. Already losing in the polls, the Republicans were being blamed for the shutdown by a polling margin of two to one.[186] In addition, the veto helped unify the Democratic minority and commit the administration. Robert Rubin transferred $60 billion from trust funds to keep the government running. The president showed no sign of blinking, or of giving in, saying the Democrats could take it "right into the next election."[187] Despite statements that they would be prepared to carry on the shutdown indefinitely, the Republican leadership recognized that they had miscalculated and soon initiated talks with President Clinton. Both houses were, in fact, so eager to end the shutdown that they passed a new CR within two days after the shutdown to fund the government through December 5. A later version, passed on November 19, extended the funding through December 15. This CR contained a revised set of prescriptions so critical for the future budget controversy that they deserve special attention. H. J. Res. 122 committed Congress and the president, within the current session, to achieve a balanced budget in seven years, using CBO numbers. There were several important provisos: that CBO use its most recent numbers and consult with OMB on their economic and technical assumptions and that the budget, in addition to meeting a number of Republican objectives, such as protecting future generations, assuring Medicare solvency, and reforming welfare, protect the president's priorities—funding for Medicaid, education, and the environment, and tax policies that would help working families.[188] Notable in the resolution was the unambiguous requirement of a balance in seven years with CBO numbers—and the vagueness of other commitments. The CR would seem to give a clear authorization to Republicans to hold the Democrats' feet to the fire on the budget issue. At the same time, it left open what "protecting" the president's priorities could mean.

Congress left town on November 20, pretty much exhausted by the final push to pass the reconciliation bill and the negotiation of a continuing resolution. Talks resumed, on November 28 after the Thanksgiving recess, with a negotiating team of sixteen members: eight Republicans and five Democrats from Congress and three from the administration. Almost immediately there was trouble.

One issue was over seven years versus the president's priorities. Republicans generally took the view that seven years was seven years; and John Kasich said as much on the nationally televised Lehrer News Hour.[189] For the Democrats, there was still a question of protecting Medicare, Medicaid, the earned income tax credit, and other domestic priories as opposed, say, to a large tax cut and, beyond that, of how much and in what way specific programs would be reduced. Leon Panetta, putting administration priorities first, said that as long as these critical programs were protected, the budget could be balanced in "seven years or eight years," a statement made on the "Today Show," which sounded to Republican ears like a recanting before negotiations had even begun.

Related to protection of the president's domestic priorities was an especially tricky issue of whether CBO scoring would be done before negotiations began or after they were complete. Normally, CBO scores only when there are legislative language or details very close to that—which the Republicans were prepared to provide. But the Democrats were not there and hoped to get some concession on their use of OMB estimates and/or avail themselves of the more optimistic CBO numbers that would be available in the near future. What they would not do was give up the struggle for the administration priorities in advance.[190] For Republicans, though, using their CBO scored budget against an administration proposal (which they had not seen) would be bargaining their hard numbers against soft Democratic estimates. A good argument could be made for either side. But in the politically charged and strategically tense situation at that time, such technicalities seemed to Republicans like one more ploy from a president they did not trust anyway.

Despite all the subsequent posturing and maneuvering—including the long shutdown over Christmas and New Year's and the subsequent negotiations in 1996—this fundamental difference was never resolved nor did either party move much from its original position. Casting the issue in the form of budgetary technicalities obscured the fact that the basic disagreements remained unchanged. These went to fundamental differences of philosophy or ideology and with who would ultimately prevail in the political contest. The Republicans never found a way to compromise and take home half a loaf, and the Democrats had little incentive to do so as long as they were winning the political fight.

On December 5, one day before he vetoed the reconciliation bill, Clinton announced a budget of his own, even though the new CBO numbers were not yet available. It was a retread of the June budget, with savings of $124 billion from Medicare and $57 billion from Medicaid. It used OMB figures but included a fail-safe of its own with automatic spending cuts should the projections turn out to be too optimistic.[191] This initiative, like the earlier June budget, was preceded by intensive debate within the White House, came about after some complex political calculations, and was denounced by Republicans as political posturing and based on phony numbers. As with the June budget there was a similar danger for Republicans of interpreting this event as a tactical retreat when it could be the beginning of an engagement.

CBO numbers, when they arrived, helped the administration, but not much. A rescoring of the reconciliation bill showed Medicare savings of $226 billion instead of $270 billion and for Medicaid, $133 billion instead of $163 billion. But the Clinton plan for Medicare was scored by CBO at $97 billion instead of $124 and for Medicaid, $37 billion instead of $57 billion—roughly $48 billion less than the OMB estimate. For the reconciliation bill as a whole, the Clinton budget would have saved, over the seven years, $385 billion, just over half as much as the $750 billion projected for the reconciliation bill.[192]

There was a fair amount of theatrical activity on both sides over this news, but also arguments for compromise and for getting started with some serious negotiation. Panetta and Domenici were consulting and working together and both urged continuing with the budget process. Panetta submitted a second version of the president's budget using CBO and OMB numbers and argued within the White House for putting forward a budget using only CBO scoring (Drew 1996:349). Both Dole and Gingrich wanted to extend the CR rather than break off negotiations. But the weight of opinion within the White House was against a CBO-scored budget at that time, some wishing for tactical reasons to postpone it as long as possible[193] and others, including Gore, Rubin, Erskine Bowles, Alice Rivlin, and George Stephanopoulos, thought more than enough had been conceded to the Republicans and opposed giving up any more. On December 15, the day on which the CR was to end, Gingrich and Dole were discussing a continuation when word reached the House Republican leadership—meeting in the speaker's conference room—that they were considering another CR. When Gingrich returned, he was told by his own leadership group that they had delayed too long and that there would be no CR because of Clinton's lack of good faith and failure to produce a seven year budget with CBO scoring (ibid.:350).

A final, symbolic gesture on the part of the House Republicans, immediately before the shutdown, was to pass H.R. 2621, a bill to eliminate the Treasury's power to borrow from the trust funds or redeem federal securities as a way of avoiding the debt limit.[194] The vote was 235–103, with 77 members voting "present," a telling indication of restiveness. In any event, the measure was futile since it could easily have been talked to death in the Senate. Meanwhile, Secretary Rubin expressed confidence that he could continue funding the government indefinitely.

The December shutdown lasted twenty-one days until January 5, a unique event in American history. It produced an enormous amount of staff activity, new or modified budget proposals in Congress, and a series of summit meetings at the White House between Clinton, Dole, and Gingrich and other top administration officials and congressional leaders—sometimes only principals, other meetings with staff attending or waiting in halls or the Roosevelt room.[195] One result was that the president agreed to negotiate a seven-year budget with CBO numbers. But no further progress was made on substantive issues dividing the participants, and by the end the Republican reconciliation bill was visibly dying.

Despite much positioning and meeting, the first week after the shutdown ended in a stalemate, even though Clinton, Dole, and Gingrich seemed to be seeking in good faith to end the shutdown. On Tuesday, December 19, Clinton called Dole and Gingrich with an offer for a seven-year, CBO-scored budget if they would accept his numbers on Medicare and Medicaid.[196] They returned to Congress, announcing a "breakthrough." Vice-President Gore, meanwhile, stated on TV that there was a "misunderstanding" about the CBO numbers, a statement later negated by Mike McCurry, the press secretary. Back in the House, Gingrich was shown a tape of Gore's comments and told by his senior leadership that they would not agree to another CR.[197] The next day, Leon Panetta brought a budget proposal to Congress but the meeting collapsed when he learned there was no CR to talk about. No negotiations took place, though staff aides begin working out compromises on some of the less controversial items, such as veterans, banking, and sale of broadcast frequencies.[198]

The summit meeting of December 22 was, according to various accounts, an extraordinary performance. It took place in the Cabinet Room—principals seated around the long table and staff lining the walls. With Clinton as leader, what ensued was a seminar in public policy, during which each side talked about its problems with the others' proposals, followed by a more general discussion.[199] Observers of this and subsequent sessions, described them as carefully staged, set next to the Oval Office in the Cabinet Room—an awe-inspiring environment—with Clinton attired informally as the genial policy wonk and Gore in the role of "attack dog" or "tough cop," there to intimidate and to keep his more generous partner from giving away too much. In any event, the meeting did seem to impress Gingrich with Clinton's willingness to work toward a deal (Drew 1996:357) and even Dick Armey, one of Clinton's severest critics, said, "Things are going well." Dole thought it had been a waste of time. The next "seminars" began on December 29, a week later, and ended on New Year's Eve. Negotiations were scheduled to resume on January 2.

As a last action in Congress, House Republicans assembled on December 23 and passed a somewhat more generous CR that would fund the District of Columbia government, and provide benefits for veterans and welfare recipients,[200] but otherwise continued the shutdown. After that, they adjourned and went home for the holidays.

At least the Republicans went home. The Democrats stayed and made the most of the respite and of the public relations opportunity handed them by the Republicans. Their message was that they were working while the Republicans were idle and while civil servants, national park concessionaires, Head Start workers, and other "victims" (some identified for TV reporters by Democrats) were furloughed and going without during the holiday season. And they were working hard, in both House and Senate, with plenary sessions of one hundred or more and committees for specialized topics, meeting with Panetta, Rubin, other top administrative officials and staff from OMB, Treasury, and Executive Office agencies, to see what they could do with the budgets they had developed. Newspapers and TV reporters seized upon the human interest stories. The effects upon Democratic spirits were important, in building consensus and morale in Congress and, especially at this juncture, in bringing the White House and Congress closer together.[201]

Top-level talks began again on January 2 in the Oval Office. The principal negotiators were Clinton, Dole, Gingrich, Daschle, and Gephardt, with the addition of John Engler to speak for the governors. Between negotiating sessions, Republican leaders caucused with their staff in the Roosevelt Room. Clinton staff waited in the halls or the Roosevelt Room, and met with the president, as needed, in the Oval Office. Medicaid was temporarily "off the table" as negotiators waited for a new round of governors' negotiations on January 5 that they hoped would break the deadlock.[202] Particularly notable in the White House talks was a hardening of the Democratic position—both on overall budget numbers and on Medicare policy and structural issues. As to the first, the administration, working in the interim especially with Senate Democrats, reached a budget that they could live with, which was close to seven years with CBO numbers, would protect the president's priorities, and would be supported by at least 140 House Democrats, the minimum needed to sustain a veto.[203] They could now argue convincingly that the budget would be in balance and still protect the president's priorities. With this matter assured, they turned their attention to Medicare policy, especially protection of beneficiaries and structural issues, raising questions about the premium, copays, MSAs, adverse selection, and the "privatization" emphasis of the Republican plan. These negotiations provided a needed opportunity to probe such issues. The Democrats' solicitous concern also prolonged the negotiations, which worked to their advantage.[204]

Meanwhile, complex maneuvering had been going on. The House Republicans were trying various tactics, including a short-term CR that would be sent to the White House only if Clinton submitted a balanced-budget plan.

They combined this move with a number of "targeted" appropriations to provide limited funds for critical programs.[205] Senator Dole, who had resisted the shutdown strategy from the beginning, used one of these targeted appropriations (H.R. 1643) as a vehicle to try to reopen the government. Replacing the original text of H.R. 1643 with a continuing resolution that ran through January 12 he pushed this through the Senate. This unilateral move on his part was a significant defection and seen as a first step in a capitulation.[206] His action was deeply resented by ideological conservatives; and Newt Gingrich, at the time, rejected the initiative. But House Republicans were watching the polls, and increasingly questioning the shutdown strategy. They were also bone-tired. On January 3, 54 House Republicans—many of them with federal workers in their district—voted in conference to end the shutdown. In danger of losing control of his own conference, Gingrich needed an exit strategy (Drew 1996:366ff.). With Dole taking a lead and providing some cover, Gingrich worked for the next two days for a change of strategy—in leadership meetings and lobbying membership factions within the conference (ibid.: 366–67). He proposed initially a CR that would run through March 15 but after strenuous opposition within the conference shortened that to January 26. This CR cleared the Republican conference on January 4 following, according to report, one of the great speeches of the speaker's career. At the vote, he received a standing ovation (ibid.:367).

On January 6, President Clinton presented the Congress with a budget, though not one that was strictly his own. It was the reworked Daschle budget hastily scored by CBO after Gingrich had signaled that he would accept pretty much any budget that met the formal conditions.[207] Congress then presented for the president's signature two "clean" CRs, putting the government back to work and providing continuing appropriations for a number of agencies. Though the shutdown ended, as a small irony it ended during a weekend followed by a blizzard, so workers did not return for a number of days. But the crisis was over. There were no more shutdowns.

Several factors appeared to work together in leading to the Republican decision to abandon the shutdown strategy. One was lack of progress in the negotiations and the increasing firmness in the Democratic stance. Senator Dole's own convictions and temperament, his sense of responsibility as a leader of the Senate, his presidential ambitions, and his belief that the Republicans were being outmaneuvered by Clinton were important.[208] For Gingrich and the Republican House leadership, there was a growing fear that their strategy would not work; they and the membership were weary and beginning to fragment; and they continued to lose in the polls even as Clinton grew stronger.[209]

When talks resumed on January 9, both parties had drawn closer on aggregate numbers but remained fundamentally divided on what programs to cut, on block-granting Medicaid, on Medicare "structural" issues, and on the size of a tax cut, i.e., how far to go beyond balancing the budget. The meeting soon broke up with an agreement to suspend talks for a week and reconvene on January 15. During this period, Republicans—who had earlier rejected an alliance with the Blue Dogs coalition—explored this option but concluded that they would still lack enough votes to override a veto.[210] The January 15 meeting produced nothing new. By then, little seemed to be sustaining the negotiations except a desire not to be the one who walked away. A new session was scheduled with President Clinton for January 17, but the Republicans called it off when it appeared that Clinton was not going to put anything new on the table.[211] That week, a bipartisan group began working with the president to craft a new CR to keep the government open through March 15. The process was uneventful. The CR passed on January 25, by a vote of 371–42 in the House and 82–8 in the Senate. President Clinton signed it the next day. In March, there was another CR and a raising of the debt limit. House freshmen and some of the House leadership talked about reviving the balanced-budget effort, but the struggle ended where it had begun, with the two parties divided over Medicare, Medicaid, entitlements, and the role of government.

Tom DeLay said, in accepting an end to the shutdown, "This president has jerked us around for 46 days; we'd better accept the reality that he's not going to be in agreement."[212] Much subsequent bitterness on the part of Republicans seemed to come from the perception that Democrats, and Clinton especially, were not negotiating in good faith. On the other hand, Clinton and other Democrats insisted that if there were any real concessions on the table they were prepared to deal.[213] In retrospect, it seems that both versions were correct. Democrats stalled, maneuvered, and bluffed—Clinton most artfully of them all—but they did work hard to achieve a balanced budget. At no point were they offered a deal they wanted. And once they were negotiating from strength, the terms of trade changed.

To outside observers, it was astonishing that Congress, especially the House leadership, did not accept Clinton's best offer in December, declare a victory, and come back for the rest next year. That would have given Republicans a moral edge and probably have spread confusion among the Democrats, who might even have rejected the president's deal.[214] However, such a strategy would have been at odds with the crusade spirit of the Republican House leadership and the shock troops of the Gingrich revolution. It would have required advance preparation and disruptive intraparty negotiation, weakened them in relation to the Democrats, and almost certainly have provoked a revolt among the conservative and freshmen Republicans.

From the beginning, the House Republicans characterized their collective effort as a "revolution" or "crusade," which gained much of its force from such rhetoric and the high level of mobilization. One trouble with so much emphasis upon unity, morale, and forward momentum is that it works against compromise and creates an incentive for pushing harder—both when winning and when losing as well. For Gingrich, the House Republican leadership, and the more conservative congressional Republicans in both houses, compromise without decisive victory was repugnant. In part, for that reason they had no well-considered fall-back positions or good exit strategies—only victory or defeat.

Of course, a major point is that a revolution—not just a coup—was what Newt Gingrich and the House Republicans had in mind. Therefore, it seems true, but perhaps obvious, that they exceeded their mandate and attempted too much within too short a time frame. Even so, the sheer audacity of the attempt and how nearly it succeeded are sobering topics for contemplation. Also notable was the thoroughness and political acumen with which Gingrich planned and organized this effort, the mobilized energy he was able to call forth from the House Republicans, and his capacity to move the Senate, the president, and even the country from his base as speaker.

For the kind of sweeping restructuring contemplated in 1995, a budget reconciliation was both good and bad. On the one hand, a reconciliation brought together an enormous range of programs under one heading, concentrated and coordinated efforts, and set a timetable. In addition, it reduced the importance of hearings, committees, and floor debates and, because not subject to unlimited debate, did so in the Senate as well. But in this particular case, the legislation was unbelievably complex and much harder to put together than to attack. Moreover, by including the entitlement fight and major restructuring of government along with deficit reduction, the reconciliation bill overwhelmed the legislative system's capacity for negotiation and conflict resolution with deeply divisive issues. And its procedures facilitated a deadly rhetorical attack of highlighting reductions in programs that protected the old and the poor to provide tax cuts for the well-to-do, even as its complexity and procedural hurdles gave opportunities for delay, regrouping, and coordinating an effective counterattack.

In checking the majority and providing for a cooling off, what has been elsewhere termed "constitutional politics" was especially important. A basic point is that, despite the revolutionary rhetoric in the House, the reconciliation procedures and regular order of legislative business were, with few exceptions, scrupulously adhered to both in House and Senate and between Congress and the president. That was important in providing legitimate and accepted procedures to challenge the majority—for instance, use of tactical delays, demanding committee hearings and markups however abbreviated, and stripping riders from House appropriations bills and nongermane material from the reconciliation bill in the Senate. Though more important for Medicaid than Medicare, federalism both checked and moderated policy on distribution formulas, DSH cuts, and protections for providers and the poor. The Senate remained the individualistic institution it had been, never fully joining the revolution. In this role, it strengthened the influence of federalism, gave voice to particularistic opposition to the reconciliation bill, tempered specific provisions and stripped extraneous ones, and on several occasions talked a bill to death or threatened to do so. The veto strategy was skillfully executed and decisive. It was even employed in a manner fairly close to the original constitutional notion: against an oppressive majority and to defend the office of the chief executive. That veto was protected by the strategy of holding together a veto-sustaining cohort of Democrats in the House and the development of a balanced budget with CBO scoring in the Senate. Arguably, the constitutional system worked effectively to restrain an extremist mood and an oppressive majority.

Followers and admirers of Newt Gingrich describe him as an inspiring, even charismatic leader, in some ways a genius, a man of warmth and charm but also of fire and toughness—and with flaws. His grand effort to remake the Republican Party, the House of Representatives, and ultimately the federal government is surely one of the most extraordinary political events in modern American history. He liked military analogies and, without question, it was a brilliant campaign. But he made mistakes, such as the tactical error of an early deployment of the "hammer" strategy. He also misjudged his own capacity to keep the House majority in line, especially the more conservative members of his leadership team and the House freshmen. Most disastrously, he misjudged the strength of his enemies and the resources at their disposal. He underestimated the political skill and intelligence of Clinton. Equally as bad, he misjudged Clinton's state of preparation, willingness to fight, and resources at his disposal—for instance, the June budget and defying the hammer. And he underestimated the capacity of the congressional Democrats to rally, come together quickly, and develop a countering political strategy—for instance, with respect to the rescissions bill, Medicaid, and the Daschle budget.

For all their efforts, the Republicans ended the year without much apparent gain. Except for the Contract with America, little of their program ever became law. They lost the presidential election of 1996 and nearly lost their majority in the House. At the same time, they startled the Democrats out of a comfortable complacency. They also changed the way we think about many programs, including Medicare: by bringing new ideas to the public forum, shifting presumptions, and opening a national debate on issues that had long been considered settled.

NOTES

[1] As quoted in *Congressional Quarterly Almanac,* 1995, p. 7-3.

[2] The night of the Ways and Means reconciliation markup, Democrats introduced a

substitute bill that got equivalent Part A and B savings and extended Trust Fund solvency as much as the Republican version, but it was denounced for "lying numbers" and voted down. Bill Vaughan, administrative assistant to Rep. Fortney H. (Pete) Stark. Interview, July 21, 1998. Also David Abernethy, Health Insurance Plan; formerly, chief of staff, Health Subcommittee of the House Ways and Means Committee. Interview, August 13, 1998.

[3] P.L. 97-35 (1981).

[4] Gingrich (1995); Ed Kutler, of Clark and Weinstock, formerly assistant to the speaker. Interview, October 21, 1998.

[5] As "scored" by Office of Management and Budget (OMB) or the Congressional Budget Office (CBO).

[6] Cuts made in the existing budget.

[7] *National Journal,* January 7, 1995, p. 32.

[8] *Health Care Policy Report,* January 16, 1995, p. 91.

[9] Ibid., p. 91.

[10] Ibid., pp. 107–8.

[11] One effect of these multijurisdictional task forces was to reduce comity and collaboration across party lines, either between members or staff. The bills were not perfected in detail since they seldom formed the basis for legislation; nor did they provide useful texts for negotiation.

[12] *Health Care Policy Report,* February 6, 1995, pp. 188–89.

[13] Ibid., February 27, 1995, pp. 305–6.

[14] Ibid., March 27, 1995, p. 415.

[15] Ibid., April 3, p. 523.

[16] Ibid., April 9, p. 624.

[17] Including the Budget Committee chairman was an unprecedented move; but so was the speaker's task force. Ed Kutler. Interview, October 21, 1998.

[18] Officially referred to as the "design committee."

[19] Kutler had worked in a similar capacity on health care reform in 1994. According to him, his role was "to facilitate a process," listen to the members and learn about their concerns, and to represent the speaker. Interview, October 21, 1998.

[20] Donald Young, Health Insurance Association of American, former executive director of the Prospective Payment Assessment Commission. Interview, July 29, 1998.

[21] The commissions served the new congressional majority with fairness and political neutrality as they had done for the Democrats, when they were the majority. In so doing, they provided a source of "neutral competence" not available to the Republicans from the administration.

[22] Howard Cohen, of Greenberg Traurig, formerly professional staff, House Commerce Committee. Interview, January 11, 1999.

[23] A reference to the high-voltage rail that carries electricity for subways—mortally dangerous to touch—often applied to the Social Security or Medicare programs.

[24] Especially prominent in legislating TEFRA (1982) and thereafter (cf. Smith 1992:25–26).

[25] This approach seems to follow Gingrich's leadership formula of "listen, learn, help, lead"—an adaptation of Edwards Deming, whom he deeply respected and admired (Gingrich 1995:44ff.).

[26] John Rother, vice-president for public affairs, AARP. Interview, September 10, 1998.

[27] The Senate Republicans had their own ways of communicating the message to lay off. Cf. p. 123.

[28] The AMA took the position that Medicare beneficiaries (and patients generally) should take more responsibility for their own health care. The association also favored the private sector over government, especially single-payer approaches to payment.

[29] Chip Kahn acknowledged that some of these provisions were "sweeteners," intended to be inducements for advocacy groups such as the AMA; but he insisted that they stood on their own merits as well. Charles N. Kahn III, chief executive officer, Health Insurance Association of American, formerly chief of staff, Ways and Means Health Subcommittee. Interview, October 14, 1998.

[30] On the other hand, the American Society of Internal Medicine, which stood to gain by the new payment method, wanted it phased in earlier. Alan R. Nelson, executive vice-president, American Society of Internal Medicine. Interview, July 29, 1998.

[31] For some time there was a "gold rush" mentality accompanied by strong defenses of the profit motive in managed care.

[32] Julie Goon, vice-president for governmental affairs, American Association of Health Plans. She reported being favorably impressed with Newt Gingrich's inclusive approach and the imaginative quality of his "modernization" proposals. She said, by way of a personal appreciation, "I know that's he's a deeply flawed man; but when he's on, he's a genius." Interview, December 8, 1998.

[33] James D. Bentley, senior vice-president, American Hospital Association. Interview, November 18, 1998.

[34] Herb Kuhn, vice-president, Federal Relations, American Hospital Association. Interview, November 10, 1998.

[35] Ibid.

[36] Ibid. For a brief time, the Federation of American Health Systems (FAHS), an organization of for-profit providers, joined in the campaign but was split off by some concessions.

[37] Cf. Congressional Quarterly Almanac, 1995, pp. 7-4, 7-5.

[38] Herb Kuhn. Interview, November 10, 1998.

[39] Especially Frank Luntz, Bob McInturff, and Linda DiVall. (Johnson and Broder 1996:577–78).

[40] *Congressional Quarterly,* February 11, 1995, p. 403.

[41] Ibid., p. 404.

[42] *National Journal,* February 11, 1995, p. 357.

[43] In 1990, President Bush had gotten maneuvered into raising taxes—breaking his "no new taxes" pledge and possibly costing him the election in 1992.

[44] Statement by Van Doorn Ooms, former chief of staff, House Budget Committee. As quoted in *Congressional Quarterly,* February 11, 1995, p. 404.

[45] National Journal, March 18, 1995, p. 700; David Nexon, minority chief of staff for Health, Senate Labor and Human Resources Committee, says that after the 1994 election he went to OMB and told them that they should start preparing a veto memo on Medicare.

[46] For some reason, often phrased in terms of values they would "fall on their swords" to protect.

[47] Medicaid linked with welfare, for instance, was more difficult to defend.

[48] Jeanne Lambrew, Office of Management and Budget. In 1995, special assistant to the deputy assistant secretary for Health, DHHS. Interview, August 3, 1999.

[49] Ibid. Interview, August 3, 1999.

[50] According to David Abernethy, it made no difference whether Democrats had good policy arguments and numbers to go with them since the House Republicans were not listening. Interview, August 13, 1998.

[51] Bill Vaughan. Interview, March 21, 2000.

[52] For instance, liberal Democrats like Richard Gephardt and Henry Waxman were of this view. In the administration, so were George Stephanopoulos and Gene Sperling. Cf. Stephanopoulos (1999:343).

[53] "Triangulation" involved taking a position between Democrats and Republicans, adopting some Republican issue positions, but with modifications that showed Democratic policy positions to advantage.

[54] The Coalition, or "blue dog" Democrats, were a group of twenty-two conservative House Democrats, mostly from the South and West, who sought to develop a compromise budget. They came together early in 1995 and were influential in budget negotiations during 1995 and 1996. Their name is a play on the "yellow-dog" Democrat—one who would vote for a yellow dog, so long as the dog was a Democrat. The Blue Dogs claimed they had been starved and choked so long that they turned blue. *National Journal,* January 6, 1996, pp. 18–19.

[55] Chris Jennings, deputy assistant to the president for Health Policy. Interview, June 9, 1999.

[56] Chris Jennings. Interview, June 9, 1999.

[57] Except for Social Security, which had been excluded from consideration along with defense.

[58] One contribution to American political slang that emerged from this period was "mantra," meaning the slogan used to put across the message: for example, "slashing Medicare to provide tax cuts for the rich"; or a tax cut to "return money to the people who earned it." A historic precedent is V. I. Lenin's distinction between propaganda and agitation, and the importance of slogans to help connect the two.

[59] Judy Feder. Interview, October 28, 1998.

[60] The use of career civil servants in this capacity raises an issue of how intimately or continuously career civil servants should be involved in an intensely political process of this nature. The political appointees were aware of this issue and made efforts to protect and, to an extent, insulate the career officials. Ibid.

[61] *Health Care Policy Report,* June 19, 1995, p. 961.

[62] *Congressional Quarterly,* June 17, 1995, p. 1715.

[63] Jack Ebeler. Interview, January 6, 1999.

[64] *Health Care Policy Report,* June 19, 1995, p. 962.

[65] *Congressional Quarterly,* June 17, p. 1715.

[66] Ibid., p. 1719.

[67] Formerly an aide to Senator Daschle.

[68] Republicans claimed that they had been treated even more shabbily when they were in the minority. Some Democrats agreed with them on this point.

[69] David Abernethy said that he and Chip Kahn communicated frequently by e-mail. Howard Cohen collaborated on a number of occasions with the minority staff.

[70] See, for example, some of the testimony by advocacy groups (U.S. Congress 1995a, 1995c).

[71] According to Bill Vaughan, a feat of David Abernethy's. Interview, July 21, 1998.

[72] See note 23.

[73] *Congressional Quarterly,* May 29, 1995, p. 1399.

[74] Ridge Multop, senior economic adviser, House Democratic Policy Committee. Interview, December 18, 1998.

[75] Ibid.

[76] Both Dole and Phil Gramm, presidential candidates, had lobbied strenuously for a tax cut. Dole said, during an NBC "Meet the Press" interview on April 17, that he had assurances from Domenici that "there would be room" for a tax cut in the Senate bill. *Congressional Quarterly,* April 22, 1995, p. 1115.

[77] *Congressional Quarterly,* May 6, 1995, p. 1230.

[78] Ibid., May 13, 1995, p. 1302.

[79] Ibid., May 20, 1995, p. 1403.

[80] This title had a counterpart in that given to Medicaid: The Medicaid Transformation Act.

[81] A point made by Ed Grossman, House legislative counsel. Interview, December 3, 1998.

[82] To illustrate the importance and the difficulties of getting parts and the whole to work together, Ed Grossman used the example of a Thanksgiving dinner at which a number of new in-laws arrive for the first time. Some of the parts are old and some new; but they all have to be fitted into new relations and the whole made, somehow, to work harmoniously.

[83] Paul Ellwood and Alain Enthoven, leaders in promoting managed care and principals of the "Jackson Hole Group," which espoused a "defined benefit" version of managed competition.

[84] James Capretta, senior policy analyst, Senate Budget Committee. Interview, February 17, 2000. Also, cf. Feldman and Dowd (1998) and Reischauer et al. (1998:75–124).

[85] Kathleen Means, Patton Boggs LLP. Formerly professional staff, Health Subcommittee of the Ways and Means Committee. Interview, September 15, 1998.

[86] P.L. 97-248 (1982).

[87] *Health Care Policy Report,* September 18, 1995, p. 1443; see also Physician Payment Review Commission (1995:Ch. 5).

[88] This provision recognized the problem of risk adjustment, but would seem to leave the question of what to do about it up to "the Secretary" without a clear mandate or authorization.

[89] Julie Goon. Interview, December 8, 1998.

[90] Mary McGrane, senior director for government affairs, Rhone-Poulenc-Rohrer Foundation; formerly professional staff, House Commerce Committee. Interview, December 2, 1998.

[91] Howard Cohen recalled "all of us" (both from Ways and Means and Commerce) working on the AAPCC and likened it to a program of simultaneous equations that kept "crashing" because of state variations. Interview, January 13, 1999.

[92] Under which the insurer (in this instance, the federal government) would pay only a set amount for each beneficiary, for instance, some percentage of an average premium as with the FEHBP, rather than paying some percentage of a "defined benefit" as with the traditional FFS Medicare program.

[93] *Health Care Policy Report,* September 25, 1995, pp. 1529–30.

[94] The Senate version, much kinder to the hospitals, was adopted in the conference.

[95] Herb Kuhn. Interview, November 10, 1998.

[96] Dan Nickleson, Cleveland Clinic Foundation. Interview, August 5, 1998; see also Smith (1992:52–53).

[97] *Health Care Policy Report,* August 7, 1995, p. 1244.

[98] Linda Fishman, American Association of Medical Colleges. Interview, November 23, 1995. Fishman observed that, in 1995, the House was closing some corporate tax loopholes. These provided offsetting funds. Otherwise, the reductions might have been more drastic.

[99] Deborah Steelman. Interview, June 22, 1999.

[100] In addition, the trust fund substituted a highly visible fund for subventions that had previously had low visibility—which is good from the standpoint of public policy, but might not be for medical schools. Richard Knapp, Linda Fishman, American Association of Medical Colleges. Interview, November 23, 1995.

[101] A rate paid to health plans serving Medicare patients that is based in part upon costs and revenues from the plans commercial business.

[102] *Health Care Policy Report,* September 25, 1995, p. 1520.

[103] James Bentley. Interview, November 18, 1998.

[104] For instance, the Mayo Clinic.

[105] Julie Goon. Interview, December 8, 1998.

[106] Negotiated regulation or "neg-reg" had been used to promote agreement in aviation and environmental matters, but not much for health care. No one seems too certain who first suggested the idea—Ed Grossman and Kathy Means were among those credited. Once neg-reg was mentioned, it was quickly adopted.

[107] Kathy Means. Interview, September 18, 1995.

[108] Ed Kutler. Interview, October 21, 1998.

[109] Removed on a procedural notion because they were "extraneous" to the deficit reduction objective of the reconciliation.

[110] Kathy Means. Interview, September 18, 1995; also Julie A. James, Health Polity Alternatives, formerly Senate Finance Committee staff. Interview, August 19, 1998.

[111] This was quickly changed to more culturally sensitive language.

[112] Congressional Budget Office Cost Estimate for H.R. 2485, October 18, 1995, p. 3.

[113] A price index based on the goods and services providers purchase to produce their particular product, such as a unit or bundle of services.

[114] Congressional Budget Office Cost Estimate for H.R. 2485, Table 2.

[115] In simplest terms, payment under the Medicare Fee Schedule is determined by assigning a "resource based relative value" to particular services or procedures and then multiplying that by a "conversion factor" to express the relative value in monetary terms. That, in turn, is increased by the annual update percentage. A reduction of 20 percent in the conversion factor would be onerous; but in addition, a return to a single conversion factor would reduce payments for high-priced specialties. However, the changes were not to become effective until 1997.

[116] Bill Vaughan. Interview, June 21, 1998.

[117] David Abernethy. Interview, August 13, 1998.

[118] Congressional Budget Office Cost Estimate for H.R. 2485, Table 1.

[119] When President Clinton argued for the same approach in 1997 he was roundly

criticized by Republicans for resorting to "smoke and mirrors," showing how much politics depends on whose ox is gored.

[120] Speaking of the Ambulatory Patient Groups, ProPAC said, "Various methods to control the volume of ambulatory services in the hospital setting, as well as in other sites, should be explored." (Prospective Payment Assessment Commission 1995:50).

[121] *Health Care Policy Report,* April 24, 1995, p. 671.

[122] Donald Young. Interview, July 29, 1998.

[123] 691 F. Supp. 1487, 1988.

[124] Congressional Budget Office Cost Estimate for H.R. 2485, p. 8.

[125] *Health Care Policy Report,* September 15, 1995, p. 1537.

[126] Congressional Budget Office Cost Estimate for H.R. 2485, p. 18.

[127] Supported by both Rep. Bill Thomas and Sen. Judd Gregg, key figures in Medicare policy. Health Care Policy Report, May 1, 1995, p. 697.

[128] For instance, Gail Wilensky, chairperson of MedPAC. Interview, January 5, 1999.

[129] Sequestration, which is a kind of fail-safe, had been a familiar device since Gramm-Rudman-Hollings of 1985. As noted above, the Medicare Fee Schedule had used a similar device from its inception in 1995; and the Medicare Preservation Act included another fail-safe for the medical education trust fund.

[130] A $2000 reduction in average capitation payments over seven years and the loss of several subsidies.

[131] An amount by which CBO estimates that provider behavior will compensate for the penalty reductions by shifting costs, increasing volume, raising prices, etc.

[132] Robert Reischauer, Urban Institute; formerly executive director, Congressional Budget Office. Interview, December 4, 1998.

[133] Congressional Budget Office Cost Estimate for H.R. 2485, p. 20.

[134] Robert Reischauer. Interview, December 4, 1998.

[135] Named after *Senator Byrd,* this rule, followed by the Senate, seeks to exclude extraneous provisions from a reconciliations bill. It defines "extraneous" and sets up procedures for enforcement. Any senator can invoke the rule and it requires a supermajority of sixty Senators to override it. Since it applies to conference reports the rule indirectly can apply to the House. Sometimes referred to as a "Byrd bath."

[136] *Health Care Policy Report,* January 23, 1995, p. 109. Senator Hatch, the primary sponsor, preferred a stand-alone bill.

[137] Ibid., March 10, p. 436. The original bill limited punitive damages in civil actions. But actions for punitive damages are rare; and the House wished to extend this limit to all noneconomic damages, especially pain and suffering.

[138] Ibid., May 8, 1995, p. 733.

[139] Ibid., May 15, 1995, p. 782.

[140] For example, *American Medical News,* the AMA weekly sent to its members.

[141] *Health Care Policy Report,* May 8, 1995, p. 473.

[142] See the testimony of D. McCartney Thornton, counsel to the DHHS inspector general, as cited in *Health Care Policy Report,* October 23, 1995, pp. 1762–63.

[143] Ibid., October 9, 1995, p. 1660.

[144] Ibid., October 23, 1995, p. 1761.

[145] This was particularly welcome to HCFA, since it provided a funding source for such activities other than the HCFA general administrative fund, which historically had gotten a meager appropriation.

[146] The Racketeering Influenced Corrupt Organization Act was passed in 1970 to provide additional resources in the fight against organized crime and criminal conspiracies. It granted broad powers and was often attacked in the courts on constitutional grounds for overbreadth and vagueness.

[147] *Congressional Quarterly Almanac,* 1995, p. 7-5.

[148] Ibid., p. 7-7.

[149] For instance, Bill Vaughan, legislative assistant to Representative Stark. Interview, June 21, 1998.

[150] *Congressional Quarterly Almanac,* 1995, p. 7-9.

[151] Julie James. Interview, June 29, 2000.

[152] *Health Care Policy Report,* July 31, 1995, pp. 1198–99.

[153] Julie James. Interview, June 20, 2000.

[154] *Congressional Quarterly Almanac,* 1995, p. 7-10.

[155] Laurie Rubiner, National Partnership for Women and Children, formerly legislative assistant to Sen. John Chafee. Interview, July 2, 1999.

[156] Julie Goon made the point that balance billing would be needed as a rationing device with so many new plans and the range of options they provided. Interview, December 8, 1998.

[157] Congressional Budget Office Cost Estimate, Title VII, subtitle A, October 20, 1995, p. 14.

[158] *Congressional Quarterly Almanac,* 1995, p. 7-11.

[159] Julie James said that the Senate "got rolled," i.e., lost points to the House. She attributed this result largely to Packwood's resignation and Senator Roth's lack of preparation and lack of interest in the non–tax side of the reconciliation. Interview, August 19, 1998.

[160] With acknowledgements to Elizabeth Drew (1996).161. Ridge Multop. Interview, December 12, 1998.

[162] *Congressional Quarterly,* May 20, 1995, p. 1400.

[163] Cf. *Business and Financial Practices of the AARP,* Hearings before the Subcommittee on Social Security and Family Policy of the Committee of Finance, United States Senate, 104th Congress, 1st session, June 13 and June 20, 1995. Senator Simpson made it clear that the intensity of his scrutiny would be proportional to AARP's lobbying efforts.

[164] *Congressional Quarterly Almanac,* 1995, p. 7-9.

[165] Bill Vaughan. Interview, July 21, 1998. He also stated that "not ten members" understood how the MedicarePlus mechanism would work.

[166] The idea of HCFA or the Medicare program as a "prudent purchaser" of quality health care was being pushed by HCFA and various outside groups. Cf. "Democratic Medicare Plan for the 21st Century," U.S. Senate, unpublished, October 2, 1995; see also Etheredge (1995a); Cybele Bjorklund, legislative assistant to Rep. Peter Stark, formerly staff of Sen. Edward Kennedy. Interview, November 11, 1995.

[167] *Congressional Quarterly,* June 17, 1995, p. 1720.

[168] Jack Ebeler. Interview, January 6, 1999; Chris Jennings. Interview, June 9, 1999.

[169] Cybele Bjorklund. Interview, November 11, 1995.

[170] *Congressional Quarterly,* June 17, 1995, p. 1770.

[171] Jack Ebeler. Interview, January 6, 1999; Chris Jennings. Interview, June 9, 1999. "Double-M, Double-E" referred to "Medicare-Medicaid and Environment-Education."

[172] Three House Democrats switched to the Republican party in 1995; also six Democratic senators announced that they would not run for reelection in 1996.

[173] Drew (1996:306); also Robert Reischauer, as quoted in *Congressional Quarterly,* September 2, 1995, p. 2611.

[174] Ibid., September 9, 1998, p. 2712.

[175] Ibid., September 23, 1995, p. 2865.

[176] Ibid.

[177] Ibid., September 30, 1995, pp. 2972–73.

[178] Ibid., October 21, 1995, p. 3187; *Health Care Policy Report,* October 23, 1995, p. 1753.

[179] *Congressional Quarterly,* October 28, 1995, p. 3284.

[180] Ibid., November 4, 1995, p. 3357.

[181] Cf. Robert Reischauer as quoted in *Congressional Quarterly,* November 18, 1995, p. 3505. Reischauer also said that Clinton "would be giving away the store" were he to adopt CBO scoring at that point.

[182] *Congressional Quarterly Almanac,* 1995, p. 7-11.

[183] Ibid. Gingrich said: "We don't get rid of it in round one because we don't think that's politically smart, and we don't think that's the right way to go through a transition. But we believe it's going to wither on the vine because we think people are going to leave it voluntarily." Parsing these sentences, the pronoun "it" seems to apply to both HCFA and FFS Medicare.

[184] Ibid.

[185] *Congressional Quarterly,* November 11, 1995, p. 3441.

[186] Ibid., p. 3503.

[187] Ibid. One aide said, "We were watching the polls, too, and would have opened up real fast if we were losing." Jack Ebeler. Interview, September 11, 1998.

[188] As reported in *Congressional Quarterly,* November 25, p. 3598.

[189] Ibid., p. 3597.

[190] Elizabeth Drew quotes Dan Meyer, Gingrich's chief of staff, as saying the Republican strategy would force Democrats "to come a long way in our direction" (1996:345).

[191] *Congressional Quarterly,* December 9, 1995, p. 3721.

[192] Ibid., December 16, 1995, p. 3792.

[193] Drew quotes one White House aide as saying, "What the Republicans didn't realize was that the longer we held out the better it would be for us

[194] *Congressional Quarterly,* December 16, 9995, p. 3793.

[195] Bruce Vladeck, then HCFA administrator, remembers the White House mess being closed. Principals were fed, he recalls, but for Medicare and Medicaid staff people, "some Budget Committee people found a box of Doritos." Interview, February 8, 1999.

[196] *Congressional Quarterly,* December 23, 1995, p. 3877.

[197] They did pass a "rifle shot" CR, funding veterans benefits, but otherwise left the government without funds.

[198] *Congressional Quarterly,* December 23, 1995, p. 3877.

[199] Drew (1996:357); Howard Cohen. Interview, May 19, 1999; Bruce Vladeck. Interview, February 8, 1999.

[200] Meanwhile, the Medicare and Medicaid program continued to pay out benefits.

[201] Ridge Multop. Interview, December 12, 1998; Bruce Vladeck commented that this was the first real coming together of the Democratic administration and Congress

and that it was an essential prerequisite for the successful budget reconciliation in 1997. Interview, February 8, 1999.

[202] *Health Care Policy Report,* January 8, 1996, p. 41.

[203] Ibid.

[204] Henry Waxman, for instance, described the talks—which made no progress on substantive issues—as "remarkably detailed . . . at a level of detail that we probably wouldn't get into in a conference committee."

[205] *Congressional Quarterly,* January 6, 1996, p. 56.

[206] Ibid., p. 64.

[207] Drew (1996:368). According to one account, John Hilley gave Clinton the Daschle budget, which had been scored by CBO. This was the budget shown to the Republican negotiators. One staff person said that they "never could get the numbers to run" on the Clinton budget. Some believe that the Republicans knew that the budget they were accepting was the Daschle budget but had no desire for further confrontation. Barry B. Anderson, Jefferson Solutions, formerly, Office of Management and Budget. Interview, December 9, 1998.

[208] Sheila Burke, Kennedy School of Government; formerly chief of staff to Sen. Robert Dole. Interview, January 5, 1999.

[209] According to Drew (1996:360), Gingrich was especially disturbed that, as they sank in the polls, Clinton was rising even faster.

[210] *Congressional Quarterly,* January 13, 1996, p. 90.

[211] *Health Care Policy Report,* January 22, 1996, p. 91.

[212] *Congressional Quarterly,* January 6, 1996, p. 13.

[213] Chris Jennings. Interview, May 30, 2000; also Richard Gephardt, saying that this is "not game playing, not stalling . . . there are fundamental differences." Quoted in *Congressional Quarterly,* January 6, 1996, p. 13.

[214] Robert Reischauer believed congressional Democrats would have been much embarrassed had the Republicans done so, and might have even refused the deal. Interview, December 4, 1999. Newt Gingrich and a number of senators proposed doing just that, but failed to get support from other Republicans.

5

A Year of Transition—1996

For Medicare and Medicaid, the year 1996 was something of a nonevent, an interlude between a historic battle and a major, though not grand compromise. But it was also a year of transition, moving on from partisan confrontation to wary collaboration and diminishing the scope of conflict so that compromise came more easily in 1997. This process of transition is interesting in itself and illustrates, as well, additional modes of legislative activity and policymaking that our tax dollars help support.

An important factor at work in 1996 was exhaustion: physical tiredness, a lack of fresh, attractive policy options, and a diminished zest for combat. After a policy effort[1] of the scale and intensity of BBA 95, leaders and staff needed a respite as well as time to develop new options. As one policy activist put it, people wanted "to get the bad taste out of their mouths" left by the acrid disputes of 1995.[2]

Nineteen ninety-six was a presidential election year, a factor that always modifies the legislative agenda and that year more so because of the events of 1995. Incumbents like to avoid big risks and want to demonstrate their usefulness to their constituents—so this was not a year for another shutdown and would be a propitious time to pass some legislation. In 1996, Democrats had a new confidence, more unity, and a sense they had a message that worked. For their part, Republicans needed to hold their political base and demonstrate to the rest of the country that they could get something done. In addition, Robert Dole and four other senators, including Phil Gramm, were seeking the Republican nomination for president. In a word, the political outlook was quite different in 1996: Democrats in a stronger position to bargain and Republicans not as well positioned or unified and in need of tangible results.

Time was a binding constraint in 1996, especially for a reconciliation strategy. The previous year's agenda had spilled over into the present, so that Congress was still struggling with 1995 appropriation bills and budget negotiations until late April. In an election year, Washington politicians need to get to the home district for the campaign. For that reason, October 1, which also marks the end of the fiscal year, was a nearly absolute deadline. Quite apart from changes in the political climate, time alone ruled out a reconciliation on the scale of 1995, especially if it had to allow time for a veto strategy at the end.

In 1996, as in 1995, there was both a reconciliation strategy and an "incremental" one.[3] But the reconciliation bill was much less ambitious in scope and was divided into three parts, taking the least controversial part first. While the reconciliation effort eventually failed, it had the important consequence of separating Medicaid from welfare reform and, in effect, reduced both the scope of conflict and some of the partisan intensity earlier associated with Medicaid. On the incremental side, both House and Senate developed insurance reform bills, parts of which were eventually combined into the Health Insurance Portability and Accountability Act of 1996 (HIPAA). For the Senate bill, also known as Kassebaum-Kennedy, the original intention was to do a "clean" bill with a maximum of bipartisan support and without controversial additions. In the House, the approach was deliberately "aggregative," putting together a number of bills from various committees, including, in this instance, some elements—most notably medical savings accounts, medical malpractice reform, and fraud and abuse—that had been lost with the 1995 veto. As with the reconciliation, this aggregative strategy also failed. This outcome made the HIPAA episode relevant in another way for the bipartisan compromise of 1997. Including the fraud and abuse provisions in HIPAA and stripping out the less popular add-ons (MSAs and malpractice reform) limited aggregative strategies in 1997 and increased the appeal of a bipartisan compromise.

The legislative efforts of 1996 illustrate both successes and failures in developing health care legislation under conditions of divided government and a less mobilized politics. This transitional phase may well have been essential to create the conditions for the bipartisan BBA of 1997. From another perspective, it shows how pragmatism, institutional adaptability, and the checks and balances of the American system can work to reduce partisan mobilization, get beyond an impasse, pass some constructive legislation, and reopen paths to bipartisan collaboration.

I. THE THREE-PART RECONCILIATION

A primary factor that led to the three-part reconciliation strategy was the continuing effect of the 1995 confrontation over BBA 95. Negotiations and activities related to BBA 95 continued into March, including new budget strategies, additional debt limit extensions, and an unfinished omnibus appropriations bill (H.R. 3019). Tactics and rhetoric from the previous year carried over as well, needing to be adapted or even abandoned, depending upon current circumstances. There was a legacy of recrimination and "I told you so" among House Republicans and between them and Senate Republicans. Provision needed to be made for the major blocs of legislation that had earlier been combined in the reconciliation bill and that now stood alone. Unfinished legislative business created a huge backlog and took time and energy away from efforts to cope with the current year and the election. It also left legislators with strong policy convictions chafing for a way to work through to some more constructive resolutions.

An item of growing importance was the more favorable economic indicators of 1996. As early as mid-1995, the economy was visibly improving. By March 1996, the deficit was reported as falling for the fourth year in a row. CBO projected a deficit of $140 billion, the lowest (as percentage of GDP) in nearly twenty years.[4] Health care costs were also moderating,[5] with both Medicare and Medicaid baselines repeatedly revised downward. These developments took some of the urgency out of deficit reduction and made more limited strategies such as extending trust fund solvency or reducing the deficit more attractive, especially to Senate Republicans and to House moderates.

Late in January, a halting "stand down" or deescalation began, marked especially by the continuing resolution (CR) of January 25, which extended the debt limit increase through March 15, and by President Clinton's conciliatory State of the Union address on the same day. Both sides called for bipartisan collaboration. The House Republican leadership said that it was abandoning confrontational tactics and would concentrate more on legislation and deficit reduction packages that both sides could agree upon. The president said, two times in the course of his address, that "the era of big government was over" and expressed support for balancing the budget, as well as for tax cuts and reductions in entitlement spending.[6]

Although the rhetoric was changing and both sides were backing off from another confrontation, they remained deeply divided over the budget. The White House and the Congress—especially the House Republicans—reaffirmed earlier priorities. The House Republicans announced plans to turn their last budget offer into a "Balanced Budget Act II," and pass that some time in March.[7] President Clinton's February 5 budget was a twenty-page summary of his last, best offer in January with little that was new.[8] The administration's detailed budget would not follow until March 19, which would make it that much harder for the Republicans to make good on their own threat.

Until mid-February, the Republican leadership and various other coalitions attempted to piece together a budget that could get enough bipartisan support to pass. At one time, there were six different budgets, including a bipartisan proposal from the National Governors' Association (NGA) that, it was hoped, might break the deadlock on Medicaid. In the House, there was a leadership proposal, developed from the vetoed reconciliation bill of 1995, and another

moderate Republican proposal. There was an offering from the Blue Dog
Democrats in the House and a Breaux-Chafee budget in the Senate, which at
one time had strong support from the White House and a good chance of passage. Also in the Senate was the Daschle budget, left over from 1995.

With this number of proposals, it would seem that there might be a winning coalition, yet the basic divisions remained—especially over entitlements
and tax cuts. As before, what one side must have, the other side could not or
would not give. This was nicely illustrated by the ultimate opposition of both
Democratic and Republican leadership to moderate, bipartisan efforts, mostly
because of the threat of losing or dividing their own political base. Not surprisingly, one way this tension got partially resolved—it being an election
year—was in the appropriations bills then being considered, which began to
sprout various popular add-ons as compensations.[9]

A second option, being pursued along with the development of alternative
budgets, was to work toward more limited savings and concessions on entitlements with separate bills that could be tied to short-term debt limit extensions. This approach, supported by Newt Gingrich and John Kasich, was a
logical next step, following the collapse of the reconciliation talks.[10] It became
the major interim strategy for the House Republicans as hopes for crafting
some kind of alternative budget waned in early February.[11] Meanwhile, the
omnibus appropriations bill—needed to close out the current year's funding—provided some additional leverage, in the form of week-long CRs to
keep agencies and programs operating, but on reduced funding. The strategy
was to moderate the demands somewhat, keep the pressure on the president
by continuing the reduced funding, and set a deadline backed by the threat of
a shutdown and/or default.

The one major application of this strategy was in connection with a bipartisan report on welfare and Medicaid being developed by the National Governors' Association. Bolstering their efforts at entitlement reform with that
report, and keeping pressure on the president, the Republican plan was to
condition a long-term raising of the debt ceiling on acceptance of legislation
based on the report. For a number of reasons, this plan failed: because the governors took too long and their proposal was not workable; because the debt
limitation linkage was not likely to survive a Senate filibuster;[12] and because
the House Republicans were bluffing and Democrats were less afraid of
another shutdown than the Republicans were.[13] But the details of this process
merit closer examination because they illustrate one way in which controversial issues can be disaggregated and "cooled out."

Medicaid and the Governors' Proposal

In any major restructuring of Medicaid, the National Governors' Association
would be prominently involved, both in the development and the ultimate

approval of the proposal. Republican governors had been a major driving force behind both welfare and Medicaid reform; and the Republican Governors' Association had been deeply involved in developing the various block grant proposals and distribution formulas (see p. 54ff) in 1995. So it was not untoward, though perhaps foolhardy,[14] for the governors—in this instance, three leading members of the Republican Governors' Association—to offer their help in negotiating a Medicaid compromise before the December 15 shutdown. Both Clinton and the Republican leadership seized upon this offer, which led in turn to the formation of a bipartisan, six-person NGA task force that worked, off and on, to produce an eventual compromise proposal that was reported at the NGA meeting in early February 1996.

Even though the ultimate issue for the task force remained entitlements vs. block grants, both Republicans and Democrats made efforts to avoid this controversial symbolism and work incrementally toward accommodations with which each side could live. In this, they were largely successful—at least, in satisfying themselves. Without too much difficulty, the task force was able to agree upon a mandated benefits package and accept federal definitions of eligibility—except for disability, which would continue to be defined by states, subject to DHHS review and a 90 percent maintenance of effort requirement. States would gain much more flexibility. Amount, scope, and duration of benefits would be up to them. Waivers would no longer be required for state cost-saving strategies, such as managed care or community-based services. The Boren amendment would be repealed; and individuals could sue over Medicaid payments only in state courts. The entitlement issue was dealt with by providing for an "umbrella" fund that could be tapped on a per person basis if there were a "demonstrable need," such as a recession or unexpected population growth.[15] Finally, in what was seen as a crass and self-serving move, the task force proposed that matching for states be lowered from 50 to 40 percent[16] and that states remain free to impose provider taxes and draw down DSH money as before.

The task force recommendation was unanimously adopted by the NGA. Elsewhere, the reviews were mixed. Democrats still did not see in this proposal the "assured, guaranteed, meaningful benefits" they were looking for. John Kasich objected that the governors were working for themselves, not helping Congress save money. But Tom DeLay lauded the proposal as a vindication of Republican principles, and added that it would become a part of BBA II.[17] The Senate Finance and the House Commerce committees scheduled hearings and put staff to work turning the proposal into legislative language.

The hearings and the negotiations that followed illustrate the difficulty of moving from an agreement in principle to workable legislation as well as some problems with reliance upon an outside group consensus, i.e., the NGA. Democrats complained that the supposedly "bipartisan" NGA proposal benefited Republican governors disproportionately and that Democratic committee staffs were being excluded from the development of the legislative text. Republicans were concerned about the 40 percent match, the use of provider taxes,[18] and the absence of a cap on the "umbrella" fund. Orrin Hatch, for the Senate Judiciary Committee, warned that the repealing of a federal cause of action for Medicaid beneficiaries and providers might be unconstitutional.[19] And, early on, there were concerns about CBO scoring—that savings would fall far short of projections or not be scorable because of the open-ended nature of the funding.[20]

One of the most difficult tasks was to turn the six-page governors' proposal into legislative language. The Republicans had more or less drifted into working with the NGA in this allegedly bipartisan effort. But the governors were painfully slow in making up their collective mind, so that many details of the plan remained in process. Some vital features were not articulated or ignored important constraints of the legislative process. The congressional hearings sharpened partisan differences, adding yet another problem for NGA and committee staff seeking to develop proposals and language agreeable to a putatively bipartisan NGA task force and the increasingly polarized congressional committees.

An illustrative example was provided by the difficulties in scoring the "insurance umbrella" fund, intended to compensate states that might be hit by unexpectedly heavy Medicaid caseloads—because of migration, economic recession, or AIDS. Neither Republicans nor the CBO liked the open-ended character of this fund, derisively characterized as an " entitlement for the States."[21] After struggling with the formula for a month, the NGA task force submitted a new proposal to Congress only to have the Commerce Committee staff reject it on the grounds that it was unworkable and could not be scored.[22] Ultimately, the Commerce staff abandoned the governors' approach and fell back on the earlier methodology of 1995, only to have Democrats complain that this step violated the bipartisan agreement. The episode at least illustrates why legislators should be cautious about delegating their work to outsiders.

After the hearings, Republican leaders in both House and Senate struggled with a critical decision of how best to move the Medicaid and welfare proposals: whether as stand-alone, single bills, tied to a long-term debt extension, or as part of a reconciliation bill or bills. Initially, the most expedient approach seemed to be including Medicare, with welfare, in the long-term debt negotiations. With this strategy in mind, another short-term debt limit extension was passed on March 7—to give both Congress and the White House additional time. By then, however, the debt ceiling strategy seemed less promising: congressional Democrats were resisting it; the president was threatening another veto;[23] assembling a majority for a long-term extension would be difficult; and the governors' proposal had done little to diminish partisan differences within the Congress.[24] Beside all that, Senator Nickles (R., Okla.), chairman of the Senate Policy Committee, confirmed what House Republicans already believed—that the Senate would not pass such a resolution.[25] That same week, and rather abruptly, the Republicans abandoned the debt limit strategy, except for minor, noncontroversial add-ons, and announced that Medicaid and welfare would be taken up together, either as free-standing legislation or as part of a reconciliation bill.

With an April 15 deadline for a budget resolution approaching, the outlook for the Republican majority was not promising. The legislative agenda was far behind schedule, with the previous year's appropriations unfinished, a budget resolution not likely before early May, and few legislative achievements to show for an election year. The party was less unified than in 1995. The Senate was vigorously contesting for a greater role in legislation and the budget, and the Democrats and the president were more unified, had a message, and were fighting back. Early in the month, CBO confirmed what Clinton had claimed in his budget message: the lowest deficit (as a percentage of GDP) since 1979.[26] Then, a week later, another drop in the Medicaid baseline was noted.[27] In effect, savings had become harder while the urgency of deficit reduction diminished.

When the House and Senate committees finally cleared the long-delayed budget resolutions on May 9 and 10, they were in outline mostly a repeat of 1995, except that the numbers were much closer to Clinton's final proposal. As a prudent election year concession, the Medicare premium was left at 25 percent. One reason for the delay was a debate within the Senate over whether to seek for Medicare anything beyond extending trust fund solvency.[28] Also unresolved until the very end was how to package the reconciliation bill: whether to have one bill or divide it into two or three separate bills and how to order them. Underlying this debate was an issue of whether and how far to go in seeking an accommodation with the president or, in the alternative, whether to develop a veto strategy.

The approach adopted in the budget resolution was to have three smaller reconciliation bills with Medicaid and welfare paired to go first and, if that were successful, to be followed by Medicare, and then a tax reduction bill. A reconciliation strategy was attractive both for its action-forcing features and because it was not subject to filibuster in the Senate. And the tripartite division would peak issues less and minimize risk.[29] Medicaid and welfare were combined because the governors wanted it that way and to raise the stakes for President Clinton. If he vetoed the bill, he could be pilloried for a do-nothing policy on welfare and for going back on his own campaign promise to "end welfare as we know it." If the veto were overturned, he would lose on both welfare and Medicaid. Medicare went next because it was seen to be the more difficult and also to pay for the tax cuts in the final bill. Few Republicans thought there was much chance of passing all three bills, though there was more hope for at least the first of these. Nevertheless, they moved quickly to complete the welfare and Medicare bills, reporting them out on May 23.[30]

Almost immediately both Democrats and Republicans began shifting to a veto strategy. Congressional Democrats and Democratic governors denounced the plan as partisan and lacking guarantees. Leon Panetta, White House chief of staff, described the linkage as a "poison pill" strategy aimed at provoking a veto. And the president, in one of his weekly radio addresses, made clear his intention to veto the bill.[31] For Republicans in both House and Senate, the issue quickly became whether to stick with their initial strategy of linking Medicaid and welfare—risking a veto and the loss of both Medicaid and welfare for this session—or to separate them and, with fair certainty, save at least the welfare reforms.

Over much of the next month this issue was intensely debated in both the House and Senate. Within the House, opposition to the linkage was led by Republican conservatives, especially members of the Ways and Means Committee, who sent a letter signed by fifty-four members to Newt Gingrich and Trent Lott,[32] asking that welfare and Medicaid be considered separately.[33] Their argument was that the Medicaid bill was going nowhere and that welfare reform was too important an issue to lose. Besides, as the letter phrased it, there should be "no place to run and no place to hide," for any (e.g., President Clinton) who do not support "true" welfare reform.[34] The impatience of House Republican conservatives had been vividly revealed a day before by a 216–211 House vote on the vitally important budget resolution conference report—which survived only because of a strenuous last-minute intervention by Newt Gingrich, who got four members to switch their votes.[35] On this particular issue, the ire of conservative Republicans was directed at various "sweeteners" that Gingrich and the House leadership had added to appease Senate moderates; but it was abundantly clear that loyalty from the House Republican conservatives could not be assumed. Shortly thereafter, the House leadership decided to postpone a final vote on the linkage issue until July 8. In the interim, a second letter in favor of separation was signed by ninety-five House Republicans and sent to Lott and Gingrich.[36]

During this period, House Republicans had moved closer to an agreement on welfare and were increasingly loath to see their bill vetoed along with Medicaid. President Clinton signaled that he would like a welfare bill he could sign; and moderate Democrats in both House and Senate favored a separation. But the Republican Governors' Association lobbied vigorously to keep welfare and Medicaid together, arguing that the two programs needed to be administratively coordinated and that Medicaid flexibility was key to welfare reform.[37] The Senate leadership stayed with the linkage, despite mounting discontent among House Republican conservatives.

According to one account, an important factor in the Senate's continuing support of the linkage was reluctance, during a presidential race, to have Clinton claiming credit for brokering a successful deal and thereby diminishing the importance of Dole's leadership.[38] At the same time, Republican enthusiasm for Medicaid reform was waning both in the House and Senate because of concessions made by the Senate Finance Committee, the prospect of a difficult conference, and an impending veto. On July 11, two Dole letters were released: one, asking Speaker Gingrich and Majority Leader Lott to pass a welfare reform bill; and a second, urging President Clinton "to sign a real welfare reform bill that most of our nation's governors can support."[39] It was a move characteristic of Dole, who preferred real options and accomplishments to ideological posturing. It may have also have been an act of generosity and statesmanship. According to an aide, Dole did not wish to be seen as an "impediment" to welfare reform, even though there was some disadvantage for him.[40] In any event, whether Dole's letters were occasion or pretext, the Republican leadership released their Dole letter and announced the splitting of welfare and Medicaid.

By then, the Congress had less than eight legislative weeks until its scheduled October 4 adjournment date. It was a time for winding up business, proclaiming whatever victories there were, blaming the other party for defeats,[41] and getting on the campaign trail. On August 1, Congress passed the welfare bill, which was signed into law by President Clinton on August 22.[42] The Health Insurance Portability and Accountability Act,[43] passed on August 2, was signed by the president on August 21. These successes revived some tentative interest in Medicare reform, which was quickly abandoned because of the crowded legislative agenda and memories of the partisan divisions created by the 1995 controversies. Medicaid reform was dead for the year. For that matter, block granting or fundamental structural change in Medicaid was a dead issue for the foreseeable future. One small footnote: the welfare act—the Personal Responsibility and Work Opportunity Reconciliation Act of 1996—contained a provision that preserved Medicaid eligibility rules for AFDC mothers and children—a small victory for Medicaid defenders.

II. THE HEALTH INSURANCE PORTABILITY AND ACCOUNTABILITY ACT

The Health Insurance Portability and Accountability Act of 1996 (HIPAA) was one of those small legislative events that—like some minor military engagements—was more significant historically than anticipated. It was unique in being the first important bipartisan health legislation to make it out of committee in the 104th Congress and the only significant bipartisan health legislation to become law in over two years. From the text, HIPAA would seem both insignificant and noncontroversial. Yet it was caught up in larger ideological conflict and high politics—including the presidential campaign.

It eventually passed, but only after weeks of wrangling over the appointment of a conference committee and Dole's departure from the Senate.

HIPAA deals primarily with reform of the small group and individual insurance market, not with Medicare or Medicaid. At the same time, some of its provisions—dealing with fraud and abuse and with medical savings accounts—were part of the vetoed Medicare Preservation Act of 1995 and were important for later Medicare legislation. Also significant is the fact that these and other items, such as medical malpractice reform, were dealt with or reviewed in 1996 rather than 1997, making later compromise easier. In addition, HIPAA illustrates particularly well two similar and sometimes mixed modes of legislation variously termed "incremental" or "targeted," and "aggregative."

The term "incremental" or "targeted" as generally used both in the House and Senate contrasts smaller, topically specific bills with more comprehensive legislation, for instance, a health insurance tax deduction in contrast to an omnibus budget reconciliation bill. In 1995 and 1996, House and Senate budget reconciliation strategies were heavily influenced or dominated by the leadership and the budget and authorizing chairmen. Both houses also had incremental or targeted health care initiatives, dealing with such items as insurance reform, patient protection, child health, and mental health benefits. Such legislation often had a lengthy gestation and originated with and was shaped by the legislative committees. Under the Republican majority, though, it was sometimes coordinated by a health care task force composed mainly of chairmen and subcommittee chairmen from the substantive committees.[44]

With intense partisanship, House and Senate differences, divided government, and the possibility of a presidential veto, a strategy commonly used was to aggregate[45] a package of bills in a manner calculated to enhance their passage or reap political and symbolic gains from a defeat. The Medicaid-welfare combination—and later separation—was a case in point. Various kinds of sweeteners, bargaining chips, and "poison pills" could be added. Illustrative of this maneuver were some of the separate proposals, for example, medical savings accounts and medical malpractice reform, that figured, along the way, in HIPAA. Either of these could be a "sweetener," necessary for gaining the support of an important interest group, committee members, or a faction needed for a legislative majority. Either could also be a "poison pill," assuring rejection by the opposing party or a second chamber or eliciting a presidential veto, and, if handled skillfully, shifting the blame. Each could also be a bargaining chip, put on the table only to be given up, with suitable rhetoric, for some positional gain or quid pro quo. Of course, aggregative strategies could be bipartisan and benign, but they could also be cunning traps, calculated to lure the unwary and achieve political advantage. In this form, they involved deception and dissimulation, making it difficult for outsiders to understand or sympathize with such stratagems.

The major parts or "incremental" elements centrally important in legislating HIPAA were small group and individual insurance market reform; fraud and abuse; ERISA[46] amendments and small business purchasing pools; medical savings accounts; and medical malpractice reform. All of these had a history. They had been included in the vetoed Medicare Preservation Act of 1995 or were part of the incremental health reform packages for that year. Before that, they had been taken up, in one way or another, in the health care reform debates of 1993 and 1994. The fraud and abuse provisions had been extensively developed in an even earlier bill by Senator Cohen. The bipartisan Bentsen-Durenberger insurance reform bill, which passed the Senate in 1991, had many features in common with HIPAA. The only comparatively novel contribution was the medical savings accounts, but these had figured as one alternative for individual coverage in the Republican minority proposal for health care reform and had been strongly supported as an independent option by Senate conservatives such as Phil Gramm, Trent Lott, and John McCain.

Since these proposals had been around and had a legislative history of sorts, there were committee drafts, often hearings, and institutional memory that substituted to some extent for more deliberate and systematic consideration. Moreover, such proposals could be crafted fairly quickly, making possible new permutations and new strategies. One drawback to this kind of procedure, though, was that some provisions found their way into aggregative bills without ever having been thoroughly vetted or worked up into proper legislative language during their entire history.

Kassebaum–Kennedy (S1028): The Health Insurance Reform Act

The immediate background for Kassebaum-Kennedy was not 1995 and the Balanced Budget Act of that year, but 1993–94 and health care reform. In the Senate, as well as the House, there was a view—shared to a large extent by Republicans and Democrats alike—that a number of worthwhile health care reforms got trashed during that period, leaving many persistent deficiencies without a remedy. Early in 1995, along with the big agenda of deficit reduction and remaking the government, there were smaller, incremental strategies for health care reform: including insurance reform and attempts to increase access to health care. One continuing problem left unresolved by the collapse of health care reform in 1994 was what to do about the large number of uninsured, forty-one million in 1995, and increasing then, at a rate of about one million a year.

Dealing with the insurance market is not the easiest thing to do. Health insurance is an arcane business, involving a diverse and highly regulated industry, the complexities of ERISA, and sensitivities about federal and state jurisdiction. Partly for this reason there were sharp partisan and ideological differences, especially over whether to get into individual insurance at all[47] and how much to regulate as opposed to relying on tax credits, MSAs, or other nonregulative approaches.

On health matters, the Senate Finance and Labor and Human Resources committees share jurisdiction in much the same way that Ways and Means and Commerce do in the House. Finance deals with health care funded by a specific tax or trust fund (e.g., Medicare and Medicaid) and Labor and Human Resources with a broader range of health care issues, including access to health care and health care insurance. While many bills can be crafted to fall under one or both jurisdictions, insurance has normally been the province of Labor and Human Resources. There were other reasons for a lead role by this committee. One was that Nancy Kassebaum, the chairwoman, and Ted Kennedy, the ranking member, both had strong interests in health insurance[48] and a tradition of bipartisan collaboration. Another reason was to keep the bill out of Finance, where there would be incentives, both because of committee jurisdiction and the interests of specific members, to move toward tax credits, as opposed to regulation, and encumber the bill with a medley of add-ons that would generate partisan controversy.

The initiative came from Senator Kennedy and his staff, who sought a reform proposal that could be done on a bipartisan basis. Their first venture was the Hatch-Kennedy bill to modify the Child Care and Development Block Grant. This received strong bipartisan endorsement but was ultimately lost in the welfare reform conference. As this ill-fated legislation was in process, Kassebaum was approached on insurance reform and welcomed the joint initiative.

To assure bipartisan collaboration and improve the chances for passage, the strategy was to maintain a low profile and keep the bill as "clean" as possible, not do a large package with controversial add-ons. Even though Kassebaum knew, for instance, that Dole had in mind a larger and more partisan bill on the subject, she did not keep him informed of her own plans. Senate supporters of the Kassebaum-Kennedy bill engaged, furthermore, not to seek the addition of extraneous amendments—an agreement that was strictly honored.[49] They also rounded up more than the usual number of endorsements—all the members of the committee and, ultimately, more than fifty senators. The one day of hearings, except for some controversy over medical savings accounts, was more like an anointing or blessing than a critical examination. The bill cleared the committee on August 2, with a unanimous vote.[50]

Most elements of the Health Insurance Reform Act were standard for this kind of insurance proposal. Fundamentally, the legislation provided for guaranteed issue and portability for group plans and for limited group-to-individual portability.[51] Exclusion on grounds of a preexisting condition by an employer or a group plan for more than a twelve-month period was barred. Nor could group plans use health status as a basis for denying coverage either to an employer or employee. Individuals losing their group coverage were guaranteed access to individual plans under specified conditions—so called group-to-individual coverage.[52] The bill also extended some guarantees to employees who became disabled and to their family members; provided some incentives for insurance purchasing pools; and had some encouraging language on medical savings accounts.

Despite a resolve to keep a low profile and seek bipartisan approval, two provisions in the bill were quite controversial. One was the inclusion of MSAs, pushed by Bill Frist (R., Tenn.) a physician and freshman senator, and adopted by the Labor and Human Resources Committee with a party-line vote of 9–7.[53] The other was group-to-individual portability, a provision strongly urged by Senator Kassebaum. Even though this guarantee was limited by a requirement of previous membership in a group plan and exhaustion of other available coverage, it met with sharp opposition from the insurance industry and from individual senators. The insurance industry especially feared the dangers associated with individual enrollment—which lacked the risk-spreading advantages of large plans and tended to attract subscribers with unknown, probably high-risk profiles. They also feared the intrusion of federal regulation. A number of senators shared this concern and wondered whether it was prudent for the federal government to be venturing again, after fifty years, into a field as traditionally "local" and difficult to regulate as the individual health insurance market.[54]

After S 1026 cleared the committee, with unanimous approval, Senator Kassebaum asked Dole, as majority leader, to schedule floor time for debate. Then she waited—for almost a full year. The reason given was "holds" put on the bill by conservative senators acting partly in response to objections coming from the insurance industry, especially the HIAA.[55] It was also true that Kassebaum-Kennedy was not well received by conservatives, especially because of its regulatory features. Furthermore, it was a bipartisan compromise bill in an election year when partisan credit-claiming was at a premium. Dole had no particular reason to promote this bill, either as majority leader or as a presidential candidate guarding his right flank. Nevertheless, both Kassebaum and Kennedy knew how to make life hard for a majority leader—through dilatory motions and holds of their own. Dole finally did promise Kassebaum floor time but not until some time after February in the next session, when voting on bills resumed.[56] For the time being, S 1026 was stalled.

The House Initiatives

The bill that ultimately emerged from the House in 1996 was both incremental and aggregative in nature. It combined bills from several committees and proposals that had been introduced repeatedly and modified incrementally over time. To complicate the narrative further, these bills were also elements of an incremental legislative strategy, which in this context meant getting lesser bills passed in addition to or in default of a larger, reconciliation effort.

Most of the proposals that eventually became part of the House bill in 1996 had an earlier history. They were components of the incremental strategy developed early in 1995 by the House Republicans and later incorporated into BBA 95, which President Clinton vetoed. Medical savings accounts, medical malpractice reform, and fraud and abuse legislation fall under this category. Reform of the private insurance market was not included in the BBA of 1995, but bills were developed that year in the Ways and Means and the Economic and Educational Opportunities committees, and there had been earlier attempts to deal with this particular issue.[57] As the Republican majority cast about for attractive initiatives—in an election year and after the shutdown— reform of the private insurance market quickly emerged as having both a wide appeal and a possible use as a vehicle for other legislation.

Several events combined to heighten the visibility of insurance reform and prod the House into action. President Clinton, in his State of the Union address on January 25, praised the bipartisan Kassebaum-Kennedy initiative, adding that fraud and abuse legislation would also be desirable.[58]

Shortly thereafter, on February 5, Senator Dole indicated that the remaining holds had been withdrawn, so that S 1028 could be scheduled for floor time—though not until April 15, over two months away.[59] Meanwhile, Bill Gradison, president of the Health Insurance Association of America (HIAA), urged the House to pass some insurance reform that would not have the group-to-individual feature of the Senate bill.[60] By early February, with the budget dispute less consuming, there was time and opportunity for more modest health care reforms. That same week, Newt Gingrich told an AARP audience that three House committees would be taking up health insurance reform, with a bill expected to pass in the spring.[61]

Other than the obvious need for legislation in an election year, other considerations provided additional incentives for the House to act. One was the probable failure of another reconciliation bill, whatever form it might take. That outcome would raise the stakes for passage of some small bills, not part of a reconciliation. Another motive was to "get ahead of the curve," in other words, to have House bills and proposals ready when the Senate bill arrived, so they could attach to it high-priority items of their own and bargain to advantage in the conference.[62] According to several reports, Senate conservatives were also appealing to the House to give them something with which to fight Kassebaum-Kennedy in the Senate.[63]

As traditional for Republicans with multijurisdictional bills, another task force was appointed, chaired by Dennis Hastert (R., Ill.), then the deputy whip. Other members were the chairmen and health subcommittee chairmen of Ways and Means, Commerce, and Economic and Educational Opportunities. Unlike the speaker's task force of 1995, however, these committees drafted their own bills. The task force members then sought to merge the separate committees' bills into a joint product to be submitted to the Rules Committee for final amendments and a "rule" governing the floor debate.

The Ways and Means draft proposal provides a good illustration of the aggregative process at work. As previously noted, the elements of this draft already existed. The core of the proposal was a bill (H.R. 1610) drafted early in 1995 that provided group-to-group portability—but not group-to-individual portability. At the time, the Health Subcommittee was drafting a broader proposal (H.R. 1234), which, along with other measures, barred use of preexisting condition as a ground for denying insurance coverage. As these drafts were under consideration, the Commerce Committee was developing a version that included a carefully conditioned form of group-to-individual insurance, and the Economic and Educational Opportunities Committee was promoting MEWAs (multiple-employer welfare arrangements) that would facilitate risk-pooling for small employers. Both of these contributions became part of final House bill when the several committee drafts were merged.

Beside providing guarantees to the insured, the Ways and Means draft sought to make health insurance more affordable and accessible in two different ways. One was through tax relief, raising the self-employed deduction for health expenses from 30 to 50 percent and making long-term care insurance deductible. The other approach was medical savings accounts, vigorously touted by conservative Republicans, especially from Texas, as a way to promote competition, foster thrift, and make health care available to the small employer and self-employed. But these provisions would cost money and fell under PAYGO budget rules, i.e., required offsetting revenues or expenditure reductions.[64] So the Ways and Means proposal added, only slightly amended, the fraud and abuse provisions from BBA 1995, made additionally attractive in 1996 because of more generous scoring by CBO.[65] And Republicans in both Ways and Means and the Commerce committees urged that medical malpractice reform be included as another important money-saver. It eventually was added, but only after later Rules Committee amendments to the three-committee product.

The Ways and Means bill, with modifications drawn from the two other committees,[66] incorporated the main elements of the final House bill. Aggregating the various provisions as it did, H.R. 3103 advanced several avowed objectives as well as some not so publicly advertised. It broadened the insurance reform initiative from protecting the insured to include some help for the uninsured in the form of tax relief and more accessible policies. Reducing fraud and abuse and malpractice judgments, in addition to offsetting expenditures, would also slow the rise in health care costs and, as a consequence, make health insurance less expensive. At the same time, the medical savings accounts and malpractice reform (and MEWAs) would increase political support, especially among Republicans, and help win over conservatives who feared that insurance reform was becoming too regulative. And, not to be missed, this bill would be an important showpiece in the Republican effort to pass as much as possible of the Balanced Budget Act of 1995 in incremental packages carried forward by suitable legislative vehicles.

One effect of this aggregative approach was to unify partisan opposition around a counterstrategy. In the Commerce Committee, for instance, Democrats objected to malpractice reform as an obvious "poison pill."[67] John Dingell, ranking Democrat on the committee, attacked the fraud and abuse provisions, arguing that they were not strong enough, would make successful prosecutions more difficult, and were primarily included to offset the costs of features such as medical savings accounts, which were not within the jurisdiction of the Commerce Committee and were objectionable to Democrats.[68] Henry Waxman offered as an amendment a bill that closely resembled the Senate's Kassebaum-Kennedy. The amendment failed, but Democrats began to unify increasingly around support for a "clean" Kassebaum-Kennedy bill, without any of the House add-ons. The White House also expressed its desire for an insurance bill without "controversial" and "potentially harmful" elements such as the MSAs, limits on malpractice awards, weakening of fraud and abuse provisions, and the ERISA amendments in favor of MEWAs.[69]

Floor action on H.R. 3103 changed nothing of substance but it did increasingly center attention on Kassebaum-Kennedy as a viable alternative to a veto. The House bill passed on March 28 by a vote of 267–151, though a Democratic substitute closely resembling Kassebaum-Kennedy failed by 192–266, a much smaller difference.

Kassebaum-Kennedy and Election Year Politics

As subsequent developments showed, Senator Dole might have saved himself much trouble if he had simply postponed debate—as many thought he would—until Kassebaum-Kennedy ran out of time toward the end of the session. However, he had promised floor time in 1995. Senator Kassebaum was insistent and Dole preferred not to arouse her ire or resentment.[70] In addition, he faced a crowded agenda in an election year and both Kassebaum and Kennedy, the cosponsors, could be formidable obstructionists.[71] Moreover, Dole had not done well in the New Hampshire primary and his campaign could benefit from a generous and statesmanlike gesture. For any or all of these reasons, Dole announced an end to the holds with assurances of floor time after April 15, 1996.

Though a minor bill, Kassebaum-Kennedy was of symbolic importance, as the only health care measure likely to be passed in an election year and as a demonstration of achievement through bipartisan collaboration. For the bill to succeed, both Kassebaum and Kennedy were convinced that it had to be free of controversial additions; and since August 2, 1995 when the Labor and Human Resources Committee approved the bill, its supporters had faithfully kept the "no amendment" pledge. Meanwhile, bipartisan support for this strategy had been growing, with approval by House Democrats and the president and endorsements by an impressive array of twelve major national advocacy groups including the AARP, the AHA, the HIAA, the National Association of Manufacturers, and the ERISA Industry Committee.[72] The AHA not only mounted a media campaign in support of the bill but, in an unusual move, sought endorsements by sixty or more senators so that it would be proof against a filibuster.[73]

But Kassebaum-Kennedy was not without strong opposition. Republican supporters of the House bill appealed to their party colleagues in the Senate to support the House version. Even as the House bill was being passed, a group of conservative Republicans in the Senate announced that they would try to amend Kassebaum-Kennedy on the floor with add-ons from the House bill. These included some of the most controversial provisions such as medical savings accounts, medical malpractice reform, and insurance pools along with various tax benefits. Among this group of senators were Trent Lott, three others from the Senate leadership, and Phil Gramm and Don Nickels from the Senate Finance Committee.

For Dole, it was a dangerous situation. The chances of success in amending Kassebaum-Kennedy were slim. Yet he was the Senate leader and, as the leading contender for the Republican presidential nomination, the party's titular head as well. In this situation, he could ill afford to have a large distance or an open break between himself and the Senate conservatives. So, he went out on a limb, announcing on April 17, the day before the floor debate, that he, along with Senator Roth, chairman of Senate Finance, would seek a floor amendment to include the controversial House MSA provision.[74] To increase support for this amendment, he put in a number of attractive tax measures, such as increasing the health expense deduction and adding long-term care. Fraud and abuse provisions drawing upon language from Senator Cohen were also included along with some revenue offsets.[75]

His venture turned out to be both embarrassing and costly. The MSA provision was successfully stripped from the bill in a dramatic floor vote with Vice President Al Gore present as the tie-breaker if needed. The vote was close, 52–46. To make defeat more bitter, it was another victory for bipartisanship, with five moderate Republicans joining the Democrats, even after Gore had allowed Dole extra time to change some votes.[76] It may also have been a clumsy mistake, since Dole could have himself sponsored the popular tax amendments and left the MSAs to some one else, especially if the advance vote-counting had shown the closeness of the issue.[77] As it was, Dole got little credit, suffered a humiliating defeat, and looked the part of a mean-spirited partisan rather than a statesman for sponsoring the MSA "poison pill."[78] Compounding his injuries, he followed the defeat with dark mutterings that the House-Senate conference committee would be in a "strong position" to change the MSA outcome—tipping his hand and inviting a counterstrategy.[79]

Some amendments did pass. With the MSAs stripped, almost all of the Dole-Roth package passed unanimously, including the tax benefits and fraud and abuse provisions. An important bipartisan amendment sponsored by Pete Domenici and Paul Wellstone was a provision for mental health "parity," which would have required health insurance plans to provide coverage for serious mental illness at least equivalent to that for physical illness. A significant amendment that failed, proposed by Senator Jeffords, would have set $10 million as a minimum limit for life-time caps on payouts from employer-sponsored health plans. Senator Kassebaum approved the concept, but said that the measure did not belong in a bill on insurance reform. It was tabled by a vote of 56–42.[80]

The Senate delayed a final vote until April 23 to allow Sen. Connie Mack to return from his father's funeral. By then, Kassebaum-Kennedy had sixty-five cosponsors. On April 23, as scheduled, the Senate voted unanimously (100–0) to approve the bill, a unanimity that covered over many differences and belied the controversy that was to follow.

The controversy over the MSAs and other add-ons in the House bill quickly shifted to the House-Senate conference. Vice President Gore, after the earlier Senate vote on MSAs, had warned that the president would veto a bill with MSA provisions in it.[81] Senator Kennedy took the lead in objecting to Dole's proposal for a conference of seven Republicans and four Democrats, which he said would enable Dole to "stack the deck" with conferees who did not represent the Senate's position on MSAs.[82] Behind this move on Kennedy's part lay a strategy of using delaying motions and prolonged debate to tie up the conference process and force preconference negotiations over the more controversial provisions in the House bill.[83] This tactic enabled Kennedy and the Senate Democrats to exert pressure on the Republican majority because it effectively held their one health bill hostage while time pressure and the need to start full-time campaigning increased with each passing day. It also made Dole seem ineffectual, as he struggled to get a relatively minor bill passed and, at the same time, campaign for president.[84] With the conference on hold, negotiations between principals and their staffs in the Senate and House over disputed provisions in the two bills continued throughout May, June, and all of July. As a result, several of the major obstacles to an agreement were whittled down or largely bargained away, including the insurance pools and medical malpractice. Meanwhile, Senator Dole announced, on July 12, that he would leave the Senate to devote full time to campaigning for the presidency.

How much Dole's decision was motivated by the Kennedy conference strategy and his other efforts to hobble Dole's Senate leadership efforts[85] during the campaign year is unclear. Dole probably would not have wished to return to the Senate if he lost the presidential race. Moreover, he was accomplishing little in the Senate and suffering in the opinion polls the longer he stayed. Some Democrats believe, though, that Kennedy's campaign drove Dole out of the Senate and may have substantially influenced the outcome of the 1996 presidential election.[86] In any event, the episode shows some of the unexpected dynamics of a controversial aggregative bill in a presidential election year.

The medical savings accounts continued to be the major sticking point. In a deal with Bill Archer, chairman of Ways and Means, Kassebaum agreed to allow MSAs, but only as a trial program. But Archer insisted on a large-scale trial that would phase in more general eligibility.[87] For Democrats, this looked too much like a sliding two-step into a full MSA alternative, not a trial or demonstration. Talks reopened after Trent Lott took over as majority leader on July 12, with Kennedy negotiating directly with Archer. Eventually a resolution was achieved, providing for a reduced trial of not more than 750,000 enrollees and a condition that Congress would have to vote affirmatively for the program to be continued after four years. This final step was a procedural oddity in one respect, with Kennedy—the ranking member of Labor and Human Resources—negotiating directly with Chairman Archer of Ways and Means over a measure affecting taxes. It also represented another victory for bipartisanship, since the final compromise was worked out by a bipartisan group of staff aides drawn from the House, Senate, and the White House.[88]

After all of this maneuvering, the conference was routine and anticlimactic. Trent Lott quickly appointed a representative group of five senators. In the conference, there was little remaining to disagree about. Mental health parity and malpractice reform were dropped.[89] The House adopted the conference report on August 1 by a vote of 421–2 and the Senate followed on August 2, voting 98–0. On August 21, President Clinton signed the Health Insurance Portability and Accountability Act into law—the first federal statute to make health insurance coverage more portable and continuous, covering an estimated 25 million workers.[90]

III. REFLECTIONS

With respect to the larger themes of Medicare and Medicaid politics, 1996 was a year of modest accomplishments: a Medicaid initiative that sputtered and died, and Medicare largely ignored except for fraud and abuse. Yet it had some important consequences—both direct and indirect—for each of these programs, especially in diminishing the scope of future conflict.

Related indirectly to Medicare, HIPAA dealt with several topics that had figured in the Balanced Budget Act of 1995: medical savings accounts, malpractice liability, and fraud and abuse, along with an assortment generally labeled "administrative simplification." Medical savings accounts were put on a trial basis and, so far, have stayed on that footing. Malpractice liability was stripped in the Senate and, to date, no serious attempt at federal legislation has been revived. The fraud and abuse provisions of BBA 95 were largely incorporated into HIPAA, though moving slightly on some issues toward the more moderate Senate version. Aside from passing important fraud and abuse provisions and making a start on administrative simplification, another important contribution of HIPAA was to remove a controversial issue from the agenda, medical malpractice, and establish a temporary truce with respect to the other, the medical savings accounts. In effect, the least controversial measures passed, leaving behind two unattractive items commonly regarded as poison pills, not winsome elements in any future reconciliation package.

For Medicaid, it was a year of "cooling out" as Congress and the National Governors' Association struggled once again to find some formula that would work fiscally and satisfy politically. As both the deficit and the Medicaid baseline continued to decline and the administration progressively liberalized its granting of Medicaid waivers, governors had less and less enthusiasm for a Medicaid block grant. Once welfare and Medicaid were separated, the local fires heating this issue died down. Six more months of frustration in seeking a solution, program numbers that belied a "crisis," little prospect either of a bipartisan solution or of prevailing with a veto strategy, and the Medicaid issue faded into the background.

Sometimes problems tend to diminish with time, especially when the economy is growing. For both Medicare and Medicaid, the improving economy and Medicare and Medicaid baselines removed much of the urgency about the deficit and program costs and, with that, much of the semirevolutionary campaign psychology that had characterized 1995. On a more substantive level, appeals to abolish or radically restructure these programs lost much of their ideological support so that, the following year the policy debate was more moderate and bipartisan initiatives were, if not in fashion, at least not regarded as oddities.

From the experience of 1996, it is hard to conclude much about aggregative legislative strategies. It was an exceptional year, much affected by the apocalyptic legislative struggles of 1995 and by a presidential campaign in which the leading Republican contender was also the Senate majority leader. At the same time, there were three different examples of this strategy during the year, and it seems to be a distinctive kind of behavior associated with divided government and controversial health and social policy, so useful to consider briefly.

The three-part reconciliation with welfare and Medicaid linked was one example of aggregation, deliberately calculated to take the easiest first and try to pull along Medicaid amendments with welfare reform, the latter having both strong symbolic appeal and potential for blame-shifting (Weaver 1987). In this example, Clinton lost on welfare and the Republican Congress lost on Medicaid. It could hardly be said that the aggregative strategy worked, since Congress gained what it could have had anyway on a welfare bill and got nothing on Medicaid. Perhaps one lesson is that, like poker, you need good cards and an ability to assess the odds and your opponent.

A second example was the elaborately devised House bill, encumbered with an array of incremental initiatives that had been part of the earlier BBA 95, including at least one poison pill (medical malpractice) and various other provisions meant to be bargained over in conference. Something was actually gained: fraud and abuse and administrative simplification were included, along with MSAs as a trial demonstration. But the controversial provisions lost initially in the Senate after which tricks on one side led to tricks on the other—Kennedy's strategy of delaying the conference—which finally got about the same result, at some political cost to Republicans generally and Senator Dole in particular. In this instance, an intricate, infernal machine damaged those using it. On a more positive note, though, this episode revealed again the importance of the Senate and its procedures in checking partisanship and majoritarian politics.

The third example was the Kassebaum-Kennedy bill or HIPAA. Even though its sponsors were determined to keep it a clean bill, free of extraneous, tactically calculated additions, it became the vehicle for a major fraud and abuse section, a number of administrative reforms, and an MSA trial demonstration. Measured in number of pages or probable future importance, the fraud and abuse provisions considerably outweighed the original insurance reform bill. One important difference is that, with the exception of the MSAs, these provisions had strong bipartisan support. The MSAs, which did not, were kept alive but whittled down to an experimental initiative—which, given its one-sided partisan backing, may not have been a bad outcome.

It would be a mistake to see this aggregative or incremental legislative politics as either unimportant or pathological. On the contrary, it is a creative adaptation of traditional kinds of behavior that provides an alternative to gridlock or partisan warfare. It helped mediate a transition from angry confrontation to a more constructive mix of partisan skirmishing and bargaining with increased opportunities for bipartisan collaboration. As part of HIPAA, Congress enacted the fraud and abuse legislation, an important leftover from BBA 95. It also provided enough small victories so that partisans could live with the result. While it was not pleasant to observe, it may be an alternative to something worse and a step to something better.

NOTES

[1] A useful concept employed by Gail Wilensky, Project HOPE, chair of MedPAC. Interview, January 5, 1999.

[2] Jack Ebeler, Robert Wood Johnson Foundation; formerly deputy assistant secretary for health, DHHS. Interview, January 6, 1999.

[3] As the term was used in Congress, "incrementalism" was a legislative strategy, not a method of decision-making. It might refer to any bill short of a major statute or reconciliation bill: (1) a minor change or addition to an exiting statute; (2) a narrowly topical or "targeted" bill; or (3) an aggregation of smaller bills combined with a political strategy in mind. It seldom had the meaning given to it by Lindblom (1950).

[4] *Congressional Quarterly,* March 29, 1996, p. 752.

[5] *Health Care Policy Report,* February 12, 1996, p. 265.

[6] *Congressional Quarterly,* January 27, 1996, p. 211.

[7] *Health Care Policy Report,* January 29, 1996, p. 127.

[8] *Congressional Quarterly,* February 10, 1996, p. 350.

[9] Ibid., March 16, 1996, p. 685.

[10] *Health Care Policy Report,* January 29, 1996, p. 127.

[11] *Congressional Quarterly,* March 2, 1996, p. 537.

[12] *Health Care Policy Report,* March 18, 1996, p. 466.

[13] *Congressional Quarterly,* March 25, 1996, p. 782.

[14] As Ray Sheppach said, "When you haven't enacted anything, you think it's a hell of a lot easier than it is." Interview, June 16, 1999. He added that both the Congress and the governors felt "used" and "distrustful" of each other as a result of this experience.

[15] *Health Care Policy Report,* February 12, 1996, p. 119.

[16] Especially pushed by states like New York with high Medicaid payments and poorer states that had difficulty in meeting the match.

[17] *Health Care Policy Report,* February 12, 1996, p. 230.

[18] Especially Rep. Greg Ganske (R., Iowa). Ibid., February 26, 1996, p. 313.

[19] Ibid.

[20] Ibid., March 4, 1996, p. 368.

[21] Ibid., February 19, 1996, p. 278.

[22] The governors' proposal had an umbrella fund that would be phased down over time to meet deficit reduction targets (supported by Republican governors). But it also provided that the federal government would have to share in the costs of increased caseloads within a given state (supported by Democratic governors). Commerce Committee staff argued that this scheme revived "per capita caps," which Republicans had earlier rejected; also that governors would not sign off on this plan until they knew how much money they would be getting. The GAO said that it could not model the governors' scheme without more reliable data on how many pregnant women or persons with disabilities would be eligible. CBO delayed scoring, but warned that the proposal might well cost the federal government more rather than saving money. Ibid., April 1, 1996, pp. 554–55.

[23] *Congressional Quarterly,* March 2, 1996, p. 538. Apparently, the veto threat was credible. Newt Gingrich remarked at the time on the "fairly bizarre new development, where on a regular basis, the Clinton administration threatens to close the government." Ibid., March 23, 1996, p. 782.

[24] Ibid., March 9, 1996, p. 607.

[25] *Health Care Policy Report,* March 18, 1996, p. 466.

[26] *Congressional Quarterly,* April 6, 1996, p. 938.

[27] Medicare inflation was also down—in 1995, the lowest rate of increase since 1972. *Health Care Policy Report,* February 5, 1996, p. 213.

[28] Ibid., May 6, p. 763.

[29] However, Senator Daschle did raise a point of order against this strategy, arguing that the third bill—which would cut some taxes—violated the Byrd Rule. Republicans disagreed and his motion was voted down on a party-line vote, 47–53. The issue could have been raised again, even after the conference report, so that it posed some significant risk. *Congressional Quarterly,* May 4, 1996, p. 1450.

[30] *Health Care Policy Report,* May 27, 1996, p. 885.

[31] Ibid., June 10, 1996, p. 992.

[32] The new majority leader in the Senate.

[33] *Health Care Policy Report,* June 24, 1996, p. 1044.

[34] Ibid.

[35] *Congressional Quarterly,* June 13, 1996, p. 1653.

[36] *Health Care Policy Report,* July 1, 1996, p. 1081.

[37] Ibid., June 24, 1996, p. 1045.

[38] *Congressional Quarterly,* June 22, 1996, p. 1761.

[39] *Health Care Policy Report,* July 15, 1996, p. 1155.

[40] Sheila Burke, Kennedy School of Government; formerly, chief of staff for Senator Dole. Interview, January 5, 1999.

[41] Cf. the Republican party platform, which claimed credit for passing HIPAA and blamed President Clinton for blocking programs to restructure and "save" Medicare and Medicaid. *Health Care Policy Report,* August 19, 1996, p. 1332.

[42] P.L. 104-193.

[43] P.L. 104-191.

[44] In the House, John Kasich, chairman of the Budget Committee, was often a member of such task forces.

[45] See note 3.

[46] Employment Retirement Income Security Act of 1974.

[47] Since the McCarran-Ferguson Act of 1945 (P.L. 15) exempting insurance companies from federal antitrust laws, insurance had been, for practical purposes, regulated by the states alone. Republicans especially were reluctant to break this fifty-year tradition.

[48] Kennedy's strong interest in health is well known. But Kassebaum had sponsored an important insurance bill during health care reform. David Nexon, Kennedy staff. Interview, October 20, 1998.

[49] With the exception of a few innocuous "sense of the Senate" amendments. *Congressional Quarterly Almanac,* 1996, p. 7-25.

[50] Ibid.

[51] "Guaranteed issue" required plans to accept qualified applicants; "portability" meant that insured persons could move to a new plan, for instance, when employed by another firm; and "group to individual" required plans to insure individuals who had lost their group insurance—a controversial feature because of the potential for adverse selection.

[52] The insured person must have had previous group coverage and been without coverage for eighteen months and exhausted short-term expedients, i.e., typically the eighteen-month COBRA mandatory extension of coverage.

[53] *Congressional Quarterly Almanac,* 1996, p. 7-25.

[54] Claims were made that such legislation would increase costs of insurance and might actually reduce coverage, although the American Association of Actuaries disputed this contention.

[55] "Holds" are used by senators to delay or postpone floor action or nominations. Since they carry an implicit threat of delay through a filibuster, they are generally honored. The senator(s) may be seeking more information, a concession, or only some more time. The use of "holds" has increased dramatically in recent years. They are supposed to be temporary, but may extend indefinitely. Senator Kassebaum asked one senator to explain the reason for his hold. He said he had forgotten the reason. *Health Care Policy Report,* December 18, 1995, p. 2195.

[56] Sheila Burke. Interview, January 5, 1999. David Nexon. Interview, October 20, 1998.

[57] Especially during health care reform: a bill by Sen. William Cohen (R., Me.) and a bipartisan effort from Senator Bentsen (D., Tex.) and Senator Durenberger (R. Minn.).

[58] *Health Care Policy Report,* January 29, 1996, p. 128.

[59] Ibid., February 12, 1996, p. 232.

[60] Ibid., February 5, 1996, p. 179.

[61] Ibid., February 12, 1996, p. 232.

[62] Howard Cohen, Greenberg Traurig, formerly professional staff, House Commerce Committee. Interview, January 13, 1999.

[63] Ed Kutler, Clark and Weinstock, formerly personal aide to Speaker Newt Gingrich. Interview, October 21, 1998.

[64] PAYGO, or pay-as-you-go, is a requirement of the Budget Enforcement Act of 1990 that requires legislation that either reduces revenues or increases mandatory spending above the baseline to be completely offset by revenue increases or reductions in mandatory spending. If not fully offset, a PAYGO sequester will be triggered.

[65] Helen Albert, Office of the Inspector General, DHHS; formerly chief investigator, Senate Special Committee on Aging. Telephone interview, June 18, 1999.

[66] Especially the "multiple-employer welfare arrangements" (MEWAs) and group-to-individual protections. Health Coverage Availability and Affordability Act of 1996, H.R. 3070, Title I, Subtitle B. Part 2. Also, *Health Care Policy Report,* April 1, 1996, p. 564.

[67] Howard Cohen pointed out that it could also be a bargaining chip: "We'll take this out if you'll take that out." Interview, January 13, 1999.

[68] *Congressional Quarterly,* March 16, 1996, p. 706.

[69] *Health Care Policy Report,* April 1, 1996, p. 563.

[70] Sheila Burke. Interview, January 5, 1999.

[71] Senator Kassebaum was at the time holding up a bill that Dole needed. Vicki Hart, director of legislative and federal affairs, Verner, Liipfert, Bernhard, McPherson and Hand; former assistant to the majority leader. Interview, October 27, 1998.

[72] *Health Care Policy Report,* March 11, 1996, p. 415.

[73] Ibid., April 15, 1996, p. 654.

[74] Sheila Burke. Interview, January 5, 1996.

[75] *Health Care Policy Report,* April 22, 1966, p. 692.

[76] Two did, William Cohen and Bill Frist. *Congressional Quarterly Almanac,* 1996, p. 6-33.

[77] Interview, David Nexon, October 20, 1998.

[78] Ibid.

[79] *Health Care Policy Report,* April 22, 1996, p. 692.

[80] Ibid., p. 694.

[81] Ibid., p. 692.

[82] Ibid., April 29, 1996, p. 725. The Senate tradition is that conferees should broadly represent the Senate's position.

[83] David Nexon. Interview, October 20, 1998.

[84] Apparently, one of Kennedy's contributions to the presidential campaign was to hamper and harass Dole. David Nexon and Sheila Burke. Interviews. See also Walsh (1997).

[85] For instance, on the minimum wage bill (Walsh 1997:80–81).

[86] The week that Clinton signed both HIPAA and the minimum wage increase into law was "the worst week of the campaign," according to Scott Reed, Dole's campaign manager. Ibid., p. 81.

[87] *Congressional Quarterly Almanac,* 1996, p. 6-38.

[88] Vicki Hart. Interview, October 27, 1998.

[89] Though mental health parity was later passed in a scaled-down version as part of VA-HUD appropriations.

[90] *Health Care Policy Report,* August 26, 1996, p. 1365.

6

Medicare and Medicaid, 1997

As in 1995, the Medicare and Medicaid legislation were parts of a budget reconciliation, though the political environment was much changed. The 1997 legislation, made possible by a temporary bipartisan consensus, was moderate in philosophy though far-reaching in its objectives. Beyond that appreciation, views about BBA 97 differ markedly. The Medicare legislation, for instance, has been viewed as the most sweeping change in the program since its inception, but also as mostly "incremental."[1] One observer thought that Clinton, in his eagerness to get a deal, fundamentally compromised Medicare and the principles of social insurance (Marmor 2000:147). Another said that Congress had largely enacted Clinton's health care plan for him.[2] The process itself has been described as a classic Rostenkowski[3] type of reconciliation in which the stakeholders got just enough to keep them from bolting the coalition. But also notable was the enthusiasm with which both Democrats and Republicans walked away claiming victory. In a word, the issues and the legislative developments of 1997 were complex and people disagreed about their significance and how to characterize them.

There was, for a time, a genuine spirit of bipartisan collaboration that shaped both the Medicare and Medicaid amendments of 1997. Why it came about, the differences it made in the legislation, who benefited from this bipartisan collaboration, and how important or recurrent this behavior is likely to be in the future are topics that need consideration. Moreover, the nature of bipartisan behavior differed considerably as between Medicare and Medicaid. The Medicare legislation seemed to represent a grand compromise, but settled little. Rather than working out differences, it walled them off and avoided them, planting the seeds for future confrontations. With Medicaid, by contrast, partisan differences and principled compromise played a larger role, producing legislation that made significant and creative additions to the program and may have created the framework for a lasting settlement.

The legislative developments of 1997 provide two differing examples of what bipartisan collaboration on major health care legislation might look like—rare as it is these days—as well as revealing some of the conditions that make it more likely or prevalent. It also illustrates two modes of behavior. One, characteristic of Democrats in these particular episodes, can be termed "institutionalizing the future," meaning preempting future policy choices by institutionalizing certain activities, either through administrative organization, rulemaking, or settled contract arrangements. The other is "postulating the future," often characteristic of the Republicans, meaning here investing the "market" or the private sector with mythical (unproven, imagined) powers of problem-solving. As we shall see, each of these tendencies is a natural response to the situation in which Democrats and Republicans find themselves in our present system of divided or weakly majoritarian government. And though they are less in evidence with bipartisan collaboration, they are a major reason why such collaboration is less effective than it could be.

I. THE CONTEXT OF EVENTS IN 1997

In accounting for the difference between 1997 and 1995, participants in events during those years cite a good many factors that could be grouped under almost as many headings. In the most general terms, both Republicans and Democrats—for their various reasons—wanted a deal; and the economic and political circumstances were favorable. But it is helpful, for understanding how exceptional the circumstances were, to particularize these broad assertions.

The election of 1996 changed little in number of seats held or formal possession of office, but its effect upon the mood of politics was profound. The reelection of President Clinton meant not only four more years in control of the White House, but some vindication of his domestic policies and an opportunity to devote more attention to the legacy he would like to leave behind. Democrats had attempted, like the Republicans in 1994, to nationalize the local election campaigns and pillory the Republicans for their record on Medicare, Medicaid, the environment, and education. While this attempt was only partly successful, it did reinforce the message that attacks on these priorities were a dangerous business. In the House, although the Republicans lost only nine seats, they no longer had a majority commanding enough to govern if there were even a minor defection within their own ranks. Among incumbents, moreover, the group that lost most heavily was the conservative freshmen. And those returning from the campaign were bringing a message that their constituents were tired of bickering and wanted to see more constructive attitudes and working together with the opposition to accomplish something.[4] In the Senate, the Republicans gained slightly, especially in the South—which would mean an even larger role for the Senate in relation to the

House. In any event, the House revolution and the kind of mobilization politics that characterized that period were over, for the time being. Even Newt Gingrich thought it would be better to wait for another election before attempting again an initiative resembling the Contract with America.

Early in the new year, the economy and other key indicators were quite favorable. For the previous three years, the deficit had been declining. In mid-January, CBO reported more good news, lowering its deficit projections for the year 2002 by a third.[5] Even better was the prospect for Medicaid. The Treasury Department reported that Medicaid spending for 1996—projected to grow 9.7 percent annually—actually increased only 3.3 percent.[6] In December 1996, the Urban Institute predicted that Medicaid spending could drop by as much as $94 billion by 2002 without any further intervention. This amount was more than the Medicaid savings proposed by either the president or the Congress.[7] For Medicare, the news was not as good—only $15 billion less projected with the Medicare trust fund still expected to go broke by 2001.[8] Even here, the numbers were headed in the right direction, and the fact that the trust fund was not doing worse was considered to be a favorable indication.

These changes did not, in fact, make savings easier, since dropping baselines meant that there was less excess to cut. But they did signify that the total amount needed was smaller and that the task itself might be less urgent and the means less drastic. The fiscal arguments for radical restructuring of either Medicare or Medicaid, for instance, lost much of their appeal. With this change of economic circumstance, political discourse tended to move away from the inflammatory rhetoric of block grants, Medicare "bankruptcy," and tax cuts for the rich. Moreover, increasing trust fund solvency or even a moderate tax cut seemed within the realm of the achievable. These tendencies created an environment in which a bipartisan politics of the possible could emerge, even though of limited scope and duration.

Another important difference in 1997 was that some learning had taken place over the preceding two years. Republicans had learned how different governing was from being in the opposition[9] and how difficult it was to pass legislation dealing with entitlements as well entrenched and as institutionally complex as Medicare and Medicaid. They had discovered that President Clinton was a wily and dangerous opponent who knew how to capitalize on their mistakes, and that it was bad tactics "to charge the president's machine gun nest frontally."[10] Republicans had also developed a healthy caution about being the first with a controversial proposal. Meanwhile, Democrats had learned how to make the most of their defensive resources and about what Republicans had to have to hold their own base and explain themselves to their constituents. Among significant indicators of the changed political climate was Clinton's "preshopping" of his 1998 budget with Republican leaders and the early initiation of bipartisan budget talks between Democrats and Republicans before positions hardened around specific budget proposals.[11]

Another factor, particularly relevant for a reconciliation strategy, was that the scope of the effort—and with that, the amount of political conflict—was greatly reduced. Lacking the revolutionary fervor that characterized 1995, there were few Republicans insisting that reconciliation should be used to remake the federal government or even to take on entitlements. Arguments for restructuring Medicare or transforming Medicaid lost much of their force. Moreover, some of the hot items from the past—such as medical savings accounts, malpractice reform, or Medicaid block grants—had been dealt with or considerably cooled in the interim.

Leadership difficulties were important in the House, arising especially from concern about Gingrich's role as speaker. In addition to doubts about the wisdom of his policies, there was increased grumbling about his style of leadership—which seemed less suited for the more prosaic politics of divided government. He was reelected speaker by a narrow margin of three votes. His prestige was further damaged by a House Ethics Committee investigation and censure of his use of campaign funds. In July, an attempt to unseat him was narrowly averted and left the House leadership divided and distracted.

One effect of these leadership difficulties in the House was to move the conduct of legislative business back toward the traditional role of the committees and committee chairs. In 1997, despite a major reconciliation, there was no talk of a speaker's task force like that of 1995. Indeed, the inclination of Congress was much more to wait for the president's proposal and then take up their own position. With this more traditional dispensation, committees originated most of the proposals and wrote the legislation. Chairmen of the committees of jurisdiction played a larger role in determining priorities and in conference negotiations. And with House leadership no longer so prominent in setting a Republican agenda, Senate leadership and priorities became more important, a shift that further strengthened the role of traditional institutions.

Different personalities were important in 1997. In general, Congress found the *troika* of Erskine Bowles, Frank Raines, and John Hilley agreeable to deal with. In the House, Newt Gingrich was much less influential. Bill Thomas and Pete Stark, respectively, the chairman and ranking Democrat of the Ways and Means Health Subcommittee, had come to share a mutual regard for each other's competence and integrity. And in the Senate, William Roth, who succeeded Bob Packwood as chairman of the Senate Finance Committee, cared mostly about taxes and was content to leave health policy to those interested in it.

These various circumstances tended either to encourage or make possible a return to a familiar kind of bipartisan collaboration and to the give-and-take negotiation generally characteristic of legislation under conditions of divided government. But some of these circumstances seem so special and almost unique—such as the declining deficit and baselines and the storms that preceded this relative calm—that it prompts a question about whether 1997 was a return to normalcy or one brief moment of calm in the midst of continuing partisan strife over Medicare, Medicaid, entitlements, and the role of government. Even as Congress adjourned in 2001, there seemed to be no clear answer to this question.

II. THE BUDGET RESOLUTION: SETTING STRATEGIC LIMITS

The budget resolution of May 2 was essential to the success of the budget reconciliation of August 5 in more than the usual sense that it set the big numbers on entitlements, discretionary spending, and tax cuts. This resolution was a novelty in its own right: its main outlines developed by an advance summit between administration staff and congressional aides and then between the principals. The participants not only agreed on budget numbers but also reached an accord on entitlements and program substance that bounded conflict and structured issues. It was primarily a deal between the president and the Republican leadership, with minimal participation by congressional Democrats,[12] so that it was bipartisan, but not an example of party collaboration within Congress. Still, it greatly facilitated future bipartisan cooperation and passage of the reconciliation. How this came about is an instructive example of assessing opportunities and moving to capitalize on them, as well as a study in the prerequisites for bipartisan cooperation.

In the first weeks of the new 105th Congress, there was talk about a budget deal and considerable speculation about how it could be done. On the Democratic side, the newly reelected president was in a position of relative strength and thinking about legacies to pass on from his second term.[13] Deficit reduction was a priority for Democrats as well as for Republicans. And seven years had elapsed without passing a reconciliation bill, so that programs such as Medicare and Medicaid had a cumulative need for changes in program structure and authority, including some that had been part of the vetoed BBA of 1995.[14] Republicans needed a victory, preferably one that would ratify some of their signature priorities such as balancing the budget, tax cuts, and reducing the role of federal government. On the other hand, they had been severely mauled over Medicare and Medicaid in 1995 and failed in another reconciliation attempt in 1996. They wanted a budget deal in 1997. They were weary, concerned about their own leadership, and knew how difficult another reconciliation fight could be. So rather than take the lead in initiating a reconciliation attempt, they were disposed to let the administration go first.

Unlike his minimal and defensive response in 1995, President Clinton moved quickly to put forward a proposal of his own. The strategy was risky, since it would concede much and Republicans might simply come back for more. House Democrats, and especially Richard Gephardt, feared that

Clinton, like George Bush in 1990, would surrender too much. On the other hand, if he made a reasonable offer, picked his fights carefully, and the Republicans lacked persuasive counterproposals, the scheme might work. In any event, it was the kind of challenge that Clinton liked, and early in 1997 was probably the best time.[15] Another part of his strategy, as it unfolded, was to concede the Republicans just enough to keep them from developing a budget of their own. The logic was that if Republicans felt compelled to develop a budget independently, that would polarize and harden bargaining positions. Unless and until they did so, though, the administration's proposals would tend to become the basis for compromise.

The president's budget proposal that was released on February 5 had not only been worked out in considerable detail, many of its proposals had been discussed in advance with Republicans. Particularly with respect to Medicare, a figure of $100 billion savings by 2002 was pretested as a likely compromise figure.[16] In an unusual gesture, the administration shared its Medicare proposals with Republicans prior to the budget release and solicited their comments.[17] Clinton also indicated in advance statements that his proposal would address such Republican priorities as a balanced budget, extending trust fund solvency, and restructuring of Medicare.[18] While not entirely happy with all that they heard from the administration, some congressional Republicans, including John Kasich and Bill Thomas, praised Clinton for the gesture, and Thomas said that it improved prospects for a Medicare agreement.[19]

The president's Medicare proposals were remarkable especially for the elements of political strategy implicit in them. The proposals were, by and large, solid policy and politically defensible—which was important, since most of them were ultimately adopted. But, they also combined "triangulation"—a co-opting of Republican proposals—along with a selective defense of Democratic priorities. While soothing, the political rhetoric was deceptive in its strategic significance. And there were gimmicks, easing the pain of deficit reduction.

Like the Republicans, the president's budget would "preserve and improve" Medicare, and extend trust fund solvency five years through 2007. It would preserve Medicare, i.e., save $100 billion over five years ($136 billion in six years) by slowing the growth of provider payments and maintaining the Part B premium contribution at 25 percent. Medicare would be improved by giving beneficiaries more choices among private health plans and making Medicare more efficient and responsive to their needs. The president would "work with" Congress on a bipartisan basis to address the health care needs of the baby boom generation.[20]

A close reading of these statements indicates that what was unsaid can be as important as what was said. The president associated himself with most of the Republican goals. However, saving was to come from providers, not beneficiaries. Private health plans enhance choice for the beneficiary and improved management makes the program more responsive to their needs—those are their main purposes, not to foster competition or contribute to private sector strategies. The budget document expresses a concern about the impending baby boomer crisis—now the major theme in Republican Medicare policy—by saying that the president "also wants to work with the Congress on a bipartisan basis" on this matter, i.e., not right now and only on a bipartisan basis.

The president's budget also had some reconciliation gimmicks in it. One was the proposal, considered earlier in 1995, to transfer from Part A to Part B expenses for home health visits that did not originate from a hospital stay—"saving" the Hospital Trust Fund about $86 billion over five years.[21] The $86 billion would not be counted toward total savings nor would it affect the beneficiary premium but—and this was the point—it would directly bolster the trust fund and extend solvency.[22] This move weakened Republican trust fund rhetoric and made the growth of hospital expenditures seem less serious than it was. Another such gimmick was a fail-safe scheme that would have imposed expenditure cuts across the board in the fourth and fifth years (2001 and 2002), first on discretionary spending and then on entitlements, if Congress and the president were unable to agree on a way to meet the deficit reduction targets. No specific mechanism for implementing the cuts was prescribed. This particular cost-saver, even though scored by CBO for $9 billion in total savings from Medicare and Medicaid,[23] was seen as a contrived and egregious example of the "back loading" (deferring reductions) that characterized the budget as a whole. Robert Reischauer, a former CBO director, commented that CBO regarded 68 percent of savings in the last two years as a reasonable limit. Clinton's budget had more than 75 percent in 2001–02, which would fall due after he left office.[24]

The Medicaid proposal was less important in 1997 and initially less controversial. With the dramatic and continuing decline in Medicaid expenditure growth, the budget called for only $22 billion in savings over five years, to be achieved through reductions in DSH payments ($15 billion) and the implementation of per capita caps ($7 billion).[25] Flexibility for the states "to design their own Medicaid program" was a principal theme, including freedom, without securing federal waivers, to implement managed care plans, to provide in-home and community-based long-term care, and to selectively extend coverage for children. The Boren Amendment would be repealed. The other important theme was a selective increase in coverage. This included bridging coverage for the working poor and buy-in programs for the working disabled. Most important under this rubric was a major initiative to extend health care coverage to an estimated five million older children through grants to the states, expansion of Medicaid, and support for school health centers. Not directly related to either Medicare or Medicaid, but a gesture in the direction of small business and the self-employed, was a program to encourage voluntary health-purchasing cooperatives. This initiative would provide $25 million in grants to the states to be used for technical assistance and setting up cooperatives that would be allowed access to the FEHBP.[26]

The Republican response to the president's budget was mixed. From past experience, they had reason to be wary of offers from the president and a reflexive impulse to feel for their wallets. They thought the savings inadequate and were suspicious of the scoring by the HCFA actuary. They also disliked the gimmicks, especially the Part A/Part B "switch"[27] and the Clinton fail-safe. Yet their predicament was difficult. Using CBO numbers, they would need $300 billion in savings, over and beyond those in the Clinton budget, to afford Republican-size tax cuts of $200 billion or more.[28] Both John Kasich and Pete Domenici had warned that might not be doable. In any event, another Republican-only reconciliation was a daunting prospect. Moreover, other lead items in the Republican legislative agenda for the year—for instance, a balanced budget amendment or the term limits proposal, left over from the Contract with America—were unlikely to pass. They could ill afford to turn this potential opportunity into another loser. Accepting an unpleasant reality, Republicans in both House and Senate joined in their praise of the president's initiative, though adding the familiar refrain of failing to use CBO numbers and not going far enough. Pete Domenici and John Kasich thought it a good basis on which to begin discussions. Both Trent Lott and Dick Armey said they preferred working with the Clinton budget to creating a separate Republican version, and two conservative senators, Phil Gramm and Don Nickles, acknowledged the reality of divided government and said there was no real alternative to working with Clinton.[29]

The legislative career of the Clinton budget began in a bipartisan spirit, after which it settled into a familiar adversarial groove or rut. In an unusual gesture, Clinton came to Capitol Hill to explain the budget to Newt Gingrich, Trent Lott, and other leadership figures.[30] For several weeks, John Hilley, chief legislative liaison, and Frank Raines, OMB director, met with Budget Committee chairmen and members to discuss the budget and hear their concerns. The House Ways and Means and Senate Finance committees treated the budget as "alive on arrival" and held hearings on its provisions, but deep partisan differences soon emerged. The budget did not save enough or allow for a sufficient tax cut. Nor did it deal with structural reform, assure long-term solvency, or provide for the baby boom generation. It also relied too much on budget gimmicks.

By the first week in March, the Clinton budget was in trouble. Late in February, CBO estimates showed Clinton's Medicare proposal not producing savings of $100.2 billion, but falling $19 billion short, with Medicare savings $15 billion less than estimated and health benefits costing $4 billion more. For Republicans, this sounded like "same old, same old." The gap could, in theory, be erased by the fail-safe in the plan, but this device was another source of controversy. Without the Part A to Part B transfer, moreover, the trust fund would not last until 2007 but only until 2003, one year longer than under current law. Other Republicans expressed concern about the back loading, the amount of savings being taken from HMOs, and the absence of structural reforms. John Kasich and Newt Gingrich called upon the Clinton administration to produce another, more serious budget and the House passed a non-binding resolution to that effect. OMB Director Frank Raines countered that if Republicans did not like the administration budget, they should produce one of their own—not something, however, that either he or the Clinton administration wished to happen.[31]

Among possibilities considered for bridging the "gap" between the Clinton budget and the Republicans were a reduction in the long-term capital gains tax, which was eventually adopted, and a lowering of the consumer price index (CPI), which was not. The CPI was used especially to index tax brackets and to calculate cost-of-living adjustments (COLAs) for Social Security and other benefit programs. It was generally acknowledged to be about one percentage point too high and talk of a "correction" had been going on for some time. But an adjustment of 0.8 to 1 percent downward would increase taxes slightly and reduce COLAs significantly. So, it was a lever of enormous power and of great political sensitivity. Recognizing that this issue was controversial, Republicans urged the president to appoint a commission to come up with recommendations. For a time, Clinton seemed to favor this quick road to a settlement, but the proposal ran into strong, unified opposition from liberal Democrats, trade unions, and the AARP. With this kind of protest coming from his political base, Clinton said that he was disinclined to appoint such a commission.[32]

During this period, Republicans were having troubles of their own—especially in finding a formula with which to move ahead. One proposal, floated by Newt Gingrich and Tom DeLay, called for deferring tax cuts and starting with budget balancing, rather as they had planned to do in 1996. This drew fire in letters from conservative House and Senate Republicans, who wrote that tax cuts were an article of faith and that their constituents deserved tax relief now, not sometime in the future. Dick Armey, the House majority leader, rebuked Gingrich for going public with proposals that should have been discussed first in party councils. Senate Republican leaders, including Trent Lott and Finance chairman William Roth also disapproved.[33] John Kasich saw little prospect for a Republican budget and favored a coalition with the Blue Dog Democrats (see Chapter 3) Even Pete Domenici, the pragmatic negotiator, was giving up hope. Despite this disarray—or perhaps because of it—Dick Armey and Trent Lott announced they were planning to go ahead and would have budgets ready to report out by the middle of May.[34]

The budget process had stalled not so much over partisan differences as over the risks for either side of going first and the lack of a consensus proposal to serve as a basis for negotiation. Neither the president nor the congressional

Republicans were willing to yield much, or anything, to the other party without significant gains in return. As the announcement from Armey and Lott indicated, though, a critical decision point had been reached at which positions would harden and the political struggle would escalate unless there were some form of detente and an opportunity to cut some deals.

During the week of March 17, following Newt Gingrich's proposal to defer tax cuts, President Clinton invited Pete Domenici, John Kasich, and the ranking Democratic members of the budget committees to meet with him at the White House to discuss ways to break the budget impasse and narrow the gap between the two sides. By one account, the president's initiative was prompted by Newt Gingrich's proposal on tax cuts and the openness to negotiation that this move seemed to indicate.[35] That interpretation of events was a major reason for the Republican conservatives' angry reaction and strong protest in favor of a immediate tax cut. It seems more likely that Clinton and the administration understood full well that there would be some tax cuts and that, at most, Gingrich's proposal served as a pretext for a timely gambit.[36] In any event, in Clinton's words, they "agreed on a goal" of seeking an agreement and "a schedule to start discussion."[37]

Bargaining sessions at this level are usually called summits, and they do not have a good reputation. In 1990, the first President Bush not only lost on the deal, but broke his "no new taxes" pledge, which was commonly regarded as a major reason for his electoral defeat in 1992. And in 1995–96 Clinton stalled to such advantage that Republicans ultimately had to settle for no deal at all. In this present instance, though, there were favoring circumstances. Both parties had strong motivation to reach a deal, and each had a sense for the strength and will of the other. Both understand that if an escalating conflict were to be avoided, the time for aversive measures was at hand. Moreover, the process was well planned and managed in ordered steps from the first initiative through each subsequent stage.

For the budget talks, which began on April 8, the congressional delegation was broadened to include, in addition to budget chairmen, the chairmen and ranking members from the House Ways and Means and the Senate Finance committees. Heading the delegation from the White House were Chief of Staff Erskine Bowles, OMB Director Frank Raines, NEC Chairman Gene Sperling, and Legislative Affairs Director John Hilley.[38] On the first day, as a gesture of good faith, the White House offered to add $18 billion more in Medicare cuts to restore the savings to the $100 billion originally put on the table.[39] Otherwise, little happened in this initial round: four days were spent in reviewing Republican and administration policies and differences with respect to entitlements, discretionary spending, tax cuts, and new spending. Congressional representatives expressed gratification at the relative openness of Raines and Hilley; and Pete Domenici said that he thought a good beginning had been made.[40]

During the next week, neither side was putting concrete proposals on the table. In fact, House Democrats criticized Clinton for conceding too much, and Republican conservatives as well as Appropriations Committee members were urging the Budget Committees to get busy on a budget of their own. But no one was walking away from the negotiations, and there were important indications of flexibility on various points. Republicans talked little about entitlements or restructuring Medicare and more about lowered expectations for a tax cut. The administration considered the possibilities of a capital gains tax cut, an income-related premium for Medicare, and per capita caps for Medicaid. It was a "politics of assurance," cautiously inching toward a middling compromise point, seeking assurances (and evidence) that the other party was also moving and in relatively good faith.

The Republicans—not having developed a budget of their own—needed, at this point, to prepare for negotiation and for the possibility that the negotiations might succeed. This meant that they had to reach some collective judgments about what could be given up in exchange for what, and to think fast about alternative budgets and tax schedules. It also meant bringing along other party leaders, committee chairs, and the members. In this respect, summits are a particular problem since they involve semisecret negotiations with the political enemy after which the party loyalists are asked to be happy with the result. In the Senate, this maneuver was not especially difficult because the Senate was generally more comfortable in dealing with the White House and already had a well-supported Breaux-Chafee budget that was close to the administration proposal. In the House, though, a number of Republicans fundamentally opposed any deal with the White House and many were deeply committed to tax cuts and reducing the size of government. These Republican members, in particular, had to be asked to lower their expectations drastically. During this week, there was a great deal of explaining, and seeking and giving assurances. Some, like Dick Armey, the majority leader, got assurances directly from the White House, specifically that a large tax cut would be part of the final deal.[41] For the Republican members, John Kasich, accompanied by Tom DeLay and John Boehner, met with small groups throughout the week to explain the budget alternatives, give assurances, and ask for support— essential steps in preparing for eventual passage of the budget deal.[42]

A summit put the minority party—in this instance, the Democrats—in the unenviable situation of being shut out of the most important budget deliberations but then expected to support the president politically whatever he, with the opposition party, may have decided about entitlements and discretionary spending. In 1997, the White House worked successfully with Senate Democrats through John Hilley, who had been a former staff aide to Tom Daschle, the minority leader. In the House, though, relations with Minority Leader Richard Gephardt and the liberal Democrats were particularly strained because they were generally not consulted and often feared that "their" president was negotiating away the hard-fought gains of a generation. As a small footnote to history, some Democrats continued to support the president in 1997 partly because of White House outreach to the House and Senate during the winter of 1995–96 and the reservoir of trust and good will that had been established then.[43]

For Republicans, especially in the House, the important priorities were balancing the budget, a major tax cut, reining in entitlements, and reducing the size of the government. For a variety of reasons, they had to settle for some relatively modest tangible gains and for a budget process that sought much less in the way of structural changes than was the case in 1995 or even 1996.

One huge factor was the booming economy—which meant that all sorts of numbers, such as higher revenues, lower payouts for unemployment and Medicaid, and reduced interest payments on the debt, were going in the right direction. A common estimate is that two-thirds either of the deficit or of deficit reduction is the economy. Throughout this period, the deficit projections, whether those of CBO or OMB, kept coming down. This meant, of course, that a sense of crisis about the deficit and entitlements driving those deficits was gone. It mattered much less, for that matter, whether the estimates or scoring came from OMB or CBO since the numbers were turning out better than either had projected.

Not only was the deficit declining, so were the Medicare and Medicaid baselines. For Medicaid, the baseline had dropped by so much that, except for DSH payments, the program virtually ceased to be regarded as a source for savings. As for Medicare, CBO reduced the baseline projections by $15 billion in April 1996 and by another $60 billion in January 1997 (Reischauer et al. 1998). These declining baselines meant that the Medicare/Medicaid budget impact was smaller—so that there was less need to reduce these program expenditures. In addition, however, there would be less there to cut, so that significant reductions would be harder to come by. CBO was still projecting the Hospital Trust Fund to be in deficit by 2001.[44] But that only strengthened the argument for moderation, since big savings would come at an enormous political cost, while extending solvency of the trust fund would be both achievable and popular on both sides of the aisle.

In budget discussions, the White House made clear some of its vital interests, in addition to the amount and sources of budget savings. Block-granting Medicaid, for instance, was not an option. Also not to be considered were Medicare structural changes like those proposed in 1995: a global cap, a "defined contribution," or managed care options "independent of the central stream of Medicare dollars."[45] These constraints pretty much ruled out radical structural changes. In doing so, they also foreclosed this path as a way to achieve larger budget savings—either to reduce the deficit or to pay for a tax cut. In effect, they determined that 1997 was not going to be about ending or radically transforming entitlements—which was a limiting decision that greatly reduced the scope of conflict.

With limited prospects for Medicare and Medicaid savings, the discretionary side of the budget became even more important.[46] Since the Republicans regained control of the Congress in 1994, discretionary spending had been targeted in part because entitlement cuts—Social Security, Medicare and Medicaid—were difficult to get. Furthermore, cuts in the discretionary budget had a symbolic or ideological importance. Though discretionary spending was only 17 percent of the budget,[47] it funded almost every federal agency with the exception of defense, including those Republicans had sought in 1995 to defund, privatize, or hamstring administratively (Drew 1996:256–57). Therefore, Republicans pushed hard in this area, seeking with a number of different methods more than twice the $79 billion in savings that Clinton had proposed.[48]

For several reasons, savings from discretionary spending were not a hopeful prospect in 1997. One reason was a number of urgent or popular spending demands, such as $5 to $10 billion to renew rental contracts for Section 8 low-income housing; $15 billion or more to support the International Monetary Fund; and a bill with strong bipartisan support to fund highways, airports, and transportation infrastructure. Clinton's budget proposal included additional spending for environment, education, and other vote-getting programs politically costly to oppose. A supplemental bill for flood relief and Bosnia peacekeeping, though not part of the current budget, would sop up billions in needed offsets. All things considered, it would be hard to squeeze out much more than the $79 billion offered by Clinton without risky heroics such as writing an appropriations freeze into the budget resolution. This was urged by conservative senators Phil Gramm and Don Nickles, but rejected by Pete Domenici as an ineffectual gesture.[49]

Although congressional Democrats and Republican hard-liners both felt they were being sold out and complained of the concessions, there was not much enthusiasm for challenging the summit. Already two weeks past the April 15 statutory deadline for a budget resolution, the pressure of time was important, especially if the Republicans were to change course and develop a budget of their own. There were renewed demands for going their separate way, but a Republican budget at this point would have been difficult to put together. The time crunch, further delay in the appropriations cycle, the prospect of another extended confrontation with the president, and the huge down-side risks associated with this venture made it seem, by then, exhausting and imprudent, maybe impossible. With a margin of only twenty votes in the House, a majority-only budget was unlikely. And there were enough differences with the Blue Dog Democrats to make a coalition budget unacceptable to Republican conservatives.[50] Even if a House Republican budget could be hastily assembled and passed, there was still the Senate, where the Breaux-Chafee alternative was a moderate, bipartisan compromise not too different from the president's offer. Indeed, a telling point with many House Republicans was that they could do as well with the president as they could with the

Senate. And pervading everything in Congress was a general tiredness and a reluctance to mobilize for another major confrontation.[51]

As the negotiations moved into a third round of talks on April 28, help of a sort appeared unexpectedly with a CBO communication that the deficit over five years would be about $114 billion lower than previously estimated.[52] For the negotiators, this windfall unsettled deals already made and extended the negotiations, but it did allow for some sweeteners that made the whole package more attractive both to conservative Republicans and to congressional Democrats. About $64 billion was allocated toward further deficit reduction. Another $24 billion enabled the negotiators to eliminate a reduction in the CPI, which was unpopular both with Democrats and Republicans. The per capita caps for Medicaid went out.[53] And some relatively small amounts were earmarked for health care for children, transportation, and Clinton's welfare-to-work amendments.[54]

Like most deals that work, both the Republicans and the administration could claim a victory, both got what was essential for them, and there were, so far, no major defections. For the Republicans, there was a balanced budget in five years and ten years of trust fund solvency. They also got a net tax cut of $85 billion over five years and $250 billion over ten years, including cuts in capital gains and estate taxes. For Clinton, there were concessions in discretionary spending that would allow continued subsidies for low-income housing, a tax credit and deduction for postsecondary students, and added expenditures for environment and welfare. Reductions in Medicare and Medicaid spending were pegged at his budget figures of $115 billion from Medicare[55] and $15 billion from Medicaid, but with a child health benefit, estimated by CBO to cost $6.8 billion over five years. Most of the health benefits lost in the welfare reform legislation were restored.[56] The Part A/Part B switch remained, though with some beneficiary liability. Medicare savings were to be generated primarily with the traditional Part A and Part B cost savers, without major structural changes or a spending cap. For Medicaid, savings would come almost entirely from hospital DSH payments, without per capita caps or other structural changes.

Least satisfied were conservative Republicans and liberal Democrats. The conservative Republicans objected that their party was betraying its fundamental principles with this bipartisan compromise. Senate Democrats gave the deal, at most, two cheers. Most discontented were the House liberal Democrats, especially Richard Gephardt, objecting to tax cuts favoring the wealthy and spending cuts or lack of benefits for the poor. Support for the deal was broad, backed by a majority of Democrats in both House and Senate. But that support was also shallow, especially in the House. At one point, during floor debate on the budget resolution, an amendment that would have added billions of new dollars for highway construction was moved by Bud Schuster, chairman of the Transportation and Infrastructure Committee. This amendment, a potential deal-breaker, was defeated by a perilously small majority,

214–216, with Democrats voting 3–1 in favor.[57] A similar attempt in the Senate, sponsored by John Warner (R., Va.) and Max Baucus (D., Mont.) was also defeated.

Despite its initial fragility, the budget deal survived intact through the Budget Committee markups, floor debates, and, eventually, the conference. It was modified in some particulars, mostly in ways that built upon the main principles underlying the consensus. It was a serious move toward bipartisanship in which each side made some genuine concessions and it bought in return a period of collaborative politics. To return to our main topic, with respect to Medicare and Medicaid, it bounded controversy, provided important assurances, got rid of some hot issues, and developed language that would enable partisans to work together despite their differences of principle.

With the summit agreement as a guide, the budget resolution moved through Congress expeditiously and with little difficulty. The agreement was reported to the House and Senate on May 2. After the initial euphoria subsided, there was a period of uncertainty and haggling over the meaning of some of the provisions, especially tax provisions.[58] Resolutions in both houses moved quickly to markups on May 16 and 19. With one day of debate, the House approved its resolution on May 21 by a vote of 333–99—with 132 Democrats voting in favor, easily satisfying Clinton's promise to back only a resolution supported by a majority of his party's caucus.[59] The Senate passed its resolution on May 23 by a vote of 78–22, with 14 Republicans and 8 Democrats voting against the measure.[60] Congress was in recess over Memorial Day, but approved the conference report on June 5.[61]

The budget resolutions added little of substantive importance for either Medicare or Medicaid beyond the provisions already in the summit agreement. There would be two reconciliation bills, as requested by President Clinton, one to balance the budget and a second with the tax amendments. Reconciliation scoring would follow CBO numbers. The summit numbers on Medicare and Medicaid savings and additional benefits were accepted. The $16 billion earmarked for child health survived. In the three days of Senate debate, a number of amendments were offered supporting increased expenditures for highway projects, welfare benefits, and child health. A major new initiative, which almost passed, was the Hatch-Kennedy proposal for a $0.47 per pack increase in the cigarette tax, which would yield $30 billion in additional revenues—$10 billion of which would be devoted to further reduction of the deficit and $20 billion to child health.[62]

III. THE BUDGET RECONCILIATION

According to the official schedule, the reconciliation process began with the passage of the budget resolution conference report on June 5. This report "ordered" the authorizing committees in both House and Senate to report back proposals implementing their reconciliation spending reductions by June 13. Deadlines for the tax bill were June 1420.[63] These dates were aspirations—subject to revision because of legislative workloads or unresolved issues. In this instance, the House Commerce and Ways and Means committees reported early, though the Senate Finance Committee, held up over Medicaid and child health issues, did not report until June 18. These prosaic facts have a background.

Early in 1997, there was a general expectation, considerably strengthened by President Clinton's budget message and his reaching out to Congress, that there would be a reconciliation bill. Authorizing committees in both House and Senate were working, more or less, with that presumption in mind, reviving and modifying old proposals and bills or developing new ones that fit with a reconciliation strategy. The budget summit encouraged that process and greatly facilitated the work of the authorizing committees by narrowing the range of alternatives, getting a number of refractory and highly charged issues off the table, and setting realistic, consensus budget targets.

Important in this context was the continuing shift in the House from leadership-driven to committee-centered for the reconciliation—more like the balance typical for ordinary legislation. In 1997 there was, for instance, no speaker's task force like that of 1995, nor even a Medicare or Medicaid task force of the more modest traditional variety. The authorizing committees were much more the centers of activity—which gave them a larger role in deciding how to fulfill the mandates of the budget resolution.

The authorizing committees had been over much of this same ground in 1995 and 1996, albeit in different circumstances. As a result, there was a presumption or tacit agreement that some of the concessions fought over and staked out then by provider and beneficiary advocacy groups could be regarded as starting points or even close approximations to a final deal in the reconciliation negotiations of 1997. It was generally understood, for instance, that there would be a PSO option in the Medicare Choice program, some redistribution of HMO payments, and increased flexibility in structuring Medicaid programs, etc., and the range of options associated with such issues had been considerably narrowed so that the principle itself was less at issue and pragmatic accommodations were easier to reach. It was important, too, that most of the principals and the staffs had been through the earlier cycles, had the language and the formulas, and knew the moves.

Because of the political context, this was an unusually constrained reconciliation. Both the summit and the budget resolution went beyond the norm in specifying how much particular programs could be cut and in ruling out substantive changes.[64] Committee chairmen are used to contesting, amending, or even ignoring such restrictions; but in this instance there was an added constraint—not to spoil a rare opportunity by upsetting an arduously bargained and carefully constructed agreement. Furthermore, the president had given clear indications that he meant to be involved in the reconciliation process up to the end, from the work of the authorizing committees to the final conference. Time was important. The summit had put the budget process two weeks behind schedule and the conference was likely to a lengthy one. Especially with respect to Medicare and Medicaid, any attempt to deviate substantially from the agreements would provoke controversy and further delay the reconciliation process. There were good reasons, therefore, to be businesslike and pragmatic, and get the deals done within the constraints established. Only a few diehards were spoiling for a fight—people were weary from two years of confrontation and wrangling and longed to be constructive. All together, these circumstances meant that committee members and staff had to concentrate on what they could get done.[65]

Medicare

A curious feature of the reconciliation in 1997, as contrasted with 1995, was that Medicare was not highly controversial, and particularly not so in the House. A child health program that originated in the Senate generated more partisan excitement than Medicare. With respect to Medicare, the most controversial proposals originated in the Senate, such as one to raise the age of Medicare eligibility to sixty-seven. This relative quiescence with respect to Medicare in the House is attributable in part to the summit and budget resolution that took a number of the most controversial items off the table. But the bipartisan comity associated with Medicare in 1997 owed much to the Ways and Means Health Subcommittee, and efforts there to craft the best bill possible within the established constraints.

In this particular circumstance, "best" meant not strategically or politically best, but a bipartisan, consensus bill that would be substantively sound and technically competent. This decision was made in advance of the budget summit, although prudent calculation would also indicate that any comprehensive Medicare bill in 1997 would probably have to meet the summit constraints. The agreement owed much to the Republican subcommittee chairman, Bill Thomas, who took pride in his Medicare expertise and had a serious respect for good policy, and to Pete Stark, the ranking Democrat on the subcommittee, who shared in this attitude. Transforming this worthy objective into a bill owed much to Chip Kahn, the subcommittee chief of staff, who stayed on to see a Medicare reform bill to completion, and to Bill Vaughan, Stark's administrative assistant, who was a source of expertise, institutional memory, and constructive suggestions.[66]

It was understood from the beginning that the subcommittee was working toward a major reform of Medicare and not just meeting budget cutting targets. The administration and congressional Democrats shared this objective with the Republicans since it had been seven years since the last major reconciliation and there was an increased need for a legislative vehicle to enact all sorts of needed changes, both large and small.[67] As was traditional with Medicare legislation, the House Ways and Means Committee, i.e., the Health Subcommittee, took the lead and major responsibility for producing a comprehensive version of a bill, for worrying more systematically about general principles, and for keeping track of small parts.

One obstacle to a sound, bipartisan Medicare bill was the legacy of the past: committee members who were ignorant of Medicare and partisans who distrusted the other side. In a gesture that in retrospect seems obviously right for the occasion but showed boldness and faith in rational inquiry and the power of education, Bill Thomas and Chip Kahn scheduled a comprehensive set of hearings to review Medicare policy, learn about the problems, and promote consensus on remedies.[68] These hearings began early, immediately after the president's budget proposal of February 5, which was given serious attention in an initial hearing. Over the next three months, thirteen hearings were held, covering every major aspect of the Medicare program. With oral testimony restricted to invited guests only, the hearings set a high standard for relevance and policy expertise. They were well attended by members and were supplemented by briefings from congressional staff agencies and by seminars conducted by Chip Kahn for the members' legislative assistants.[69]

The subcommittee had an abundance of technical resources and expertise to draw upon in addition to its own staff. As in 1995, the directors and staff of ProPAC and PPRC provided technical information, data, and projections for Part A and Part B and other Medicare topics under consideration. More occasionally, congressional staff agencies—the CBO, the GAO, and the CRS—supplied technical studies, data on trends, and expenditure projections. This time around, the majority and minority staff collaborated extensively, sharing information and critiquing proposals. The administration cooperated in working out acceptable compromises and brought in HCFA staff to help draft some of the technical provisions.[70] Given the time constraints, an enormous amount of technical information and expertise was assimilated. The committee wrote its own legislation—none of it was drafted by interest groups or a task force.[71]

In developing the legislative proposal, the subcommittee worked from the Medicare Preservation Act of 1995, removing its most controversial elements and modifying other provisions in the light of subsequent political and technical developments.[72] Under the first category, the fail-safe and look-back feature, the defined contribution philosophy, and the notion of "two HCFAs" came out. The major new addition was an array of prospective payment systems covering pretty much the entire spectrum of outpatient and postacute services. Also new was Medigap regulation and a PPO addition to the MedicarePlus health plans. The secretary was directed to develop a managed care risk adjuster. A small addition was made to the fraud and abuse legislation established by HIPAA. There were some new demonstrations, and a provision making the Program of All-inclusive Care for the Elderly (PACE) a permanent Medicare option. HCFA got some minor additional authority to help implement its new prudent purchaser initiative, and a small list of preventive health benefits was added.

This unimpressive list would seem to indicate that not much heavy lifting was going on, and that the basic achievement of the subcommittee was to take out a few major elements and rearrange the other parts. However, the members and staff were seriously striving for a bipartisan product and to do it right. That meant that much of the previous legislation had to be rethought in the light of what a first iteration had revealed and, in addition, to incorporate minority perspectives. All the payment mechanisms were reviewed and many of them revised. With baselines dropping, expenditure reductions— though smaller[73]—were often harder to justify. Each of the outpatient prospective payment systems was a specialized and complex thicket of problems in itself. There were hundreds of minor provisions that were, nevertheless, major issues to some particular group.[74] And the legislation, as a whole and in particular, had to work both technically and politically.

Except for the fail-safe cap and the "two HCFAs" provision, the subcommittee treatment of MedicarePlus—or Medicare+Choice as it became in the final legislation—followed the original Medicare Preservation Act of 1995 closely. Many sections were included verbatim, with changes only in numbers or dates. Most of the material on marketing of plans stayed the same, except for such changes as slightly less freedom to disenroll, more time for the secretary to review marketing materials, and specifying that the secretary "may" contract with "non-Federal entities" in administering the election procedures, instead of "shall, to the maximum extent feasible" do so. The major change in plan options was to include preferred provider organizations (PPOs) and to limit Medicare MSAs to 500,000 beneficiaries.[75] Also, like the earlier legislation, the 1997 bill included quality and consumer protection standards, updated to include more patients' rights and mandated for all MedicarePlus plans.

One way in which the subcommittee bill moved significantly beyond the Medicare Preservation Act of 1995 was with respect to quality standards, patient protection, and consumer information. As noted earlier, the House bill of 1995 was favorable to beneficiaries in all of these respects. A major step in 1997 was to mandate quality assurance programs for Medicare and Medicaid managed care plans that incorporated outcome measurement and continuous quality improvement (CQI). In effect, Medicare health plans would have to meet demanding, state-of-the-art standards currently being devised in the private sector and by HCFA to address the specialized needs of quality assurance for managed care. Plans would also be required to provide quality information in their marketing materials designed to facilitate plan comparison and consumer choice. In addition to the patient protections in the earlier bill, the 1997 version added several of the proposals being currently discussed for inclusion in patient protection acts or patients' "bills of rights," such as the "prudent layperson" standard[76] for access to emergency medical care, clarifying responsibility for poststabilization care, and requiring expedited appeals from health plan decisions.

These provisions had bipartisan support and were worked out in cooperation with administration officials, mostly from HCFA. One compelling reason for the quality standards, especially for Medicaid, was a need to balance increased flexibility for state programs with standards and protections for the beneficiaries. If this prescription was good medicine for Medicaid, why not Medicare as well? In any event, as one staff aide pointed out, government was paying for these benefits, so it would seem appropriate to assure the quality of the product that was purchased.[77]

There was concern about how much competitive edge and market share managed care plans might lose from adding such options as PSOs and PPOs, constraints on marketing, and expensive quality assurance and improvement systems. As one illustration, CBO noted the factors inhibiting growth or reducing the cost-saving potential of capitated plans and lowered its estimate of savings in consideration of items such as the addition of a PSO option, increased coverage for emergency medical care, and limits on provider incentives.

In accord with the summit agreement, the five-year Medicare savings were projected to be $115 billion—with only $6.8 billion. or about 6 percent, scheduled for 1998, an election year. More remarkable than the back-loading, though, was the extent to which these savings came from "traditional" sources and had very little to do with managed care, market-type reforms, or even prospective payment systems. Over half of the total, nearly $60 billion, would come from hospitals, cuts in the physician fee schedule, and leaving the Part B premium contribution at 25 percent.[78] Net savings from managed care plans were scored by CBO at $18 billion, with almost 90 percent of that expected to result from lower growth rates in FFS Medicare, from which the capitation rates would be calculated.[79] The secretary was directed to develop prospective payment systems or fee schedules for skilled nursing facilities, rehabilitation hospitals, outpatient hospital services, outpatient therapy providers, and home health services. Total net savings from these provisions were estimated by CBO to be $23 billion over five years, but the prospective payment systems had yet to be developed. For the short term, with the exception of the SNFs, most of the significant five-year savings would come from cutting per visit and aggregate limits (home health services), limiting overpayments (hospital outpatient), or extending the physician fee schedule (outpatient therapy).[80]

The wholesale adoption of the outpatient prospective payment systems deserves comment, since it would seem to represent a concession to the administration, especially HCFA, as well as a broad endorsement of administered pricing. For years, such prospective systems had been under development in HCFA, though not generally given high priority. Leaders in the provider community usually supported this approach as rational and systematic—better than the unpredictable vagaries of an administrative nonsystem and legislative annual appropriations. In the hearings, the subcommittee members saw for themselves the jumble that time and neglect had created.[81] Prospective payment systems were generally viewed as a good thing and, at the time, pretty much the best game in town. HCFA leadership, with reservations, expressed confidence that the job could be done.[82] Various opinions have been expressed about this decision. Some Republicans believed their own priorities would have been better served by continuing to modify payment systems incrementally and monitoring progress over time.[83] Others expressed a view that HCFA was promising too much, but were content to let them bear the onus of failure. It was a move away from micromanaging payment, but without much assurance as to the successor methodology.

One important program enhancement that HCFA and the administration did not get was "prudent purchaser" authority. Introduced in the HCFA Strategic Plan of 1994 (Health Care Financing Administration 1994:25) and pushed strongly by the administrator, Bruce Vladeck, the idea was to strengthen the program by adapting private sector methods of purchasing and contracting and to take advantage of HCFA's market power as the main purchaser of government-financed health care. Many of these ideas had been around for years, but they received contemporary support from the General Accounting Office, which urged the "modernization" of the traditional FFS Medicare program and from Vice-President Gore's "reinventing" government initiative.[84] A major aim of this approach was to use tools and methods available to the private sector, and especially managed care plans, but in ways acceptable to the FFS Medicare beneficiaries. Examples would be an authority to buy medical supplies at prices available to other bulk purchasers, use of competitive bidding or a power to contract selectively, use of case-management techniques in the FFS program, and contracting with "centers of excellence," such as the Cleveland Clinic or a medical school, for all-inclusive treatment of chronic and severely ill patients.

This notion of HCFA as a prudent purchaser rather than a passive bill-payer, along with the idea of Medicare as a continuum of high-quality and beneficiary friendly plan alternatives, was central to HCFA's long-term strategy, was strongly supported by the Clinton administration, and resonated with a number of congressional Democrats. It was especially seen as important in enabling FFS Medicare, then and in the future, to cope with adverse selection and to remain competitive with HMOs and other managed care plans (Fox 1998). As noted, the subcommittee bill largely accommodated the second objective, for instance, with the addition of PPOs to the plan offerings and the quality standards and patient and consumer protection features. On the first part, though, the prudent purchasing approach, the subcommittee adopted a "wait and see" attitude, including a number of demonstrations (rather than new authority), some of them more part of the Republican agenda than the administration's. The bill did provide for an open-ended extension of the "centers of excellence" demonstration. It included another competitive bidding project to test a "market oriented pricing system" in a range of Medicare plans—this project to be accompanied by advisory committees to monitor both the plan design and its implementation. But there was no avowed recognition or adoption of the prudent purchaser concept as such.[85]

For the most part, the subcommittee preserved its bipartisan spirit and kept politically sensitive items out of the bill. Two notable exceptions were Medical Savings Accounts (MSAs) and the $250,000 cap on medical malpractice awards for noneconomic damages. MSAs were established as a demonstration project by HIPAA in 1996 for the private sector—though enrollees reaching the age of sixty-five would be allowed to continue with their MSAs under Medicare, so that the MSA option acquired an element of permanency. Bill Thomas, chairman of the subcommittee, seemed to have no particular liking for MSAs himself, but the Ways and Means chairman and the Texas delegation did, and among Republican membership there was strong support for them, especially from the Conservative Action Teams (CATs). So he proposed a "demonstration" for Medicare MSAs for 500,000 beneficiaries that would continue indefinitely and allow enrollees to retain their plans. Democrats, including the administration, objected both to the extension of MSAs to Medicare and to the permanent features of the scheme. In a party-line vote of 7–5, the subcommittee defeated a Stark amendment to cap the program at 100,000 (enough for a demonstration) and limit it to four years. Subsequently, though, Chairman Thomas agreed to a four-year limit and the White House withdrew its opposition.[86] In another party-line vote of 8–5, the subcommittee refused to strip the medical malpractice cap of $250,000. This perennial got included[87] as a result of some late and intense AMA lobbying.[88] Unlike the MSA proposal, the malpractice cap produced little stir in the subcommittee—it had been passed twice before and stripped in the Senate, so that adopting it at this stage was more ceremonial than substantive.

Two relatively noncontroversial but important items were the merger of ProPAC and PPRC into a new Medicare Payment Advisory Commission and the establishment of a fifteen-member Bipartisan Commission on the Effect of the "Babyboom" Generation on Medicare, to report not later than May 1, 1999, on how to keep Medicare solvent until the year 2030. Both of these recommendations had been in the Medicare Preservation Act of 1995 and were generally expected to be a part of the 1997 legislation.

On June 4, only two weeks after final passage of the budget resolution, the subcommittee unanimously approved its Medicare reconciliation proposals. Chairman Thomas made a speech praising the work of the subcommittee and the cooperative, bipartisan spirit that had made it possible. Pete Stark, the ranking Democrat—generally known for brickbats rather than bouquets—graciously commended the chairman and the Republican members, with special praise for Chip Kahn, the Republican chief of staff. Staff aides still speak, enthusiastically and even misty-eyed with nostalgia, about how splendid it was, working together constructively, with talented counterparts in Congress as well as the administration, and trying to do it right.

Few significant amendments were made by the full Ways and Means Committee, which passed the Medicare budget bill by a vote of 36–3 on June 9. One amendment changed the blended capitation rate for Medicare HMOs to a 50/50 local/national blend from one that was 70 percent local and 30 percent national—a change that benefited rural plans and cost the government $300 million over five years. That expense was covered, however, by an additional $300 million that, according to latest CBO scoring, the current proposals would save.[89] By a vote of 20–19, the full committee defeated a heavily lobbied provision on hospital capital payments that would have benefited for-profit hospitals.[90]

The Commerce Committee approved its bill on June 12, after committee markups that were more partisan than those in Ways and Means. With respect to Medicare, the two bills were almost identical. One important difference was in the treatment of medical education and DSH allowances that were to be "carved out" of managed care payments. Unlike Ways and Means, the Commerce Committee provided that these funds would be "targeted," i.e., paid directly to the hospitals and medical schools actually serving the low-income and uninsured patients.[91] Commerce made the Part A/Part B shift immediate, rather than phasing it in over time as Ways and Means had done. The full committee also let stand a subcommittee patient protection amendment, backed by anti-HMO Republicans and Democrats, that would allow patients and attending physicians, rather than the health plan, to set the hospital length of stay.

Floor action on the budget bill produced almost no Medicare changes. In fact, the only important, largely automatic, changes were made by the Rules Committee in assembling the rule for debate. The Commerce Committee's length-of-stay amendment was taken out in response to a CBO estimate that it would increase federal spending by $800 million over five years, and $1 billion was added to help pay for Part B premium support for Specially Qualified Low-income Medicare Beneficiaries (SLMBs).[92]

Senate.   As in 1995, the House bill was largely the template for Medicare, providing many of the policy assumptions and structural features that served as first approximations. There were significant differences with respect to one of the plan options under Medicare Choice, as it was known in the Senate; formulas for managed care payments; the Medical Savings Accounts; the medical malpractice $250,000 cap on noneconomic damages; and the emphasis put upon the long-term future of Medicare.

The mood was less hectic or partisan than in 1995 or 1996, with many proposals cosponsored and enjoying strong bipartisan support. Bipartisanship and individualism have traditionally characterized the Senate, especially with respect to Medicare legislation. Many Senators in 1995, including Republicans, had been skeptical about major structural changes in Medicare; and the 1997 summit agreement on budget parameters strengthened that attitude. There were still sharp disagreements and some proposals that attacked fundamentals of the Medicare program, but they tended to arise from particularistic concerns of local areas or professional groups and not a shared policy stance or ideology of the majority.

As with the House bill, the Senate Finance Committee draft included as options traditional FFS Medicare, managed care plans, point-of-service (PoS), PSOs, PPOs, and MSAs. The committee added a "private FFS" option that could operate with a "private fee schedule," in other words, without a Medicare fee schedule or balance billing limits. This option had been included in the House bill in 1995, but not in 1997. It had strong appeal both to physicians and to economic conservatives, but was opposed by the administration and by Democrats because it was contrary to the underlying social insurance principle of Medicare and a threat to the risk pool. When later combined with the Kyl amendment, which would allow Medicare enrollees to use their own money to pay for services from physicians who did not participate in the Medicare program, the private fee schedule initiative began to seem quite threatening. [93] Nevertheless, both of these changes found their way into the final legislation.

Senate changes in the managed care payments were not a partisan issue; but they were sharply divisive, setting urban and high-payment areas against rural and low-payments areas and threatening, at times, to become another formula fight similar to the one that erupted over the Medicaid block grants in 1995. The House formula, which was a consensus proposal worked out in collaboration with the American Association of Health Plans, was relatively generous and not highly redistributive as between rich and poor payment areas. [94] In the Senate, there was considerable sophistication about managed care and a strong awareness of how inflated and inequitable payment rates based on the AAPCC could be, especially as between counties with historically high AAPCCs and poorer or thriftier areas not so richly blessed. [95] Accordingly, the Senate version was tough on HMOs, especially urban ones, phasing out GME and DSH payments from the managed care rates, linking the update to growth in the gross domestic product (GDP), [96] and adding a special risk adjustment "tax" of 5 percent on new enrollees in managed care plans. [97] Like the House, the Senate provided for an increasing blend of local and national rates, scheduled to reach 50/50 by 2002. It set a lower minimum annual percentage increase than the House. At the same time, it gave rural and relatively poorer plans the benefit of a higher payment floor, providing that no plan should receive less than 85 percent of the national average rate. Both the House and Senate specified that these payment arrangements should be "budget neutral," which meant in practical terms that if the updates were low, other adjustments would lag.

Some measure of the comparative harshness of the Senate plan was illustrated by an AAHP study showing that, under the Senate version, urban HMOs serving about 60 percent of Medicare beneficiaries enrolled in managed care plans would experience payment reductions of 15 percent or more by 2002.[98] HMOs in Miami and New Orleans, would be hit with a 35 percent reduction in monthly capitation rates. As another illustration, CBO scored Senate managed care savings over five years at $30 billion, and the House at only $19 billion.[99]

Other topics in dispute between House and Senate were Medical Savings Accounts and the $250,000 cap on malpractice awards for noneconomic damages. Neither of these was expected to fare well in the Senate, and they lived up to these expectations. As for the malpractice provision, it had a long history of defeat in the Senate, whether as part of a product liability initiative or tucked into a reconciliation bill. If reported out of committee, it would almost certainly have been stripped from its legislative vehicle, but it was buried in the committee. MSAs had a somewhat more unusual fate. Private sector MSAs enjoyed considerable support, especially from senators in rural states, where they might be not only convenient but quite possibly the only kind of insurance available to farmers and small-town artisans. When it came to Medicare, though, Finance Committee members like Chafee, Graham, and Rockefeller strongly opposed them as a direct challenge to the concept of social insurance. Moreover, 500,000 of them, which was the number in Chairman Roth's bill, was far more than needed for a demonstration, would cost extra money, and was, properly, out of place in a reconciliation bill. MSAs did emerge from the committee, but in a radically amended form. By a vote of 11–9, the Finance Committee accepted amendments by Senator Rockefeller to reduce the maximum deductibles from $6,000 in Roth's plan to $1,500 for an individual and $2,250 for a family. Beneficiaries' out-of-pocket expenses would be capped at $3,000. A second major amendment, which had been artfully baited with sweeteners, reduced the number eligible for enrollment to 100,000. This passed the committee by a vote of 12–8. Together, these amendments cut the MSA initiative back to a number more appropriate for a demonstration and a structure much closer to traditional health insurance.[100]

A fundamental policy difference between the House and the Senate was over the long-term future of Medicare as an entitlement for an increasingly older population. In the House bill, this issue was scarcely touched upon as such, except for the establishment of a bipartisan "baby boomer" commission. In the Senate, a small cluster of amendments helped frame a continuing debate on such issues as the nature of social insurance and the Medicare entitlement, equity between the generations, and how to prepare for the demographic and technological challenges that would confront Medicare by the year 2030.

These amendments—which would have "means-tested" Medicare, gradually raised the eligibility age from sixty-five to sixty-seven, and added a $5 copay for home health visit—got broad support from a diverse group of senators. Some, like Breaux (D., La.) and Kerrey,(D., Neb.) who had served on the 1994 Bipartisan Commission on Entitlement and Tax Reform, shared a concern about the long-term fiscal integrity of Medicare. Chafee and a few other moderates thought more attention should be paid to mothers and children and less to the elderly. Fiscal conservatives, like Gramm, wanted to see more of the burden of payment for Medicare shifted to beneficiaries.

The Finance Committee's proposal raising the Medicare eligibility age to sixty-seven was promoted as consistent with Social Security, already scheduled to make this change gradually over twenty-five years, from 2003 to 2027. The Medicare amendment produced no scorable savings, but would add to long-term solvency for the trust fund. Despite a low-profile presentation, this initiative provoked strong opposition from leading advocacy groups for the aging, from business and industry, and from the administration. The major objections were that raising eligibility would lengthen the period of time without coverage for early retirees and workers discharged from down-sized industries, and that it would greatly increase the retiree liabilities of industries.[101] This provision did not survive the conference; but it left troubling questions of what considerations should determine the age for eligibility and of how much weight should be given to individual retirement preferences and industry practices.

"Means testing" the Part B deductible[102] was another proposal more interesting theoretically than a first inspection might suggest. The Part B deductible would be related to the beneficiary's income—for individuals with incomes over $50,000 or couples over $75,000, the deductible would increase by stages from $100 to a maximum of $2,160 a year. Though this provision was approved 18–2 by the Finance Committee and would affect, initially, only about 6 percent of the Medicare beneficiaries, it generated strong opposition from the House, the administration, and among beneficiary groups, over the principle itself and especially over how to administer it (see p. 229). This proposal did not survive the conference either; but it left unresolved a tension dating back to the original Medicare legislation: between social insurance (Part A) and a subsidized, voluntary insurance plan (Part B) and what should be the balance between them (Myers 1970:87).

The home health copay provided another instructive example, this time of an informal accommodation that is difficult or perilous to disturb. The

Finance Committee proposed a $5 copay for home health visits that would be capped at the same amount as the Part A deductible. With home health visits often exceeding two hundred per year, the need for some deterrent would seem obvious. At the same time, studies showed that these high-use beneficiaries tended to be the poorest and sickest, for whom home health visits served as a safety net and as an alternative to a nursing home.[103] Since this group had little choice, a copay did not so much deter as inflict yet one more penalty for being poor and sick. Furthermore, keeping such people in the hospital or transferring them to a nursing home was not necessarily the best solution, either for them or for the government. In other words, a $5 copay had symbolic value, but did not get at the deep-lying problems. Its loss in the conference was not mourned.

Of these provisions, the only one that was adopted was the most hortatory and had the least immediate practical significance: establishing a bipartisan commission on the future of Medicare. The House, the Senate, and the administration had all made such a proposal at various times, both as an alternative to a more substantive initiative, and as an earnest of good intentions for the future. The Senate version, much the most comprehensive, extended the time horizon to the year 2030, and asked for recommendations on the feasibility of a buy-in at age sixty-two, the impact of chronic disease and disability trends on program costs, and the funding of graduate medical education along with such staples as extending solvency and reviewing program structure. Not all of these recommendations survived, but they had a substantial effect in broadening the version adopted by the conference.

In commenting on these Senate proposals, President Clinton acknowledged that some of them might have merit—such as the means testing and the increase in age of eligibility—but said they needed to be discussed within a larger context and over a longer term in order to decide about Medicare's future.[104] This was wise counsel; but most times, and especially with reconciliation bills, present urgencies crowd out a larger vision. The Senate bill was a modest effort to counter this tendency. And despite the general view that commissions are usually a way not to act, this particular measure proved ultimately to be politically important, though not in the way most of its supporters expected (see p. 350ff).

Floor action in the Senate on June 24 and 25, despite the host of amendments offered, made little change in the Finance Committee report. A few of the amendments were adopted, some of them important and one, at least, whimsically characteristic of American legislative politics. The latter example followed upon the adoption of a bipartisan motion by Roth and Moynihan to make higher income beneficiaries pay more of the Part B premium rather than means-testing the Part B deductible—a change generally recognized as fairer to the less affluent beneficiaries.[105] Senator Kennedy moved to delay the beginning of this change for two years, from 1998 to 2000. His motion was defeated. But then—in a move to "share the pain"—Kennedy proposed that the same means test be applied to Senators themselves. This motion was adopted by a voice vote.[106]

The Senate adopted by another voice vote an amendment by John Kyl (R., Ariz.) that would permit Medicare beneficiaries to use their own money to pay for services of physicians who did not participate in the Medicare program. This amendment, seemingly innocuous and arguably appropriate for a free country, has since caused an unusual amount of perplexity and controversy.

Medicaid and Child Health

With Medicaid, as with Medicare, the summit agreement bounded and structured the work of the budget and authorizing committees, but for Medicaid, there were some important differences. Even with the budget agreements, a basic conflict remained between program flexibility and beneficiary protection and how, practically, to achieve a workable compromise between them. Another important difference was the proposal of a new child health benefit, which led to a revival, on a lesser scale, of the entitlement controversy. Also, partisanship was more salient for Medicaid, especially in the House. Despite these complicating factors, the authorizing committees, the House and Senate leaders, and the administration were able to work effectively within their negotiating framework, producing legislation that won broad acceptance and provided workable and even elegant solutions to some of the policy dilemmas.

As with Medicare, some settled understandings had developed as a legacy from the budget wars of 1995 and 1996. By 1997, no one was seriously advocating block-granting of Medicaid, except as occasional saber rattling.[107] New entitlements or "unfunded mandates" were also out of fashion. In general terms, Congress, the administration, and the National Governors' Association were agreed that greater programmatic flexibility for the states along with less intrusive forms of accountability and selective protections for beneficiaries were, in principle, the way to head. Within this consensus, it was understood that both the president and the Republicans in Congress had critical or symbolic priorities that needed to be addressed, such as the Boren Amendment for Republicans and protection of various categories of "dual eligibles"[108] for the administration. While new entitlements or mandates were, in the mildest of terms, likely to be unpopular, there was strong bipartisan support for extending insurance to the one in seven American children without health care coverage[109] and for improving and updating the standards applicable to Medicaid managed care.[110]

The budget committees' reconciliation instructions primarily set savings targets, leaving details of how they were to be achieved largely up to the authorizing committees. For the five-year period 1998–2002, the agreement required overall reductions of $17.8 billion ($13.6 billion net) over five years, with almost three-fourths of that amount delayed until the last two years. It was assumed that most of the savings would come from Medicaid DSH payments, but the exact share was not specified. Outlays totaling $4.2 billion would help low-income Medicare beneficiaries with the cost of Part B premiums and increase the matching rate for the District of Columbia and Puerto Rico. A major inclusion was $16 billion for a new program to extend medical care to five million uninsured children by 2002. The instructions specified that the money could be used for (1) standard Medicaid coverage, including outreach programs; (2) grants to the states to cover insurance for uninsured children; or (3) "for other possibilities, if mutually agreeable" (Center for Budget and Policy Priorities 1997:3). Again, details were left up to the committees. Moreover, in the House, jurisdiction over the child health program was assigned jointly to Commerce and Ways and Means, with no instructions about allocation of funds between the committees (ibid.).

In practice, the lack of specifying directives, appropriate for resolution instructions generally, led to two kinds of disputes between Congress and the administration. One was simply different views as to what had been agreed upon by the budget summit. For instance, the administration thought the agreement committed $1.5 billion to help low-income beneficiaries pay for increased Part B premiums. House Republicans said that the commitment was only to offset increases resulting from the Part A/Part B shift in home health services;[111] another example was the restoration of disability benefits to legal aliens—questioned in a House Budget Committee fact sheet released after the summit.[112] A second kind of dispute arose from differences over how money would be saved. Governors, for example, wanted less cut from DSH money and argued that their "flexibility" savings (e.g., Medicaid HMOs) could offset the reduced savings. CBO disagreed with the governors' estimate of the flexibility savings. Would this NGA interpretation violate the spirit of the summit agreement? Whatever the right answer, such issues were an important part of the ongoing negotiations during the reconciliation process, requiring continuing engagement by the administration and leading to charges and countercharges of "deal-breaking" by the parties.

One welcome achievement of the budget summit was to drop the "per capita cap" proposal that the administration had earlier supported (see pp. 60, 179). By this time, it was no longer seen either as an important guarantee for beneficiaries or a needed brake on Medicaid spending. Besides, getting rid of it obviated a source of controversy and spared Congress another formula fight. Dropping it, though, created another problem, since CBO indicated that, without the per capita caps, savings attributable to DSH reductions would have to be offset (reduced) by 25 per cent, making the Medicaid savings target considerably harder to achieve.

Both the Medicaid and child health legislation in the House were Commerce Committee products, developed in traditional legislative fashion. At one point, Newt Gingrich had formed a task force, charged with drafting legislation to counter the Senate Hatch-Kennedy proposal,[113] but this initiative soon dwindled. The budget resolution assigned jurisdiction over child health to both Commerce and Ways and Means and, for a time, there was something of a turf war between the two committees over the allotted child health funds, but the Ways and Means tax credit proposal was eventually dropped. Essentially, Commerce developed the bill, with hearings, minority staff participation in drafting sessions, and substantial bipartisan collaboration in the markups. There were a number of party-line votes and "60–40 deals," but with significant efforts to accommodate the minority.[114] In general, as with the Ways and Means Committee, it was a return to committee-centered policy.

For Medicaid, the approach agreed upon by the budget summit and incorporated in the budget resolutions of House and Senate was to compensate for or soften state flexibility reforms with beneficiary protections. This approach represented, in part, the wisdom of experience—beaten into people by the 1995 and 1996 battles. There was a widespread consensus that nothing else was going to work. At the same time, the changes being proposed for Medicaid amounted, cumulatively, to an extensive transformation of the program as well as a shift toward a new philosophy. And people disagreed, especially the House Democrats, about how much flexibility was a good thing and what protections were essential.[115] Therefore, what was claimed under the heading of state flexibility or beneficiary protection had to make good policy sense, and the statutory embodiments of these two concepts needed to be well matched, not just subsumed. It was also important that this approach be deeply shared and that it persist throughout the reconciliation process.

In the Commerce bill, "State Flexibility" is the first and longest chapter, providing broadly for greater freedom in utilizing managed care options, more flexibility in payment methodologies and in extending eligibility or modifying benefits, and relieving states of a number of administrative requirements.

One of the least controversial but potentially most important of the flexibility amendments was allowing states to provide benefits through managed care plans, including primary care case management, without a Section 1915(b) waiver, and to limit beneficiary choice of plans to a maximum of two plans. Accompanying this provision was elimination of the 75/25 restriction on risk contracts, which required managed care plans to limit their enrollment of Medicare and Medicaid patients to not more than 75 percent of the total.[116] In addition, the threshold amount for managed care contracts requiring the secretary's prior approval was raised from $100,000 to $1 million.

An important change in payment methodology was repeal of the Boren Amendment, which required states to pay rates to hospitals, nursing facilities, and intermediate care facilities for the mentally retarded that were "reasonable and adequate" to cover the costs of "efficiently and economically operated facilities." In place of a legislative standard enforced by lawsuits, the committee substituted a public notice and comment procedure for setting rates. Despite some strong views that the Boren Amendment was still needed to protect not just hospitals but the elderly poor and mentally retarded patients, and that providers might find public rate-making a poor substitute,[117] repeal of the amendment was supported in the administration proposal and had acquired symbolic and emotive content that made it especially popular with governors and with House Republicans.

Together, these two amendments nicely illustrate a major problem with the Medicaid legislation. Lifting the waiver requirement for MCOs frees states to manage with greater freedom. Repealing the Boren Amendment moves in the same direction, but also takes away an important and enforceable protection for providers and, indirectly, for specially vulnerable populations, such as the elderly and disabled. In Medicaid policy, these people are described as "dual eligibles" and they are for Medicaid pretty much what the 10 percent or so of high-utilization beneficiaries are for Medicare: they are costly, often difficult to treat, and bill-payers, including some states and MCOs, like to avoid responsibility for them. The thrust of policy, both in the House and Senate, was to balance increased flexibility for the states with essential protections for the beneficiaries—but what were essential? This category of dual eligible was, not surprisingly, a tough issue and, as with Medicare, only partially resolved.

Most of the flexibility amendments were of relatively modest, incremental proportions, providing new options for the states or easing some requirement. Incremental changes, especially characteristic of Commerce, were to give states more freedom to enroll individuals in private insurance plans and to allow them to guarantee children under the age of nineteen twelve months of coverage after an eligibility determination. The capitated Program for All-Inclusive Care of the Elderly, or PACE, was made a permanent option for Medicaid, as well as for Medicare. The requirement of prior institutionalization in order to receive habilitation services from a qualified home health or community service agency was repealed. Extension of Section 1115 waivers was also much simplified, providing that a request to the secretary for a three-year renewal, if not responded to within six months, would be deemed to be granted.

Included in these flexibility amendments were provisions that would benefit Medicaid recipients, but in several respects they would not make out so well. Most importantly, states would be authorized to impose the same cost-sharing requirements—such as deductibles, copayments, and enrollment fees—that were permitted under the Medicaid FFS program. In addition, and contrary at least to Democratic understandings of the summit agreement, the committee bill included only $500 million[118] to pay for premium increases of low-income Medicare beneficiaries, a category of dual eligible of special concern both to Commerce Democrats and to the administration. Another provision that seemed gratuitously stingy to Democrats was the phasing down of cost reimbursement for Federally Qualified Health Centers and Rural Health Clinics—providers especially important for underserved areas where MCOs often were not available.

Since the presumption was that most of the care under Medicaid would be provided by managed care plans, much of the protection that was to balance the increased flexibility accorded governors and the states would need to be achieved by regulating or otherwise affecting the behavior of these plans. That, in turn, posed a second-order problem, since the federal government did not contract with or pay these plans—the states did. For HCFA to be micromanaging health plans in fifty states and the territories did not seem prudent or even feasible.

What was particularly needed was some sensible method to delegate decisions about operating level behavior, but also to monitor these decisions and improve their quality. By 1997, the quality movement was fairly well advanced and was being increasingly accepted by industry, among health care providers, and within the government. Since 1992, state Medicaid officials, private accrediting bodies, and HCFA had been working on a Medicaid version of quality assurance and improvement.[119] A sophisticated version of quality improvement was included in the Medicare amendments of 1995 [sec. 1852(e)]. A Medicaid quality proposal had also been developed by John Dingell and Commerce Democrats in 1995 for inclusion in the Medicaid provisions of BBA I, but was sidetracked because of the press of committee business.[120] Fortunately, by this time there was a broad, bipartisan consensus that quality standards for Medicaid HMOs were a needed addition. It was understood to be part of the summit agreements on Medicaid.[121] The National Governors' Association, in its demands for greater flexibility, expressed no objection in principle, mostly a concern that they be included in the planning.[122]

In the Commerce bill, the quality standards for Medicaid were intended to be roughly midway in comprehensiveness and control between Medicare at one extreme and the child health state plans at the other.[123] State agencies were to develop and implement a "quality assurance and improvement strategy" consistent with standards that the secretary would "establish and monitor" (Section 3461). These standards would not preempt stronger ones adopted by the state, but they would have to include standards of access to care, procedures for "monitoring the quality and appropriateness of care" for a "full spectrum" of the population enrolled under the contract, "regular and periodic" examination of the quality improvement strategy, and "other aspects of care and service directly related to the improvement of quality of care (including grievance procedures and marketing and information standards." As was customary, compliance with these requirements could be "deemed" when the MCO met the standards of and was approved by an acceptable private accrediting body, such as NCQA or JCAHO.

Quoting some of the text of the committee draft illustrates the careful articulation of the provision as well as its general tone or philosophy. It requires the elements of a CQI strategy, but provides that the secretary consult with states about the standards and leaves details of implementation to the states. The language stresses the importance of a strategy, not the specific concepts or techniques of a CQI methodology in contrast, for example, with the quality provisions of the House Medicare amendments of 1995 [Section 1852 (e)] and 1997[Section 1852 (e)]. Quality improvement also extends beyond direct care to include standards of access, marketing and information, and grievance procedures.

Quality improvement was seen as central to a larger strategy. It provided, most immediately, a plausible method of delegation and of replacing Washington micromanagement with internalized standards. Assuming that many of the more enlightened state Medicaid officials and providers would buy into this philosophy, this approach could encourage emulation and help bring other states and programs up to a common standard. It might also nudge the Medicaid program closer to the standards of medical practice and provider behavior characteristic of Medicare—a long-sought objective.[124] Politically, this initiative looked good: the quality movement was growing, had good provider acceptance, and was being pushed by the administration.

At the same time, improving quality of care does not necessarily take care of patients' rights. Bills embodying "patients' bills of rights," aimed at HMOs in general, were sprouting both in the House and Senate, though just what rights should be included was much in dispute. In any event, it was good policy and good politics to acknowledge this burgeoning enthusiasm and include some of the more sensible and warmly advocated measures. The candidates chosen seemed obvious enough, but they also provided some inkling of the tricky issues and controversy likely to be provoked by patients' bills of rights.

Establishing a "prudent layperson" standard for access to emergency care was a popular idea at the time and not especially controversial, since managed care plans saw this one as pretty much inevitable. According to the Commerce version, a managed care plan would be required to provide coverage for emergency medical services, without regard to prior authorization, in the case of "acute symptoms of sufficient severity" such that a "prudent layperson . . . could reasonably expect the absence of immediate medical attention to result in (1) placing the health of the individual (including a mother and unborn child) in serious jeopardy; (2) serious impairment to bodily function; or (3) serious dysfunction of any bodily part or organ." Also included was responsibility for poststabilization care that complied with guidelines established for MedicarePlus plans under Part C of Title XVIII—a specific illustration of how Medicare and Medicaid could be brought more closely together. The Senate version added "severe pain" to the list of criteria. Not to be missed, of course, is the fact that many of these words, like "prudent," "immediate," "severe pain," and "poststabilization" are legal terms of art, which as jurists like to say, gain precision through application, but meanwhile are the occasion for uncertainty and lawsuits.

A second patient protection was the prohibition of gag rules, i.e., protocols set up by MCOs prohibiting plan providers from advising patients about courses of treatment or actions open to them that might be in the patients' interests but would undermine or work against some policy of the managed care entity—such as suggesting to a patient that he or she needs a more expensive course of treatment than the plan normally allows and then collaborating with the patient to get it authorized. Included with this prohibition was a proviso that it did not apply to an HMO that had "moral or religious grounds" against covering such a service (e.g., abortions or reproductive services) so long as the plan notified the members before or during the enrollment or within ninety days of adopting such a policy. Nor could the HMO be required to furnish counseling or referrals with respect to such services. This was one small illustration of a Medicaid issue that does not go away. Indeed, the Hyde Amendment,[125] first passed in 1976, figured prominently and repeatedly in the Medicaid debates of 1997, and was again included in the final legislation.

Another patient protection, not a part of quality assurance but oddly included in the flexibility provisions, would have required that the length of an inpatient hospital stay be determined by the attending physician (or other healthcare provider) and the patient, not, as Representative Coburn (R., Okla.) put it, by "an insurance clerk 600 miles away."[126] This provision was directed at both Medicare and Medicaid HMOs and was especially pushed by three House Republicans: Tom Coburn and Greg Ganske (R., Iowa), who were physicians, and Charlie Norwood (R., Ga.), who was a dentist. With Democratic support, it passed the subcommittee by a vote of 17–10 and went unchallenged in the full committee. But in cooler moments and with a growing realization of the incalculable effects such an amendment could have upon HMOs-which, as Peter Deutsch (D., Fla.), a supporter of HMOs, complained, "still do some good"—it was eventually dropped.[127]

One substantial addition to patient protections was to mandate a Medicaid HMO appeals process. In its particulars, this mandate combined existing practice of the better HMOs with some popular additions and some significant legal language. Plans had to provide a "meaningful and expedited" procedure for resolving "grievances" that would meet "notice and hearing" requirements. Plans had to establish a board of appeals that would include, in addition to plan representatives, consumers who were not plan enrollees and providers expert in the relevant field of medicine. Filed complaints were to be resolved in thirty days. Not included was a then popular provision for an external board or appeal to the courts. However, with the weighty "notice and hearing" language, which resonates profoundly in administrative law, as well as the consumer and specialist representation, the requirements were pretty stringent. Many HMOs had wretchedly inadequate appeals procedures, so that mandating such a requirement was important, even though it could prove burdensome and costly.[128]

A strong move toward internalized standards and institutionalizing a process of continuous improvement was a vital and well-calculated step in putting the Medicaid program on a new footing and beginning a transformation. Yet, as the example of patient protections illustrates, there also need to be checks upon organizations and attention to specific abuses. Moreover, Medicaid had a long history of marginal, fly-by-night, and even crooked operators who might not be receptive to the quality message and for whom more stringent and peremptory regulative prescriptions would be in order. A number of Democrats thought so and some Republicans as well, especially when the regulations were directed at HMOs. One approach was to raise entry requirements for new HMOs, for instance, by the quality standards themselves and by requiring Medicaid HMOs to meet the same solvency standards set by the state for private HMOs or be certified by the state as a risk-bearing entity.[129] Democratic members of the committee, particularly John Dingell and Henry Waxman, still lobbied hard for more specific regulations, especially dealing with marketing and fraud and abuse. These were eventually included, as part of the quality standards, toward the end of the markup in the full committee, after other major elements of the bill had been resolved.[130]

The marketing requirements (dealt with under the rubric of "fraud and abuse") were both tough and highly prescriptive. They aimed at setting up, within the states, marketing protections similar to those provided for Medicare HMOs. The states, consulting with a medical care advisory board, approved all marketing materials before they could be used. The secretary was to prescribe "procedures and conditions" that would ensure adequate and accurate "oral and written" information sufficient to make an informed decision. HMOs found guilty of distributing false or materially misleading materials would be barred from the program.[131] Targeting some of the more objectionable Medicaid marketing abuses, the legislation specifically required that HMOs market "to the entire service area" and refrain from "directly or indirectly" conducting "door-to-door, telephonic, or other 'cold call' approaches."

Getting gross savings of $17.8 billion dollars from Medicaid, as agreed upon in the budget summit, was a third important part of the committee's task. With the large amount available from Medicaid DSH payments and the anticipated state flexibility savings, this might seem to be a fairly easy assignment; but complications arose, with the result that even this modest total was not achieved in committee or on the floor, occasioned presidential intervention, and was ultimately resolved only in conference.

One problem had to do with overestimating savings or, put another way, with CBO scoring. For instance, the National Governors' Association, interested in preserving more DSH payments, optimistically estimated savings from the bill's flexibility provisions at $8 billion over the five years. CBO said that $2.9 billion was more like it (Center for Budget and Policy Priorities 1997:2) and later lowered this estimate to $1.8 billion.[132] This scoring, of course, made DSH savings even more important, but CBO was also critical of the committee's estimates of DSH savings and used a 25 percent "offset" in its own scoring. CBO assumed that state practices such as "Medicaid maximizing" and "intergovernmental transfers"[133] were likely to continue and, therefore, required a behavioral "offset" that would take account of lower actual savings. The 25 percent offset meant that the committee had to come up with $4 in savings to get $3—or, $20 billion instead of $15 billion. The offset was high in part because there would be no per capita cap to reduce cumulative spending. Ironically, CBO's estimate was also based in part on one of the committee's own amendments reinstating "provider taxes" that would enable states to draw down more Medicaid matching funds. Objecting to the CBO position, the committee initially reported its savings without taking into account the CBO offset and continued to argue this matter with CBO almost to the last day of the conference.[134]

Finding savings elsewhere was difficult. The child health initiative was not yet law, and so was not eligible for scored savings. State flexibility reforms were a wash—with savings offset by new expenditures. Some of these savings, such as phasing down cost reimbursement for the health centers, seemed mean-spirited and would save little.[135] One contentious measure was to allocate only $500 million of the $1.5 billion that was to provide premium support for low-income Medicare beneficiaries. This ran afoul of an administration priority that included protection of this group-along with legal immigrants who had become disabled and children of parents who had lost their SSI eligibility—as a consequence of welfare reform. The House sustained this committee recommendation, but with strong objections from OMB director, Frank Raines. The full amount was ultimately restored in conference.

Ultimately, the Commerce Committee had to rely upon DSH savings for $15.3 billion ($20 billion in actual cuts) of its total Medicaid gross savings of $16.5 billion. They did so with reluctance and with grumbling. Reading between the lines, the payment formula that was devised revealed the committee's unhappiness and almost in terms invited someone else—i.e., the Senate—to fix it. For low-DSH states (less than 1 percent of their Medicaid spending) the DSH payments would be frozen at the 1995 level. High-DSH states (more than 12 percent of Medicaid spending) would have their rates reduced by 2 percent of their 1995 or 1996 level (whichever was higher), by 5 percent in 1999, then by 20 percent in 2000, 30 percent in 2001 and 40 percent in 2002. Other states, neither high nor low, would be reduced at half the rate for high-DSH states. Among high-DSH states Texas, Louisiana,

Florida, and New York were all represented on the Senate Finance Committee. If the treatment of these high-DSH states seemed harsh, their senators could act in their behalf.

The Commerce Committee met its self-defined savings target, though its report included a homily on the pernicious effects of relying heavily on DSH payments as a source of Medicaid savings, the plight of "safety net" hospitals, and the committee's reluctance to go along with the "Administration's proposed reduction in DSH funding and the inclusion of this proposal in the budget agreement."[136] Committee Republicans defended other Medicaid expenditure reductions, such as taking $1 billion from premium support, as necessary to forestall even deeper DSH cuts.[137]

Child Health.   Along with quality standards for Medicaid managed care, another generally shared presumption in 1997 was that something substantial would be done about children without health insurance or basic health care coverage. In part, this concern grew from a recognition that, despite prosperity and continuing efforts by the states and the federal government, roughly the same number of children remained uninsured from 1989 through 1995 and that an increasing number were failing to get critical medical attention.[138] There were a number of reasons for this state of affairs, some of them not obvious. By far the most important, though, were that employers were providing less insurance or none at all and that many of the Medicaid eligibles were not being enrolled. According to a June 1996 report of the General Accounting Office (1996a), eighteen million people worked for companies with no health insurance at all and another five million for companies that covered employees but not their families. A startling fact, moreover, was that among the 10.5 million children uninsured at any particular time, 3.5 million—one-third of the group—were not enrolled by their parents or guardians because of such factors as transience, the stigma associated with Medicaid, or lack of motivation or knowledge about eligibility. A complicating factor was, paradoxically, the government's own efforts to improve matters, especially the series of incremental reforms beginning in 1986, originating mostly with the Commerce Committee and Henry Waxman (D., Calif.). These reforms greatly expanded the Medicaid coverage for pregnant women and children. This was one way of inexpensively covering a particularly vulnerable population, but it also led to "crowding out," whereby a number of the working poor opted for this "free" (to them) Medicaid coverage instead of private policies. As a result, Medicaid efforts to increase coverage seemed to gain little if any ground, while the states groaned under onerous mandates.

The various proposals being floated early in 1997 illustrate several aspects of this problem and reveal that it was by no means only or even primarily a child health problem. Senators Hatch and Kennedy, who were the first out with a child health initiative, proposed a block grant to be funded by an increase in the tobacco tax. Phil Gramm (R. Tex.), chairman of the Senate Republican health care task force, would add $3.75 billion to the Maternal and Child Health Block Grant, to be funded mostly by cuts in the Earned Income Tax Credit. This was a minimal and inexpensive alternative that found strong support among conservatives on the Senate Finance Committee. Senator Chafee, several liberal Republicans, and a number of Democrats in both the Senate and the House were working toward a plan that would expand existing Medicare coverage. President Clinton, in his February budget, however, divided his attention between children and workers. With respect to Medicaid, he proposed mainly enrolling the eligible and extending coverage for one year for children being dropped from the program, for instance, because of welfare reform. He wanted a $9.8 billion program to help pay for insurance when workers were changing jobs. Also included was a small amount, $25 million, for grants to the states to facilitate the formation of small business insurance pools.[139] Tom Daschle, the Senate minority leader, and Bill Thomas, chairman of the Health Subcommittee of Ways and Means, both favored tax credits to help the working poor afford coverage. Newt Gingrich appointed a House task force to develop a counter to the Hatch-Kennedy initiative. There was a stir of activity and concern, both in the Senate and the House, but as Chairman Thomas said at the time, "The issue has generated significantly more interest than solutions."[140]

The Child Health Assistance Program (CHAP), was the Commerce Committee's proposal for a five-year, $14.4 billion program of grants to the states. This proposal is worth reviewing in some detail since—after the House and Senate bills had gone to conference and the administration had its say—the Commerce bill was pretty much what survived with respect to child health. In structure and approach, it followed closely the block grant proposal of 1995, though suitably adapted for child health assistance. A separate paragraph on "Non-entitlement" made the point that "nothing in this title" should be construed as creating an entitlement under any state plan. Beyond that, the state plan requirements were spelled out, including submission to and approval by the secretary, a setting forth of strategic objectives, performance goals and performance measures, and methods for monitoring results, with extensive reporting to the secretary.

Although protections for beneficiaries were included, this program was intended to provide more flexibility for states and governors than Medicaid. In part, this intention resulted from a Republican preference for block grants over the expansion of an entitlement. But in Congress there was also a widely shared belief that increased freedom and grant money without too many strings attached would allow governors and state Medicaid agencies to experiment constructively with ways to increase coverage or develop new approaches to service delivery for children. One example mentioned favorably in the committee report was the Florida "Healthy Kids" program, which allowed the state to explore trade-offs between substance abuse and mental health programs.[141] Expressing this philosophy, the state plan language leaves the "strategic objectives" pretty much to the states, within the broad mission of increasing "health assistance" for poor children: there were no quality or access standards or reference to CQI methodology and data requirements. Language in the committee report suggests that the committee was doing its part by giving states the "tools they need" to expand coverage and the quality of care—with the hope (and faith) that the states would use this freedom well (U.S. Congress 1997d:603).

The intended beneficiaries were protected in a variety of standard ways required of state plans that were, in turn, a qualification for grant funding. Plans had to spell out eligibility standards. Outreach activities and enrollment assistance were mandated. A preexisting condition could not be invoked to exclude an otherwise eligible party. Child health assistance, in general, would be required to provide, as a minimum, inpatient and outpatient hospital care, physician and laboratory services, and well-baby and well-child care, including preventive and primary dental care. State plans could prescribe premiums and cost-sharing, but only if the scale of payments took a fair account of family income; and no cost-sharing would be permitted for preventive services. States would also be required to assure access to specialty care for children with life-threatening or chronic conditions

A state that qualified could receive 80 percent funding for its proposed program—with a required match of 20 percent—up to the limit of its allotment, which was based on the number of uninsured low-income children and a "state cost factor" reflecting average wages in the state. No state would receive less than $2 million a year.[142] The allotment could be spent for Medicaid coverage, group health plans or private insurance, direct services from providers, outreach activities, and other methods spelled out in the state plan. Specifically excluded was Medicaid expansion beyond 1997 limits. For this purpose, a separate fund of $2 million was provided, with a different matching rate for that option.[143] A cap of 15 percent was put upon administrative and other nonassistance expenditures. The bill included a proviso that funds directly provided by the federal government or services assisted or supported "to any significant extent" by the federal government could not be used for a match.

Committee Markup and Passage in the House. The markup for the subcommittee took place on June 10, and for the full committee on June 12. Neither produced major change, though unlike the era of good feelings that overtook the Ways and Means Committee, there was more partisan controversy and some surprises in the Commerce Committee. In the subcommittee, two managed care amendments were added. The first, from Tom Coburn (R., Okla.), a physician, was the hospital stay amendment, providing that the physician and patient would decide the length of stay, not the managed care plan. A second, from another physician, Greg Ganske (R., Iowa), added the prudent-layperson standard for emergency care. Both of these survived the full committee markup. The full committee added another Coburn amendment: the grievance procedure already described. Two other measures, sponsored by individual Republicans, would allow women enrolled in Medicaid managed care plans to designate an obstetrician-gynecologist as their primary care provider and would let states impose managed care standards that went beyond the federal ones.[144]

These developments could be interpreted as additional manifestations of a burgeoning patient protection movement. The Commerce Committee was also experiencing something of a populist revolt led by its professional health care providers, Coburn, Ganske, and Norwood. Along with these developments, a rather astonishing twist was the subcommittee's reinstating of the Boren Amendment, despite endorsement of its repeal in the summit agreement and by the president. Repeal of the amendment had not been an uncontested issue and many hospitals and nursing homes had rallied to its defense.[145] Some Republicans were also wavering on this issue. When the repeal came up for a vote in the subcommittee markup, John Dingle—veteran of many Medicare and Medicaid battles—rose to the occasion with some resonant oratory about the bad old days when nursing homes strapped grannies to their beds or kicked them out. With a number of Republicans crossing over, the repeal was defeated in the subcommittee by a vote of 15–13. It was a temporary victory. Between that vote and the full committee markup, some intense lobbying developed, with appeals to the White House saying that a number of deals were off the table if this vote were not reversed.[146] In the full committee, the Bowen Amendment was finally laid to rest by a party-line vote of 29–19.[147]

Between the committee markup and floor action in the House, some complicated maneuvering and dickering occurred, both responding to administration concerns and clearing the way for the conference. The administration weighed in with letters—including one from the president to the Budget Committee chairmen in House and Senate—expressing discontent with the DSH cuts and failures to live up to the budget agreement on such items as premium support for low-income beneficiaries, and coverage for "SSI kids" and disabled legal aliens. John Kasich and Pete Domenici met and agreed to the full $1.5 billion for premium support.[148] The House allowed states the option of covering the "SSI kids," though would not mandate it. Rather than terminate CHAP at the end of five years, it agreed to have the program evaluated for continuation. Several of these items were incorporated in the House rule governing floor debate and automatically became part of the final bill. Included in this category was the $1 billion addition to Part B premium support and dropping of the Coburn amendment on length of hospital stays. With a nice symmetry, the money saved by stripping this provision helped pay for the premium support.

On June 25, the House approved the bill by a vote of 270–162. John Dingle, ranking Democrat on the Commerce Committee, voted with the Republican majority, a testimonial to the comity and collaboration that had prevailed in the committee, despite sharp differences on a number of issues. The bill expressed a coherent policy, but also contained a number of concessions to the administration and the Democrats. A former Republican staff aide said that many issues were partisan, but that was more a matter of "who's got the gavel" than of deep divisions over policy. They added as many bipartisan measures as they could. It was an inclusive process, he said, the "most amicable" of the reconciliations he had experienced, though he added that he was referring to relations with Democrats in Congress, not those with the administration.[149]

The Senate: SCHIP and Medicaid. With respect to Medicaid and child health, Senate behavior was much the same as usual, except in one important respect. As usual, Senate Finance acted both to mitigate and tighten up provisions affecting Medicaid: to ease some of the pinch for providers, but also to add beneficiary protections and new legislation on fraud and abuse. Preceding this incremental activity, though, a bipartisan enthusiasm for child health nearly overwhelmed this routine agenda with the Chafee-Rockefeller amendment. This was a proposal to cover child health by expanding Medicaid, a step that would have made the largest single addition to entitlements since 1965. The initiative did not succeed, though it survived as one alternative, but it helped make child health a dominant agenda item for the Senate. Moreover, this episode provides a good illustration of the policy and politics involved in creating a new health grant.

A concern about increased coverage and access to health care often alternates with cost containment efforts, and 1997 was a good year to consider child health because baselines and the deficit were dropping and because an attack on this issue was overdue. Moreover, health care for children and the working poor often got well represented in the Senate, with the relatively liberal makeup of the Senate Finance Committee and Senator Chafee as chairman of its Medicaid subcommittee,[150] and Jim Jeffords (R., Vt.), a health care liberal, as chairman of the Labor and Human Resources Committee and Ted Kennedy as the ranking member

Increasing access to health care has usually been a Democratic issue; and the earliest proposals in 1997 came from Democrats: Tom Daschle's Senate minority proposal for a tax credit for the working poor that would pay 90 percent of the insurance premium for their children; and President Clinton's February budget proposal for expanded Medicaid coverage, primarily by enrolling already eligible but uninsured children. The president put $13 billion on the table for this and related Medicaid reforms, as agreed to by the budget summit. In the House, Newt Gingrich appointed a task force to counter the

Hatch-Kennedy proposal in the Senate, but the Commerce Committee developed the actual proposal as part of the reconciliation. In the Senate, though, child health evoked more interest and produced three major proposals.

The first important bill and the one with the longest pedigree, was the Hatch-Kennedy proposal, announced on March 13. This was a revised version of a bill Kennedy and John Kerry (D., Mass.) had sponsored in 1996 to modify the Maternal and Child Health Block Grant and use it as a vehicle to cover uninsured children.[151] That bill, which failed, was followed by Kassebaum-Kennedy—a successful, bipartisan effort to increase access to health care for uninsured workers. For the child health bill, Kennedy sought out Orrin Hatch (R., Utah),[152] who, despite his ideological conservatism was a close, personal friend with a strong interest in health care. In teaming up with Kennedy, Hatch said that it was "the right thing to do," despite some stiff conservative opposition, and that he and Kennedy were trying to recreate the bipartisan approach that had led to passage of Kassebaum-Kennedy.[153]

Hatch-Kennedy was a block grant to provide health insurance for children in low-income families. States could set the eligibility criteria, but had to give top priority to the poorest families; and no family with incomes below 185 percent of the federal poverty level (FPL) could be required to pay more than 5 percent of their health care costs. The money allotted could be used either to pay for child-only policies or to contribute to insurance provided by employers, but insurance policies would have to cover, at a minimum, the benefits provided by Medicaid. The sponsors made the point that their initiative was intended to complement the president's outreach efforts to the three million or more children who were eligible for Medicaid but had not been enrolled.[154] The program was not an entitlement, though it was intended to be permanent. States could participate or not, but those that did so would contribute matching funds of 10 percent to 20 percent, which would vary according to average income within the state. The proposal would be funded by a $0.43 increase per pack in the cigarette tax. This revenue source was thought to be productive enough to include an additional inducement—of another $10 billion for deficit reduction.

The first major proposal to be seriously considered, Hatch-Kennedy was also the first to fall by the way. Not surprising, even though tobacco seemed at the time fair game for any and all, a number of senators from the South and from tobacco states objected to an increase in taxes and this one in particular. Thousands of jobs would be lost. According to an analysis by the Senate Republican Policy Committee, the Hatch-Kennedy tax would cost the federal government $4 billion in lost tax revenues, including $2.5 billion for an increase in the CPI, and would cost the states another $6.5 billion in lost taxes.[155] Among cosponsors, five senators—including three of the four Republicans—supported the child health part but not the tax increase. Others, such as Jim Jeffords, the chairman of Labor and Human Resources, and

Jay Rockefeller (D., W. Va.), a member of Senate Finance, disliked the block grant feature and preferred the Chafee approach of Medicaid expansion.[156] Despite its bipartisan auspices, Hatch-Kennedy was losing support among liberals and conservatives alike. From a strategic perspective, moreover, it was a stand-alone bill increasing health care access and raising taxes: two objectives hard to reach without a powerful legislative vehicle. With the budget negotiations progressing and a major reconciliation in prospect, efforts both in the House and Senate shifted more in that direction.

Various other proposals were sprouting about this time. Arlen Specter (R., Pa.) came forward with what he termed "a distinctive Republican approach," which would have funded vouchers for children's health policies through a $10 billion, five-year program. His plan required no new taxes, and would have been financed through sale of federal broadcast spectrum assets. Against the bill, it was another stand-alone proposal. There was little enthusiasm for the vouchers, and considerable skepticism about the amount and dependability of the revenues to be gotten from selling off broadcast frequencies.[157]

Meanwhile, Phil Gramm, a member of the Finance Committee and chairman of the Senate Republican health care task force, had been working on a minimalist proposal, which he announced on April 17. His bill would extend coverage by adding $3.5 billion to the Maternal and Child Health Block Grant. Most of the funding would come from repealing the child health portion of the Earned Income Tax Credit. In addition to child health, Gramm's proposal added key Medicaid flexibility amendments advocated by the National Governors' Association. Also included was removal of any limit on the number of Medical Savings Accounts, which Gramm defended as another way in which low-income enrollments could be increased. That claim was hardly plausible, since low-income families could not afford and did not buy such policies, but MSAs were a high priority of Republican conservatives.[158] Gramm, on the Finance Committee, indicated that he expected his bill—which already had the support of Chairman Roth and five other Republican members—to become part of the leadership proposal.[159]

Gramm's initiative deserves some comment since it neatly illustrates both the persuasive features of a minimalist approach as well as some objections to it. One item is that it builds upon and strengthens existing programs, using the Maternal and Child Health Block Grant already established in fifty states and with a long history of providing primary, preventive, and specialty health care to uninsured children. This approach articulates well with Medicaid, since children identified under the MCH grant as eligible for Medicaid are, by law, required to be enrolled in that program. It would be better targeted than Hatch-Kennedy, since it would be categorically aimed at the 3.2 million children ineligible for Medicaid because their parents earn more than the Medicaid limit but are below 200 percent of the federal poverty line ($32,000 for a family of four in 1997). Gramm's version would be incremental and would foster experiment and public-private ventures at the state and local level It would spend only $3.75 billion over five years and would be much more cost-effective in reaching individual children than either Hatch-Kennedy or Chafee's Medicaid expansion approach.[160]

Aside from diminishing the Earned Income Tax Credit and the artful ploy with Medical Savings Accounts, the basic objection to Gramm's approach is that *it* was minimalist: it would not do much to promote outreach and get low-income children insured and would not move children from "poverty" medicine to mainstream health care and provide quality and access standards to protect them. Another objection was that too much of block grant funds could be spent for purposes not directly related to health care, including high-ways and football stadiums. Moreover, some health care liberals, like Chafee and Rockefeller, wanted not just to provide health care for poor children, but to extend the existing entitlement.

On April 24, as the budget negotiations were approaching a conclusion and Hatch-Kennedy was faltering, Chafee and Rockefeller announced another child health proposal. This initiative was also bipartisan, endorsed by both Hatch and Kennedy, and by nine Democrats and six Republicans. To date, that was the highest number of cosponsors. Moreover, six of them were on the Finance Committee; so that this proposal quickly became the main alternative to the Gramm proposal, which was expected to be incorporated in Chairman Roth's leadership bill.

Chafee and Rockefeller, like Hatch and Kennedy, were an interesting pair of cosponsors. Both of them came from patrician, "old money" backgrounds, with a strong sense of responsibility for the poor and the less fortunate. Both shared an interest in health care: Chafee was chairman of the Finance Sub-committee on Medicaid and Health Care for Low-Income Families and Rock-efeller was the ranking Democrat of the Subcommittee on Health Care. Both came from states for which Medicaid and health care for low-income families were vitally important. For Chafee, especially, this legislation touched upon some core values. As a matter of social philosophy, he believed that too much was spent on elders and not enough on mothers and children. He was a long-time champion of the poor and especially persons with disabilities. Further-more, he believed that health care for such people should be a protected entitlement and regarded block grants as anathema.[161] Also, Senator Chafee was formidable, both because of his personal style and his position of leader-ship among Senate liberal Republicans, especially his New England "Snow Birds."

The Chafee-Rockefeller approach to child health was clean and simple, though controversial. They would have expanded Medicaid to cover children in families earning up to 150 percent of the FPL, an increase from 133 percent of poverty. States choosing this option would receive an incentive bonus of a 30 percent increase in the matching rate for children enrolled. As in the president's bill, states could guarantee continuous Medicaid coverage for a year. Twenty-five million dollars in grants would help states with outreach efforts. Costs of this plan were estimated at $15 billion over five years, but the proposal avoided specifying how the money would be raised.[162] No additional mandates were involved. These were the simple and clean features. The controversial part was, of course, a major extension of the Medicaid entitlement adding as many as two million children to the seven million already eligible but not enrolled. Besides that, governors and states would be subject to the usual Medicaid regulations with respect to benefits, quality, access, and so forth. At 150 percent of poverty, it reached only two million more kids. So, it was an expensive program that would still leave most of the ten million low-income children uninsured.[163] Because of the technicalities of scoring, moreover, if states spent all or most of the child health funds on Medicaid expansion, that would effectively wipe out the entire agreed-upon $13.6 billion in net Medicaid savings.[164]

The budget agreement in the Senate both limited the alternatives and sharpened contrasts between them. Hatch-Kennedy was tabled on May 21 in the course of reaching the budget agreement. The resolution set $16 billion as a figure to be spent, either for Medicaid expansion or for "capped mandatory grants," leaving open the issue of which of these to choose, the possibility of a split between them, or still other approaches, such as tax incentives or block grants. Realistically, though, the alternatives were either Chafee-Rockefeller or the Gramm option in the Roth leadership bill. This was a polarizing choice, which led to a threatened insurgency within the committee. On May 22 twelve members of the Finance Committee, a majority, sent a letter to Chairman Roth supporting the Chafee-Rockefeller proposal.[165] Trent Lott was also facing serious disagreements with respect to other Medicaid proposals, such as the Medicaid DSH cuts and the failure to provide premium support for low-income Medicare beneficiaries or restore benefits for the disabled "SSI kids."

Faced with these circumstances, Lott and the leadership group did what sensible legislators often do: they put together a compromise combining ideas from both the Gramm and the Chafee-Rockefeller proposals. Included was the key provision of Medicaid expansion up to 150 percent of poverty and the 30 percent increment in the match. The block grant had a 25 percent match. It also allowed states to use the grant money for a wide variety of purposes, such as insurance, vouchers, health care services, and community, based centers. States had to opt for only one program: either the block grant or Medicaid.

The "compromise" proposal did not make the Medicaid expansionists happy, since with a block grant most states could have more money without the added protections associated with Medicaid. Reviewing a similar provision in the House Commerce Committee bill, CBO said it was "unlikely" that the states would use this option to expand coverage. Moreover, since the block grant program was traditionally one that funded limited services, like prenatal care and vaccinations, CBO believed that the temptations for states and governors to "make out" on these programs at the expense of its beneficiaries would be a serious matter.[166] Chafee and Rockefeller offered an amendment that would have allocated $12 billion to Medicaid expansion and $4 billion to the block grant program, but that was defeated in a Finance Committee vote, 9–11.[167]

At this critical juncture, the National Governors' Association, despite President Clinton's endorsement of the Chafee-Rockefeller approach, communicated their objections to Medicaid expansion[168] Following that intervention, four members of the Finance Committee withdrew their support—a change that was decisive in putting a quietus on this approach to Medicaid expansion. Characteristically, Chafee and his allies responded by developing a compromise of their own, which included accelerating an existing obligation to provide Medicaid coverage for adolescents, and specific amendments to tighten up the block grant program.[169]

A concurrent development helped to sustain the child health movement. On June 17, the same day that the Finance Committee voted down the Chafee-Rockefeller amendment, Hatch and Kennedy moved to add $20 billion more for child health, to be paid for by increasing the cigarette tax.[170] Chairman Roth ruled the amendment not germane to the markup. The vote was 11–9, a majority in favor, but not the 14 votes required to overturn the chairman's ruling. Two days later, though, the Finance Committee, meeting behind closed doors on some two hundred items in its tax package, agreed to increase the cigarette tax by $0.20 and earmark $8 billion of that for child health.[171]

Though not strong enough to impose their own version, the Chafee-Rockefeller supporters could exact important concessions,[172] which they proceeded to do with amendments during the markup and on the Senate floor. One important change was to drop the MCH block grant and, following the House Commerce approach, establish a new Title XXI, "The Child Health Insurance Initiatives," which would be added to the Social Security Act. Along with this change came some standard definitions and safeguards under Title XI of the act. In order to qualify for funds under the new Title XXI, states would have to begin extending Medicaid coverage immediately to all adolescents between fourteen and eighteen years, up to 133 percent of FPL, rather than letting the coverage phase in by 2002, as required under current law.[173] The secretary was given authority to approve the states' "outlines" for increasing coverage as well as the benefit packages they would provide. Federal matching percentages for expansion under either plan would be the same: the existing Medicaid rate with bonuses up to 15 percent for new coverage. Elaborate precautions were taken to insure that states spent money received under this title for child health: a "maintenance of effort" clause; applying

Medicaid limits on provider taxes and donations;[174] and giving the secretary authority to audit the programs. The changes obtained in this fashion amounted cumulatively to a significant difference—enough to narrow considerably the distance between the block grant and the Medicaid option and to make the Senate version the clear favorite of child health advocates.

Several other measures enhanced to benefits or beneficiary protections. One amendment protected families below 150 percent of the poverty line from more than nominal copayments.[175] Senator Chafee added to this one of the most far-reaching and potentially controversial measures: requiring states choosing the block grant option to provide health care benefits equivalent to the FEHBP standard Blue Cross/Blue Shield PPO plan, including hearing and vision services. And the Domenici-Wellstone alliance struck again, this time with a floor amendment that required full parity for mental health benefits under the block grant option.

Medicaid.   With regard to flexibility provisions, the Senate Finance bill was similar, in general outlines, to the House version. It repealed the Boren Amendment, like the House providing a public notice and comment for the rate-making procedure. The committee rejected a compromise proposal backed by Jim Jeffords (R., Vt.) that would have required that an actuary review the payment rates, but did agree to a review by the secretary after four years to determine the effect of the repeal upon access and quality of services.[176] As with the House bill, states would no longer need a waiver to enroll Medicaid beneficiaries in managed care plans, including the PACE program, though children with special needs and dual eligibles were exempt from this provision. The Finance Committee continued existing law with respect to the Federally Qualified Health Centers and Rural Health Centers (i.e., full cost reimbursement). However, with a homily on personal responsibility (U.S. Congress 1997b:172), the committee allowed limited cost sharing for services states were not required to cover, and capped states' liability for coinsurance for low-income Medicare beneficiaries at the level of Medicaid provider payments.

As in the House, the Senate Finance Committee required managed care quality standards, technically a substitute for the 75/25 formula, but also an agreed-upon complement to the flexibility provisions. Again, Senator Chafee and some of the moderates and liberals on Senate Finance were decisive. Chafee had long supported managed care quality standards and patients' rights. In 1995, he introduced an earlier version, which failed to pass. In 1997, a bipartisan Chafee-Breaux bill built upon this foundation and provided most of the quality and access standards eventually included in the Senate bill.[177]

As reported, the Finance Committee provision would require the state agency "to develop and implement a quality assessment and improvement strategy consistent with standards the Secretary shall monitor" (U.S. Congress 1997b:166). Along with this came "quality assurance data . . . the Secretary shall specify . . . regular and periodic examination of the scope and content of the quality improvement strategy," and "annual validation surveys." Also included were other aspects of care and service delivery related to quality, including grievance procedures and marketing and information standards as well as a number of specific patient and provider rights.[178]

Unlike the House bill, the Chafee-Breaux initiative went beyond quality standards to include access requirements and regulation of the enrollment process. Access requirements got rather specific, including ratios of primary care practitioners to enrollees; access to and appropriate referral to specialists; services available to children with special needs; and timely delivery of services on a twenty-four-hour, seven-day-a-week basis. Another set of provisions dealt in detail with the enrollment process, with requirements that states and MCOs provide user-friendly election materials including comparisons of plans in a chartlike form and guarantees to assure fair and nondiscriminatory enrollment, change of plan, reentry, and termination. These amendments, though not included in the committee report, were accepted in principle during the markup and legislative language was added later.[179]

These Chafee-Breaux amendments, if passed, and fully implemented, would have gone some distance toward bringing Medicaid into the mainstream of American medicine. They vexed the governors and the House Commerce Committee, though, both of which took a dim view of proliferating standards and attempting to micromanage or even closely monitor health plans at the state level, especially on such matters as enrollment procedures and the mix of provider services. Most of these amendments were dropped in conference or the House version substituted.[180]

During the markup, the committee included most of S. 865, a fraud and abuse bill dealing with Medicare and Medicaid that had been developed by Sen. Bob Graham and his staff. The Medicaid elements were assembled into a bill introduced by Senator Breaux. Among the more important statements was one that no Medicaid payment would be made for "roads, bridges, stadiums, or any other item or service" not covered under a state plan.[181] Full disclosure and $50,000 surety bonds were required of home health agencies or suppliers of durable medical equipment.[182] And authority was given to the secretary to refuse to contract with individuals or entities convicted of a felony and to impose civil monetary penalties upon providers who did deal with them.

A seemingly innocuous inclusion was a mandate to states "to provide programs to ensure program integrity, *protect and advocate on behalf of individuals,* [emphasis added] and collect data about complaints and instances of beneficiary abuse or of program fraud, waste, and abuse."[183] This was, not so obviously, a move to establish ombudsmen within the states or, at a minimum, programs for consumer advocacy. However wise or desirable this initiative might have been, it had not been generally discussed. This language passed the Finance Committee and the Senate and survived almost to the conference, but it was spotted by Ed Grossman, the House legislative counsel, and called to the attention of Commerce Committee staff. Following their objection the provision was removed.[184]

One item in both the House and Senate bills that survived the conference was language that "a person who, for a fee, assists an individual to dispose of assets" in order to qualify for nursing home care would be liable to a fine or imprisonment.[185] This egregious piece of foolishness was actually a step forward—or at least sideways—in the annals of legislation, since it replaced an earlier version in HIPAA known as the "Granny goes to jail" provision, which made the elderly individual personally liable. The 1997 version was appropriately tagged as "Granny's lawyer goes to jail" and savvy folk had fun speculating on the problems of enforcing it. Many thought it was unconstitutional on its face; and Janet Reno—then the attorney general —said that she would not allocate any funds for defending this provision should it be challenged in the courts.

The Senate, like the House, expected to achieve most of their Medicaid savings by cutting DSH payments. The original budget agreement called for $17.8 billion total Medicaid savings. CBO estimated, at the time, that the various flexibility amendments would save no more than a paltry $1.2 billion. CBO also estimated a 25 percent leakage or "behavioral offset," so that instead of $16.2 billion, actual DSH cuts of more than $21 billion might be needed.[186] Confronted with this prospect, and anticipating another nasty formula fight, Senate Finance devised an artful solution, but one that, like the House Commerce formula, left some matters unresolved.

The Finance Committee proposal was complex, but it amounted, in the main, to a scheduled reduction that was easy on low-DSH states (less than 3 percent of Medicaid expenditures), moderately hard on middle-DSH states (3–12 percent), and easy on high-DSH states (over 12 percent), except for those with large payments for their mental health "institutes"[187] or other mental facilities. Low-DSH states would have their DSH payments frozen through 2002. Middle-DSH states would be reduced by steps, for a maximum reduction of 15 percent by 2002. High-DSH states without any mental health DSH payments in 1995 would get payments through 2002 equal to their average for 1995 and 1996. But high-DSH states with mental health DSH payments would have their DSH payments for inpatient facilities reduced 20 percent by 2002, and their payments for IMDs or mental hospitals completely phased out over five years. The committee draft also directed the states to "provide assurances" to the secretary that they had developed a system for prioritizing DSH payments, but did not itself undertake that difficult and thankless task.[188]

Behind this odd-looking approach, and seemingly heartless attack on mental health facilities, lies a story. Senate Finance, especially Senator Breaux and some of the staff,[189] had been tracking the most recent DSH "scam," involving "intergovernmental transfers" (IGTs), practiced most egregiously by mental health "institutes" or facilities.[190] As documented by the General Accounting Office and the Congressional Research Service, some states—notably Maryland, Pennsylvania, and Texas—had been raking in vast amounts of DSH employing this method.

In effect, by shutting down one more state DSH scam, the Finance Committee was closing a loophole and saving a considerable amount of money. This amounted almost to "found" money, hit only a few states, and would avoid a nasty formula fight. Yet there was another side to the story. Scam or not, this money helped needy patients and supported institutions caring for the poor and disabled. Provider and advocacy groups and two states in particular, Texas and Pennsylvania, protested so strongly that John Kasich promised the matter would receive special attention in the conference. In the Senate, Chairman Roth's manager's amendment, adopted by a floor vote, delayed the beginning of the phase out by a year and changed the formula so that no state would fall below its 1995 level of funds.[191] The loophole was far from closed and the Senate had to look elsewhere for additional savings.

With respect to eligibility, coverage, and cost-sharing, the Senate bill was roughly similar to the House, but with characteristic differences. As for children, both houses would begin immediately to cover children up to the age of nineteen. Both went along with a Clinton priority to support continuous coverage for a year. The Senate did not, however, extend coverage to "SSI kids" who had lost eligibility as a result of welfare reforms. The House allowed states to provide such coverage but did not mandate it. The House also allowed "presumptive eligibility" for children; the Senate did not. On the other hand, the Senate was, in general, more protective of dual eligibles, especially the disabled (a Chafee priority). Both houses restored SSI and Medicaid benefits to qualified aliens receiving benefits before August, 1996; but the Senate added those who became disabled after 1996. The Senate also allowed a Medicaid "buy in" for disabled workers with family incomes up to 250 percent of FPL. On the other hand, the Senate adopted a measure, strongly lobbied by the state governors, that would require providers to accept Medicaid rates of reimbursement for treating dual eligibles, rather than the higher Medicare payments—a provision that saved $5 billion.

These items were relatively insignificant pieces of the vast reconciliation process. One important factor in determining their fate was conservative opposition, within Senate Finance, to increasing entitlements or a major expansion in eligibility.[192] This was countered by strong advocacy for the disabled and for children by Chafee and Rockefeller, less often by Hatch and Graham. Most of these small, specific differences were settled in the conference, some with strong lobbying from the administration.

After two days of markup, characterized by a number of strongly argued differences and close votes, Senate Finance approved both its Medicare and Medicaid reforms by a unanimous vote of 20–0. In floor action, the Senate endorsed the work of the committee. It adopted by voice vote the Chafee-Rockefeller amendments, which would have required FEHBP equivalent plans and limited premiums, deductibles, and copays for low-income families. Also by voice vote, it approved the proposal by Domenici and Wellstone for mental health parity for children's health care funded under the block grant option.[193] On June 25, the Senate passed the spending part of the reconciliation bill by a vote of 73–27—most of the Democrats objecting to the provision that would have raised eligibility from sixty-five to sixty-seven. On July 26 both houses adjourned for the weeklong Independence Day recess, with July 7 set as the date for the conference to begin.

IV. THE CONFERENCE

The summit agreement and the bipartisan budget resolution called for two separate reconciliation bills. The first, HR 2014, "The Taxpayers' Relief Act of 1997," dealt with taxes, mostly reductions, while the second, HR 2015, the Balanced Budget Act of 1997, contained the expenditure savings, roughly half to come from Medicare and Medicaid, and the rest from caps on discretionary spending and defense cuts. Like the three-part reconciliation strategy attempted by the Republican leadership in 1996, the two-part variant in 1997 was a calculated political move, this time, by the White House. It would give Democrats the option of voting for the BBA but against the tax bill, if it turned out to be skewed toward the wealthy, and it preserved White House leverage, since Clinton could champion the balanced budget act and still veto the tax package.[194]

The separation also symbolized rather effectively the importance of the tax provisions in the reconciliation process. In this instance, tax reductions rather than new taxes were most of the story, except for taxes on cigarettes and airline tickets. Even though the main business was tax reductions, these were more divisive and time consuming than Medicare and Medicaid for two major reasons. For Medicare and Medicaid some of the most controversial issues had been eliminated over time, and there had been more experience and learning about what was politically possible. With respect to the tax legislation, positions were initially less well known and tested. In addition, a number of the tax provisions—such as a child tax credit, education tax credits, new IRAs, and the corporate alternative minimum tax (AMT)—were signature items for both political parties and the president, most of them freighted with ideological overtones.

For this reconciliation, the president was in a strong position relative to the

Congress. Both sides wanted a successful outcome, but the Republicans needed it more.[195] They had behind them two unsuccessful legislative years and, within the House, were embroiled in an attempted coup to unseat Newt Gingrich as speaker. Republicans could use a victory, something they could take home to their constituents during the August recess. The August adjournment had for them both a symbolic and a practical importance, and they had already posted it as a deadline. That meant time was on the side of the president and the Democrats, who were in a better position to demur and postpone the debate beyond August into the fall. The president was enjoying 65 percent approval ratings in the polls and some of his issues, such as child care and education tax incentives, played well with the public compared, for instance, to cutting corporate and estate taxes. Another important factor was that members of the administration had been actively involved in the reconciliation process since April, so that they were at a high level of proficiency in the specialized kind of politics and negotiation that was involved.

The conference on the spending bill was initially scheduled to begin on July 7, immediately after the July 4 recess. It began formally on July 10, with an opening ceremony and a number of statements, following which it adjourned and several working subconferences were appointed.[196] The week of July 7 was important in a preliminary way, as advocates for particular policies in House, Senate, and the administration staked out some positions, put forward tentative offers, and probed for possible negotiating opportunities. An early move of strategic significance was a House resolution, instructing its conferees to oppose a Senate attempt to increase the Medicare age of eligibility from sixty-five to sixty-seven. Though this was a nonbinding resolution, it passed by a vote of 414–14. President Clinton, who had earlier sent to Congress a list of his concerns about Medicare and Medicaid provisions in the House and Senate bills, let it be known that he was firmly opposed to increasing the Medicare age of eligibility, but might be open to means-testing.[197] Senators Chafee and Rockefeller were working with John Dingell, Henry Waxman, and other allies on the House Commerce Committee to see if they could get the House to adopt language on child health friendly to the Senate position. Advocacy groups for providers or beneficiaries were taking this critical opportunity to alert or mobilize their constituencies and "to work with" congressional staff over the particulars of DSH formulas, updates, capital reimbursement percentages, and so forth.

In size and importance, this reconciliation conference compared with that of 1995 (which led to the veto) and an earlier one in 1990. It had other distinguishing features of its own. One was the prominent role of the two budget committee chairmen, Pete Domenici and John Kasich, who chaired the budget conferences for their respective houses. More commonly, because of their role in authorization and taxes, the chairmen of Ways and Means and Senate Finance would manage this part of the reconciliation conference. Also noteworthy were the Senate health conferees: Lott, Roth, and Moynihan. None of them was either expert or especially interested in health care. Senator Chafee, who usually managed for the Senate in health affairs was left out of the conference. A third unusual aspect of this conference, and of the reconciliation process as a whole, was the extent of involvement by the administration.

The year 1997 was seen as a good time for a reconciliation—a quest looking for an opportunity to happen. Serious negotiations between the White House and the Congress had begun roughly a week after March 19, when Clinton first requested a meeting with the House and Senate Budget Committee chairmen and the ranking Democrats.[198] From then until July 31, when the conference report was passed by the House and Senate, the executive branch was in a negotiating mode, similar to though not as highly mobilized as 1995.[199] Like earlier "negotiations," the activities included letters and statements from the White House and a few strategic meetings with the president; many sessions between administration and congressional principals; and enormous amounts of staff work to vet and critique proposals, brief principals, develop options, and help negotiate viable compromises. Of special importance was a collective ability to combine negotiable policies with well-timed jawboning, credible threats, and persuasive rhetoric—a natural advantage of the presidency, and a skill that both Clinton and the administration had acquired in the school of hard knocks.

The conference did most of its work in thirteen large " subconferences" of which Medicare/ Medicaid was one. Their general mode of proceeding was to have staff work over the proposals to see how much could be quickly resolved and what had to be referred back to principals, the subconference members, another subconference, or the leadership. Operating in this fashion and under pressure of time, the conferees tended to make the easy decisions first and to begin offering and counteroffering on the more intractable or divisive items in preparation for the hard bargaining that lay ahead. For instance, in the Medicare subconference, medical savings accounts (and MEWAs), medical malpractice, and means testing along with the Medicare eligibility age were deferred,[200] while they set to work on hospital payment updates, a relatively nonpartisan issue and one on which House and Senate were close to agreement. Meanwhile, proposals were being floated and offers and counteroffers proffered with respect to the eligibility age and means testing.

Within the subconferences, the minority had a relatively minor role. For an item, they were a distinct minority—only one Democrat in the Senate subconference and two in the House. They were excluded from Republican-only strategy sessions. Nevertheless, when the conferees were respected and savvy members such as Pete Stark and John Dingell, their personal force and expertise were worth a good deal. Moreover, as the Republican conference chairman, John Boehner, described the process, it was a "two-and-one-half-way talk,"[201] with the House and Senate Republicans negotiating their differences, while keeping an eye out for what the Democrats and the White House were doing. In this sense, the Democrats were quite active, reminding the Republicans of the summit agreement and seeking to develop viable alternatives that they and the president could support and use to win concessions, prevail in a close vote, or if bad came to worse, sustain a veto.

An important factor working to moderate partisanship was staff—personal and committee staff and staff from the executive agencies. Negotiations during this reconciliation conference were hurried and fluid, with new initiatives and counteroffers being put on the table, often in rapid succession. With Medicare and Medicaid, the policy issues were institutionally dense and complex, technical, and consequential so that, in practice, members—even the most knowledgeable—were heavily dependent on their staff to know what they are voting for and to work out compromises among principals, within the majority, and across party lines. The demand for numbers and programmatic expertise was both immediate and enormous, so that, regularly, expert staff from HCFA, DHHS, CBO, and OMB got detailed to work with or called in to consult with the Medicare/Medicaid subconference.[202] In fact, in this kind of situation, staff is not just "consulted," they often develop in detail a proposal or a compromise that has been agreed upon in principle. Differences between parties and between Congress and the administration are diminished and shared expertise and institutional memory can have an important influence. To put it another way, a reconciliation conference without good staff support would be risky and possibly disastrous.

Initially, Republican leaders had expected to complete the spending reconciliation bill within eight to ten days, so that it could come to the House and Senate floors during the week of July 21. That schedule was thrown off by a slow start, several divisive Medicare and Medicaid issues, and some serious disagreements over the tax bill. As a result, the Republicans who went to the White House on July 23 with an initial proposal brought a plan still unresolved on important particulars such as eligibility age, means testing, and the prescribed minimum benefits and authorizations for child care.

Throughout the month of June and into July, the administration expressed concern and pressed its views on a number of issues, such as the eligibility age for Medicare and means testing, where savings should come from, the Part A/Part B shift, premium support for low-income Medicare beneficiaries, restoring benefits to the "SSI kids" and disabled legal aliens, and the size, structure, and funding of the child health program. Most of these items were covered in the original summit agreement, though some were not. Others were subject to interpretation or reopening. As a form of politics, the process closely resembled diplomatic preliminaries to negotiation or to conflict, in which priorities are signaled, and the seriousness of the issue or ultimate intentions indicated by the rank and gravity of the speaker and the rhetoric employed. Viewed this way, Clinton and his lead team of Erskine Bowles,

Frank Raines, and John Hilley did a good job, though Democrats, especially in the House, complained that the administration left them guessing or in the dark too much of the time.

Meanwhile, the conferees continued to struggle with the massive complexities of hospital updates, managed care payment formulas, DSH cuts, and concessions for individual provider groups, such as rural clinics or teaching hospitals, while their colleagues and cohorts of lobbyists pressed their own vital concerns. Not surprisingly, the schedule slipped somewhat, though the conferees repeated their resolve to have a report ready for the president's signature before the August recess.

Prior to the meeting with the White House on July 23, Republican leadership and the conferees spent several days in closed meetings, developing a unified position as a basis for negotiation.[203] During this period, the administration, congressional leaders, and key advocacy groups were sending letters and issuing statements that served to identify priorities, stake out positions, and reassure their own followers. Republicans took a hard stand on some taxes, on the total amount and the specific benefits for child health, and on Medicare managed care options. The president stated that he would fight for $24 billion and warned against a "watered down" package for child health; offered his own version of a compromise on the means testing proposal; and sent a letter saying that a failure to restore funding for legal immigrants would be a serious violation of the budget agreement.[204]

This stage of the conference followed the pattern of conference negotiations generally, except that it was president vs. the Congress, not House vs. Senate. That being the case, the administration's decision to exclude congressional Democrats from the negotiations made sense, but it was a decision that rankled with these Democrats.[205] Otherwise, in typical conference fashion, once the Republican conferees had agreed upon their position and delivered their offer to the president, they broke again into subgroups to explain and defend their proposals and begin negotiating with the administration. As the negotiations developed, conferees, senior staff, and administration officials moved from group to group. Within these groups, behind closed doors, senior staff briefed their principals and sought to provide the numbers, policy considerations, and political intelligence needed for decisions, while outside these doors other staff from Congress and the administration mostly waited but occasionally engaged in less controversial staff-level negotiations, the vetting of new options as they developed, or working out agreements in detail.[206]

Several factors were working strongly to facilitate an agreement. Critically important was the removal, demoting, or resolving over time of a number of "deal-breakers," such as block-granting Medicaid, medical savings accounts, or dropping the premium support for SLMBs.[207] Another was the enormous investment both sides had in a successful outcome—both in the form of time and effort already expended and the potential gains for the administration and the congressional Republicans—though House Democrats were skeptical about the benefits for them. Time was especially important for the Republicans, who were eager to bring the conference to a successful conclusion before the August recess and not have to face this unfinished business upon their return to Washington.

On the first day of negotiations, July 24, administration representatives and the budget conferees explained and reexplained their positions and defended them rhetorically, without negotiating any differences. For an opening day, that was probably to be expected. In a constructive move, though, Republican negotiators set about to reduce the number of their major differences with the administration to ten issues so that serious discussions could begin.[208] Also, on the 24, the White House sent to GOP leaders a list of thirteen objectionable Medicare provisions in the draft conferees report.[209] Then, on July 26, top White House officials and congressional leaders sat down together to try to narrow their differences. Notable for its absence was the concealment of intentions, strategic gamesmanship, and blustering rhetoric that had characterized summit negotiations in 1995.

Most of this stage of the conference was occupied with the tax bill, for which positions were much less developed, and a number of high policy issues yet to be resolved. With respect to Medicare and Medicaid, there were items disputed as between House and Senate—such as the Medicaid DSH formula—but few differences of real consequence or that could not be settled with some relatively straightforward bargaining. Moreover, the mood was one of negotiation and deal-making with an expectation that, as issues got resolved, momentum would develop and the negotiators would soon be shaking hands. The steady progress made to this point on Medicare and Medicaid encouraged compromise, since, by now, neither the House and Senate nor the president and Congress were far apart on most important issues, often differing about small dollar amounts or incremental program changes. Another important point is that policy options had been well staffed, so that for a number of issues conferees could reach a comfortable compromise: by combining both approaches (Medicaid and child health), phasing in a change (Part A/Part B shift), or tilting a bit more toward the House or Senate position (child health benefits package).

A troublesome Medicare issue was the familiar Senate amendments sponsored by Breaux and Kerrey. These amendments would have raised the eligibility age to sixty-seven, means-tested the Part B premium payment, and required a $5 copay for home health visits. Of the three, the eligibility age was almost a nonstarter, since both the House and the president were strongly opposed, even with its compromise buy-in provision.[210] This proposal was eventually dropped, though it was one of the twelve items referred to the National Bipartisan Commission on the Future of Medicare.

The means testing proposal was potentially an important money saver and largely for that reason was supported by the president. A major problem with means testing, especially if administered by the Internal Revenue Service, was that it looked too much like a tax—which was repugnant to many Republicans.[211] One compromise proposal in the Senate would have had DHHS administer the program, but that option lost most of the savings. Shortly thereafter, the administration brought forward another proposal that would allow the taxpayer to determine his or her own income and send a check along with the April 15 income tax form. This option would also funnel part of the revenue through the Treasury, not the IRS, and augment the Medicare trust fund.[212] Even this sanitized version did not satisfy tax-haters like Phil Gramm, who complained that it still "looks and smells like a tax." Eventually, the administration gave up on means testing and it was dropped from the final conference report, but it provides a good illustration of how a proposal can lose in part because of lack of prior staffing and associations with the "T-word."

The defeat of these proposals left a number of legislators, especially in the Senate, distressed that so little attention was being given to issues of baby-boomer demography and the long-term viability of the Medicare program. One response would be that the reconciliation process is not a very good method for examining or discussing such issues. Congress did provide for the Bipartisan Commission in the Senate version with its more comprehensive and ambitious charge. That also proved to be a poor vehicle for thoughtful consideration (see pp. 353–54).

The child health provision, which continued to divide the conferees, provided an illustration of how a "deal-breaker" can be turned into a "deal-maker." Back in mid-June, the National Governors' Association had come out strongly against the Chafee-Breaux proposal. When this was dropped, CHIP was left as the plausible alternative, even though President Clinton argued with low intensity and volume that the conference reconsider the Chafee-Breaux approach. With Medicaid expansion sidelined, the administration was even more committed to the $24 billion increased authorization for child health and to assuring that there be a robust benefits plan.

The trouble was that the momentum seemed to be going the other way, as the House and Senate conferees, in their preliminary sessions, moved back toward the House $16 billion proposal and a more flexible benefit package.[213] As an aftermath to the Hatch-Kennedy defeat, though, the Finance Committee had agreed to increase the cigarette tax by $0.20 and earmark $8 billion of the revenues for child health. In the original plan, a cigarette tax would also allow a reduction in the airline ticket tax and the capital gains tax for real estate and fund an increase in the number of working poor who would get the $500 tax credit.[214] Of course, that decision did not commit the conference. But Clinton took a strong position on $24 billion and congressional Democrats weighed in, with Senator Daschle ruminating darkly that the August recess might have to be delayed.[215] The solution, first broached on July 24, was to transfer the cigarette tax, somewhat reduced, from the tax bill to the spending bill, which would help assure its survival and make the $8 billion immediately available. As compensation, tobacco companies would be allowed to offset this tax against their June settlement with the forty states that had sued them for tobacco-related damages.[216] Like it or not, when there is a will in Congress, there is often a way.

Benefits for the SLMBs, the "SSI kids," and the disabled legal immigrants had been pretty much resolved by this stage—but not quite. Although the amounts of money were comparatively trivial, these categories had important symbolic value, both for the Clinton administration and for Congress. Neither house, for instance, had initially authorized the full $1.5 billion in premium supplements for the low-income Medicare beneficiaries, in effect passing the issue on to the conference. The matter was dealt with, prior to the conference, in negotiations between John Kasich and Pete Domenici. With respect to the "SSI kids," House and Senate had gone part of the way, allowing but not requiring states to provide coverage. In the conference, they went the rest of the distance. Even more importantly, they also dropped a provision that would have allowed states to discontinue SSI benefits entirely, a change that would have affected as many as 345,000 aged or disabled persons.[217] The legal aliens remained a sticking point, up to a pretty explicit veto threat. In the final conference report, Congress yielded on this as well, mostly adopting Senate language, to restore coverage to legal aliens, including those who had become subsequently disabled, so long as they had entered the country by August 22, 1996.[218] The conference agreement did not, however, cover the children of these aliens, or people who became disabled during the naturalization process.

During this period, the House and Senate conferees continued to struggled with some outstanding issues that they had failed to resolve. No surprise, the two most difficult of these involved distribution formulas. Final agreement on the payment formula for HMOs continued to divide the provider constituency and the House and Senate, especially over how rapidly to increase payments for rural and relatively underpaid HMOs at the expense of those with historically high AAPCCs. This controversy was finally resolved by guaranteeing a minimum payment for all HMOs of $378 per beneficiary per month to help out rural areas and low-cost urban areas and a minimum overall payment increase of 2 percent a year, to protect the urban and high-cost HMOs. Arbitrary though it might seem, this formula represented some carefully crafted incrementalism.

The House and Senate conferees continued to tussle over the Medicaid DSH formula almost to the end, providing another example of how Congress prefers to resolve complex distributive issues. Neither the House nor the Senate had reached an elegant resolution of this issue; and their final word seemed to be, "Let the conference do it." Initially, the conference approach was to leave it to the states: let them decide which of the two approaches they preferred—

House or Senate. Twelve high-DSH states, including Texas, were not happy with either option and lobbied the conference for a more favorable formula. Congress also did some lobbying of its own and got CBO to reduce its offset from 25 to 15 percent, which meant considerably less had to be saved. The DSH cuts were then readjusted to make sure that no state would lose more than 3.5 percent of its total Medicaid funding.[219] Meanwhile, $600 million was allocated to help out four states—Texas, New York, New Jersey, and Missouri—that had a large number of low-income, uninsured beneficiaries.[220] Conferees also wrote into law the lesser of the House or Senate DSH cuts for each state. The Senate restrictions on payments to Institutions for Mental Diseases [IMDs] and other mental institutions remained. CBO scored the new DSH savings at $10.4 billion, down considerably from the $18 to $21 billion once anticipated.

The penultimate stage of the reconciliation ended with an intense weekend of discussion and negotiation, July 26–27. On Monday, July 28, Trent Lott announced from his office that a tentative agreement had been reached. Considering the number of difficult issues to be resolved, the period of time seems remarkably short. The president received this welcome news while playing golf. Trent Lott said at the time, "We gave ground, and the administration gave ground, and we found common ground."[221] It sounds easier than it was.

On July 30, after ninety minutes of debate, the House adopted the conference report by a vote of 346–85. A day later, the Senate cleared the report by a vote of 85–15. The dissenters were mostly liberal Democrats in the House and conservative Republicans in the Senate. On August 5, with flags flying and a military band playing, President Clinton signed the spending and tax reconciliation bills, calling them "a true milestone for our nation."[222]

V. SOME ACCOMPLISHMENTS

Use of the term "accomplishment" may be inaccurate or misleading, since it suggests definite achievements and the reaching of some kind of closure. That may be too positive a description of what happened. Without doubt, BBA 97 was, for Medicare and Medicaid, the most important—at least the biggest and most comprehensive—body of legislation passed since 1965. Yet with some years in which to gain distance and perspective, it would seemed to have achieved little except to make some incremental changes and put the debate over Medicare and Medicaid on a somewhat different footing without resolving fundamental differences over basic philosophy, program structure, or methods of payment and cost containment.

The reconciliation itself—considered solely as a legislative exercise—was a remarkable achievement, even though so unusual in some respects that it is hard to know what to conclude from the event. Much was owed to the past: to the BBA of 1995 that challenged the Medicare and Medicaid entitlements and created a plausible template for change; and to the "cooling out" exercises of 1996 that tempered ideology and began a shift away from mobilization politics. Of comparable importance was the summit agreement between the president and the Republican Congress that bounded controversy within a deficit reduction matrix and took off the table the most divisive issues, such as the disentitlement of Medicare or Medicaid.

Under rather special circumstances, Congress and the president put together a huge, complex, broadly acceptable, and bipartisan body of legislation from which both sides—House Democrats excepted—could walk away claiming important victories. Republicans could point to a balanced budget, a $500 per child tax credit, reductions in the capital gains and estate taxes, and ten years of solvency for Medicare along with some restructuring of both the Medicare and Medicaid entitlements. President Clinton and the Democrats could claim their part in deficit reduction, tilting of the tax cuts toward middle and lower income groups, preserving the Medicare and Medicaid entitlements, a new child health initiative, and restoration of welfare and/or health benefits for legal aliens, disabled children, and low-income Medicare beneficiaries.

Particularly striking about the Medicare and Medicaid legislation, to consider these more narrowly, is how much seemed to be determined by the numbers and policy rather than by cutting deals for specific interest groups or constituencies. For the most part, Congress and the administration were trying to hit the budget numbers and fashion a bipartisan compromise on policy. There were some "rifle shots" in the reconciliation, delays in implementation, and tinkering with formulas. The Medicaid DSH and the managed care payments were adjusted—in fact, largely designed—to address but also mitigate regional disparities, and physicians, medical schools, and Texas got some special consideration—which mostly reflected the interests of particular legislators, not the strength of the lobby. So far as the Medicare and Medicaid legislation are concerned, this reconciliation seemed, as policy, comparable or better than most reconciliation exercises and much larger in scope and programmatic effect.

It is remarkable that both Republicans and Democrats declared a win on Medicare and Medicaid. That was, in part, because the most divisive issues, such as the status of the entitlement or fundamental restructuring were taken off the table by the summit agreement. It is also true that neither confronted the major weaknesses of their own positions. For Democrats, the unresolved problem, which for the most part they walled off and ignored, was how to restructure or "reinvent" Medicare in anticipation of the long-term demographics and technological change that would, within ten to fifteen years begin generating drastically increasing costs. For Republicans, it was how to assure that the frail elderly, the chronically ill, and the "dual eligibles" would be protected and not selected against by health plans or otherwise neglected and unfairly burdened. As for cost containment, each side fudged the issues by prescribing untried or unknown solutions. For Democrats it was prospective payment systems and the "prudent purchaser." For Republicans, it was the promise of competition. Not then and not today has either side ever seriously confronted the limitations of its own cost containment strategy of choice. Both were, of course, engaged in the politically charged and action-forcing reconciliation process—not a time to be choosy or diffident about key elements of that strategy. Nonetheless, that is the point: the situation encourages one-sided solutions and dubious commitments that can mortgage the future.

Chip Kahn, who was the chief staff aide for the Medicare legislation, both in 1995 and 1997, later described to an HIAA conference on Medicare+Choice what he thought to be the most important achievements of the legislation.[223] After citing trust fund solvency and increased choice, he stressed especially expanding the types of health plan choices, comparison shopping, and reaping the quality and savings potential of managed care in order to improve benefits.[224] One comment is that Medicare+Choice was, in fact, poorly designed to foster competition, as opposed to increasing choice. Beyond that, the evidence that competition, except under special conditions, works to control costs or enhance quality for a Medicare population is spotty and often tendentious. The main point is that to base a broad strategy like Medicare+Choice upon such considerations has to be, in large measure, an act of faith, not one justified by good economic theory, empirical evidence, or demonstrations. Of course, public policy is often based upon faith, and frequently goes against the putative wisdom of policy experts. Yet, it is also true that much of the ideology supporting managed care and MSA options is uncritically invoked as though an abstract and unexamined concept of the "market" will do whatever it needs to do to make dreams come true.[225] In this sense, as mentioned earlier, Republicans often tend in health care discussions to "postulate" the future.

Bruce Vladeck, the administrator of HCFA, had both a unique grasp of Medicare politics and observed the reconciliation process in both 1995 and 1997. In reviewing the accomplishments of BBA 97, he emphasized the preservation of the entitlement with a link between FFS Medicare and managed care, the legislative structure of the Medicare+Choice option, quality standards and government control of marketing, "prudent purchasing," and the extension of prospective payment systems to cover outpatient and subacute activities. Not mentioned were private sector or competitive strategies. It was well-known that Bruce Vladeck was not a fan of managed care or private sector strategies. Beyond that, the Democrats have had, generally, a comparative advantage in regulatory and incremental approaches—they are more comfortable and also more experienced with them. As one result, when a specific proposal or legislative text was needed, for instance, for Medicare+

Choice or the outpatient PPSs, Democrats often had experience, grasp of detail, and control of the administration working for them, while Republicans were pushing for the new and untried. Of course, this advantage is at its maximum when building upon existing institutions or approaches, for instance, by extending administered pricing to the outpatient payment categories or adding quality standards and marketing regulations to managed care. In this, Democrats in Congress or a Democratic administration simply did what comes naturally, and what, in their view, would defend Medicare against being disentitled or gradually privatized. This approach tends to "institutionalize the future," to lock up some choices and to make future change difficult. The multiple prospective payment systems would be a case in point—hard to perfect and hard to get rid of.

Somewhat similar observations apply to Medicaid. Neither Republicans nor Democrats squarely addressed the critically important issue of how to provide, effectively and humanely, for the dual eligibles, especially the handicapped and frail elderly. Also, Medicaid has its own myths, which have to do not with the market, but with imaginary consequences of centralization or decentralization and how governors (or states) would use or abuse flexibility. There, too, Democrats like to regulate and Republicans to deregulate, though with fifty states and the territories there is a wealth of empirical and experimental evidence.

It would be comforting the think that BBA 97 represented some kind of return to normalcy (whatever that term now means) and to bipartisan government. As an episode of bipartisanship, it was instructive but complex. In some ways the virtual unanimity of the Ways and Means Committee on Medicare was remarkable, though it may have sacrificed inventiveness and illumination of the issues to what amounted almost to nonpartisan behavior. In this respect, the House Commerce Committee provided an interesting contrast, in which differing partisan views were combined into a product that seemed to gain from both points of view. The Senate showed itself in traditional form, displaying individualism, bipartisan collaboration, and critical review. In this sense, the institutions of government seemed to work well. Yet this was a special and possibly unique situation. It is hard to believe that legislation of this scope and difficulty could have been passed without a legislative vehicle and the discipline provided by the reconciliation bill and the leadership of the president and administration.

This observation invites a sober reflection. Most of the changes in either Medicare or Medicaid since 1982 have been enacted through the budget and reconciliation process, driven in turn by attempts to contain the budget deficit. The disappearance of the deficit for a brief period brought about an uneasy recognition that having a surplus does not necessarily make policy easy, especially for Medicare and Medicaid. A former staff person observed that when Congress and the administration each put $120 billion on the table for new health care expenditures, that provoked as much partisan wrangling as taking it off had done in 1995.[226] For Medicare and Medicaid—somewhat like the Soviet Union in foreign policy—the deficit was an important unifying force, setting priorities and encouraging discipline. The surplus is now gone, but also gone for a time—in the aftermath of September 11, 2001 and the fight against terrorism—is concern about the deficit and the fiscal discipline that made the reconciliation process work, especially as a vehicle for change in the Medicare and Medicaid programs. For these programs, the future role of the reconciliation process is uncertain; but it is worth remembering that the deficit was not all bad.

NOTES

[1] Chip Kahn, CEO, Health Insurance Association of America; formerly, chief of staff, Ways and Means Medicare Subcommittee. Interview, October 14, 1998.

[2] Robert E. Moffit, deputy director of domestic policy, Heritage Foundation. Interview, June 22, 1999.

[3] Dan Rostenkowski (D., Ill.), long-time chairman of the House Ways and Means Committee, was legendary for his ability to put together tax compromises. A key to his strategy was to give each member enough to keep him or her from bolting the coalition, but just enough, so that he would have resources to hold others and to reward faithful supporters and contributors.

[4] *Congressional Quarterly,* January 4, 1997, p. 25.

[5] The lower figure resulted, in large part, from a "fiscal dividend," interest saved as the deficit was reduced. Ibid., February 1, 1997, p. 276.

[6] *Health Care Policy Report,* January 13, 1997, p. 67.

[7] Ibid., p. 67.

[8] Ibid., January 27, 1997, p. 138.

[9] David Abernethy, senior vice-president, Health Insurance Plan; formerly chief of staff, Ways and Means Health Subcommittee. Interview, August 13, 1998.

[10] Robert Reischauer, speaking of the Republicans' position on Medicare. *Congressional Quarterly,* February 1, 1997, p. 276.

[11] Ibid., p. 275.

[12] Ranking Democrats from House and Senate Budget Committees were included, but other Democratic leaders were not, specifically Richard Gephardt and Tom Daschle, the House and Senate minority leaders.

[13] Pundits were beginning to speak, for example, about the transition from presidential campaign politics to a legacy politics, in which the president would increasingly evaluate his actions with respect to how they might affect the legacy he would leave behind. *Congressional Quarterly,* April 19, 1997, p. 896.

[14] Bruce Vladeck, Mount Sinai School of Medicine; formerly HCFA administrator. Interview, February 8, 1999.

[15] Chris Jennings, deputy assistant to the president for health policy. Interview, June 9, 1999.16. *Health Care Policy Report,* January 13, 1997, p. 64.

[17] Ibid., January 27, 1997, p. 136.

[18] Ibid.

[19] Ibid.

[20] *Budget of the United States Government, Fiscal Year 1998* (Washington, D.C.: Government Printing Office, 1997), p. 50.

[21] *Health Care Policy Report,* March 10, 1997, p. 385.

[22] Although, as Representative Thomas pointed out, since it was a charge on Part B, most of the money would come from the U.S. Treasury. Ibid.

[23] Ibid., p. 386.

[24] *Congressional Quarterly,* February 8, 1997, p. 331.

[25] *Budget of the Unites States Government, Fiscal Year 1998,* p. 50.

[26] Ibid., p.54.

[27] Even though Republicans had proposed a similar switch in BBA 95.

[28] *Congressional Quarterly,* February 8, 1997, p. 328.

[29] Ibid.

[30] Ibid., February 15, 1997, p. 406.

[31] *Health Care Policy Report,* March 10, 1997, p. 385.

[32] *Congressional Quarterly,* March 15, 1997, p. 619.

[33] Ibid., March 22, 1997, p. 693.

[34] Ibid., March 15, 1997, p. 620.

[35] *Health Care Policy Report,* March 24, 1997, p. 472.

[36] Chris Jennings. Interview, May 30, 2000.

[37] *Health Care Policy Report,* March 24, 1997, p. 472.

[38] Also included were Deputy Chief of Staff John Podesta, CEA chairwoman Janet Yellen, Donna Shalala, and Chris Jennings. Ibid., April 14, 1997, p. 575.

[39] *Congressional Quarterly,* April 4, 1997, p. 838.

[40] Ibid., p. 839.

[41] Ibid., April 19, 1997, p. 897.

[42] Ibid.

[43] J. Ridgway Multop, senior economic adviser, House Democratic Policy Committee. Interview, December 12, 1998.

[44] *Health Care Policy Report,* January 27, 1997, p. 128.

[45] Chris Jennings. Interview, May 30, 2000.

[46] Discretionary spending is outlays controllable by appropriation, in contrast to entitlements, which by statute provide for payments to "entitled" individuals—for instance, Social Security, Medicare, and Medicaid enrollees.

[47] *Congressional Quarterly,* April 19, p. 892.

[48] Ibid., p. 897.

[49] Ibid., pp. 892–93.

[50] The Blue Dog budget would have delayed the tax cut to see if deficit reduction was effective; also it did not include a change in the CPI.

[51] Bill Vaughan, administrative assistant to Rep. Pete Stark. Interview, July 21, 1998.

[52] *Congressional Quarterly,* May 3, 1997, p. 993.

[53] Republican governors especially hated them; and congressional Democrats saw them as undermining the entitlement itself.

54 *Congressional Quarterly,* May 10, 1997, p. 1052.

55 net savings of $100 billion, added benefits of $15 billion.

56 *Health Care Policy Report,* May 12, 1997, p. 731.

57 *Congressional Quarterly,* May 24, 1997, p. 1183.

58 Ibid., May 10, 1997, p. 1047.

59 *Congressional Quarterly Almanac,* 1997, p. 2-26.

60 Ibid.

61 At one point, the House proceedings bogged down briefly, but over discretionary spending, not entitlements. *Congressional Quarterly,* May 24, 1997, p. 1189.

62 *Health Care Policy Report,* May 26, 1997, p. 815.

63 *Congressional Quarterly,* June 7, 1997, p. 1304.

64 Cf. Schick (1995:Exhibit 5-5, p. 84), for examples of typical reconciliation instructions.

65 Both Chip Kahn and Bill Vaughan, key staff members, agree upon this general mood and attitude.

66 Chip Kahn. Interview, October 14, 1998; Anne-Marie Lynch, chief of staff, Ways and Means Health Subcommittee; currently Pharmaceutical Manufacturers Association. Interview, August 12, 1998.

67 Bruce Vladeck. Interview, February 8, 1999.

68 Chip Kahn. Interview, October 14, 1998.

69 Anne-Marie Lynch. Interview, August 12, 1998.

70 Donald Young, Health Insurance Association of America; formerly, executive director of ProPAC. Interview, July 29, 1998. Anne-Marie Lynch. Interview, August 12, 1998.

71 Anne-Marie Lynch. Interview, August 12, 1998.

72 Chip Kahn. Interview, October 14, 1998.

73 Ibid. Interview, May 31, 2000.

74 Ibid. Also Bill Vaughan. Interview, July 21, 1998.

75 Medicare MSAs had to be combined with high-deductible (catastrophic) insurance plans and administered under risk contracts with HCFA.

76 Making the existence of an "emergency" depend upon what a "prudent layperson" would think under the circumstances, not what the health plan representative thought.

77 Howard Cohen, Goldberg Traurig; formerly professional staff, House Commerce Committee. Interview, May 19, 1999.

78 Rather than reverting to an earlier link to the Social Security cost-of-living adjustment (COLA).

79 The Health Subcommittee kept the link between the AAPCC and capitation payments, as did the final legislation.

80 "Cost Estimate Prepared by the Congressional Budget Office," *Balanced Budget Act of 1997,* House Report 105-149, p. 1382.

81 Anna-Marie Lynch. Interview, August 12, 1998.

82 During early discussions when considering what kind of payment mechanisms to adopt, Bruce Vladeck said that HCFA could design the systems. Later, doubts about doing all the systems at once were communicated to Chip Kahn and Julie James, lead staff persons for the Ways and Means and Finance health subcommittees; but by then the decisions were locked in. Nancy-Ann (Min) deParle, Kennedy School of Govern-

ment; formerly, HCFA administrator. Interview, March 8, 1999. Also Thomas Hoyer, director, Office of Chronic Care and Insurance, HCFA. Interview, April 20, 1999. No one was then thinking about the cumulative impact of BBA 97, the HCFA reorganization, and the Y2K problem.

[83] Gail Wilensky, chair, MedPAC. Interview, January 5, 1999.

[84] This initiative connected with the Senate Democrat's theme of moving Medicare from a role of "passive bill-payer" toward that of a "prudent purchaser."

[85] The venerable, and seemingly immortal, On Lok S/HMO demonstration was renewed.

[86] *Health Care Policy Report,* June 9, 1997, p. 883.

[87] Along with a delay in the resource-based payment schedule for physician office practice expenses.

[88] *Congressional Quarterly Almanac,* 1997, p. 6-6.

[89] *Health Care Policy Report,* June 16, 1997, p. 917.

[90] Ibid.

[91] *Congressional Quarterly Almanac,* 1997, p. 6-6.

[92] Ibid.

[93] After Sen. Jon Kyl (R., Ariz.), a physician.

[94] *Health Care Policy Report,* June 30, 1997, p. 1005.

[95] Senate Finance had a history of senators like Packwood and Durenberger who were informed and interested in health care. Senator Grassley, coming from Iowa, was especially concerned about managed care in rural areas.

[96] Linking the update to growth in GDP rather than the AAPCC would result in capitation payments under the Senate bill growing at 2 percent less per year than with the House version. *Health Care Policy Report,* June 30, 1997, p. 1005.

[97] As a way of compensating for favorable selection. The 5 percent would be phased out over five years.

[98] Ibid.

[99] Ibid., p. 1006.

[100] *Congressional Quarterly Almanac,* 1997, p. 6-8. The Senate amendment was concocted by Chafee and Graham staff aides and baited with funds to support telemedicine, osteoporosis screening, and Medigap for the disabled, which the staff knew appealed to particular senators on the Finance Committee. Lisa Layman, staff of Sen. Bob Graham, formerly staff of Sen. John Chafee. Interview, August 26, 1998.

[101] *Health Care Policy Report,* July 7, 1997, p. 1043.

[102] The deductible is the amount of out-of-pocket expense to be paid before the insurance coverage begins.

[103] *Health Care Policy Report,* July 7, 1997, p. 1073.

[104] Ibid., p. 1043.

[105] Part of the savings would have been used to increase premium support for low-income Medicare beneficiaries.

[106] *Congressional Quarterly Almanac,* 1997, p. 6-10.

[107] *Health Care Policy Report,* February 10, 1997, p. 219.

[108] Individuals who, because of poverty, age, or disability, are eligible for both Medicare and Medicaid.

[109] *Congressional Quarterly,* April 12, pp. 850–51.

[110] *Health Care Policy Report,* February 10, 1997, p. 219. Governors assumed that the

changes would occur, and wished primarily to have a strong voice in deciding particular arrangements that would be included.

[111] *Congressional Quarterly,* June 14, 1997, p. 1372.

[112] *Health Care Policy Report,* May 12, 1997, p. 731.

[113] Ibid., April 21, 1997, p. 618. Composed mainly of the usual suspects, i.e., Thomas, Bilirakis, Fawell.

[114] Howard Cohen. Interview, June 6, 2000.

[115] Bridgett Taylor, minority professional staff, Commerce Committee. Interview, June 2, 1999. She believes, for instance, that the Democrats "gave away too much."

[116] Some exceptions were allowed, primarily for rural areas.

[117] Bridgett Taylor. Interview, June 2, 2000. Also Andy Schneider, Kaiser Commission on the Future of Medicaid; formerly minority professional staff, Commerce Committee. Interview, June 15, 1999.

[118] Instead of $1.5 billion. The Republicans said that the summit agreement applied only to increased out-of-pocket costs because of the Part A/Part B shift; Democrats said it covered expenses for all Medicare copays and deductibles.

[119] For more details on this process, see pp. XX.

[120] Bridgett Taylor. Interview, June 2, 2000.

[121] Howard Cohen. Interview, June 6, 2000.

[122] *Health Care Policy Report,* February 10, 1997, p. 219.

[123] Howard Cohen. Interview, June 6, 2000.

[124] Ibid.

[125] P.L. 96-123 (1976). From Henry Hyde (R., Ill.), an amendment to DHEW appropriations passed in 1976 and each year since then providing that no federal Medicaid funds can be used to fund abortions except where the mother's life is endangered or the pregnancy results from rape or incest, promptly reported.

[126] *Congressional Quarterly Almanac,* 1997, p. 6-7.

[127] Ibid.

[128] Because of litigation over coverage, for instance, some HMO executives have said that the best course for them would be to allow the coverage and reduce other coverage or raise premiums and/or copays.

[129] Which would typically bring them under strict state insurance standards.

[130] Howard Cohen. Interview, June 6, 2000. Bridgett Taylor. Interview, June 2, 1999.

[131] States participating in the Medicaid program could not contract with them.

[132] *Health Care Policy Report,* May 26, 1997, p. 817.

[133] Increasing the amount of money available for a Medicaid match by using provider taxes or "contributions" or transfers of money from local governments or other entities that received Medicaid payments.

[134] Howard Cohen. Interview, June 6, 2000.

[135] As a former Commerce staffer observed, "This was peanuts," and asked, "Who will it take from?" In some instances, "Indians on reservations that cost states not one cent." Andy Schneider. Interview, June 15, 1999.

[136] *Balanced Budget Act of 1997—Report of the Committee on the Budget, House of Representatives, to Accompany HR 2015* (Washington, DC: Government Printing Office, 1997), p. 601.

[137] *Health Care Policy Report,* June 16, 1997, p. 935. The committee did provide that DSH payments would be "carved out" of payments to managed care plans and made

directly to hospitals, but did not develop a formula for targeting these payments to the individual hospitals, a task that staff aides said would have been "politically difficult." Howard Cohen. Interview, June 6, 2000.

[138] *Congressional Quarterly,* April 12, 1997, p. 851.

[139] Ibid. February 8, 1997, p. 341.

[140] Ibid., April 12, 1997, p. 851.

[141] *Health Care Policy Report,* June 26, 1997, p. 1166. The committee report also mentions "public-private partnerships" with approval.

[142] Minus an offset for "presumptive" eligibility—persons not formally enrolled but presumed eligible and receiving benefits.

[143] An add-on of 30 percent of the difference between 100 percent and the existing Medicaid match.

[144] *Health Care Policy Report,* June 16, 1997, p. 935.

[145] Bridgett Taylor. Interview, June 2, 2000.

[146] Ibid.

[147] *Health Care Policy Report,* June 16, 1997, p. 935.

[148] Ibid., June 30, 1997, p. 1002–3.

[149] Howard Cohen. Interview, June 6, 2000.

[150] Senator Chafee had an important role in creating this subcommittee and determining its jurisdiction. Its full title was Subcommittee on Medicaid and Health Care for Low Income Families.

[151] *Health Care Policy Report,* March 17, 1997, p. 429.

[152] After Senator Kassebaum retired from the Senate in 1996, Kennedy staff approached Hatch's staff; following that, the two senators agreed upon collaboration. David Nexon. Interview, October 22, 1998.

[153] *Health Care Policy Report,* March 17, 1997, p. 429.

[154] Ibid.

[155] Ibid., May 26, 1997, p. 815.

[156] Ibid., April 26, 1997, pp. 654–55.

[157] Ibid., March 17, 1997, p. 430.

[158] Senate Majority Leader Trent Lott signaled his support on April 6 in a statement on the TV program "Meet the Nation," saying that MSAs could be used to provide child health coverage. Ibid., April 14, 1997, p. 578.

[159] Ibid., April 21, 1997, p. 617.

[160] Ibid.

[161] Laurie Rubiner, National Partnership for Women and Families; formerly legislative aide to Sen. John Chafee. Interview, June 2, 1999. Also, Lisa Layman. Interview, August 26, 1998.

[162] Rockefeller said that this omission was intentional, since they "knew from experience" that the funding source would inevitably become the issue and detract from the merits of the proposal itself. *Health Care Policy Report,* April 28, 1997, p. 652.

[163] Though at 200 percent of poverty, the "crowd out" effect would be considerable, perhaps unacceptable.

[164] *Health Care Policy Report,* June 2, 1997, p. 849.

[165] Ibid.

[166] Ibid., June 16, 1997, p. 920.

[167] *Congressional Quarterly Almanac,* 1997, p. 9-11.

[168] *Health Care Policy Report,* June 23, 1997, p. 959.

169 Ibid., June 23, 1997, p. 960.

170 Ibid., p. 959.

171 *Congressional Quarterly,* June 21, 1997, p. 1426.

172 See note 148.

173 *Health Care Policy Report,* June 23, 1997, p. 960.

174 Ibid.

175 Ibid., June 30, 1997, p. 1004.

176 Ibid., June 23, 1997, p. 961.

177 Laurie Rubiner. Interview, June 2, 1999.

178 Ibid.

179 Bruce Lesley, senior policy adviser for health, Rep. Diana DeGette (D., Colo.); formerly minority staff director, Special Committee on Aging. Interview, July 13, 2000.

180 U.S. Congress (1997b:586ff.). At one point Howard Cohen, majority staff, took Bridgett Taylor, minority staff, to task for getting too close to the Senate Finance provisions.

181 Ibid., p. 877.

182 The $50,000 surety bond was thought to be onerous by the National Association for Home Care, and likely to be especially so for small and/or nonprofit agencies. The surety provision was suggested by Sen. Bob Graham (D., Fla.) who had considerable success in his own state with a surety bond of $10,000. In his view, the main point was not insurance but to have a way of registering and checking the credentials of home care operators. Through the vagaries of the drafting process, the amount was raised to $50,000, which changed the emphasis contrary to his wishes. Bryant Hall, staff of Sen. Graham. Interview, September 2, 1998.

183 *House Report 105-217,* 1997, U.S. Congress 1997c, p. 877.

184 Bruce Leslie. Interview, July 13, 2000.

185 *House Report 105-217,* 1997, U.S. Congress 1997c, p. 883.

186 *Health Care Policy Report,* May 26,1997, pp. 816–17.

187 Institutes for Mental Disease or IMDs.

188 *House Report 105-217, U.S. Congress 1997c,* pp. 872–74.

189 Bruce Lesley. Interview, July 13, 2000.

190 For ten years or more, there had been a history of states profiting on Medicaid DSH payments with a variety of methods such as provider taxes or "contributions" and "intergovernmental transfers." Over the years the GAO and Congress would identify loopholes and seek to close them, and the states would persist with newly invented scams or modified versions of old ones. In 1991, Congress banned provider donations, restricted provider taxes, and capped DSH payments at 12 percent of program expenditures. States then began to turn to intergovernmental transfers (IGTs). States would transfer or receive payments from these institutions and provide them, in turn, with DSH payments, which the states could count as Medicaid matching funds. This tactic also allowed states to escape the "upper payment limits," which set a limit on DSH funds of 12 percent of program costs and an upper limit for individual services of the amount that Medicare would pay. In this way, states could make out handsomely, and some did, raking in vast amounts of DSH money, treating patients at little or no cost to the state, and at times even making money on them. Cf. Matherlee (2000:5–9).

191 *Health Care Policy Report,* June 30, 1997, p. 1004.

192 Julie James. Interview, June 29, 2000.

193 *Congressional Quarterly Almanac,* 1997, p. 6-10.

[194] Ibid., p. 2-24.

[195] President Clinton was concerned with his legacy. With over two years in office remaining, he could use the political credit as well.

[196] With its huge workload, the Medicare subconference began its work that same day, opening with an offer by the House conferees to the Senate. *Health Care Policy Report,* July 14, 1997, p. 1088.

[197] Ibid.

[198] Nancy-Ann (Min) deParle recalls that she married on March 22. One week afterward their executive branch task force went into action again. Interview, March 8, 1999.

[199] Described as being more like an "alumni gathering" as compared with the intense action of 1995.

[200] *Health Care Policy Report,* July 14, 1997, p. 1087.

[201] *Congressional Quarterly,* July 12, 1997, p. 1612.

[202] Gary Claxton, deputy assistant secretary for health, DHHS. Interview, May 12, 1999.

[203] *Congressional Quarterly,* July 26, p. 1765.

[204] *Health Care Policy Report,* July 26, 1997, pp. 1166–67.

[205] Chris Jennings. Interview, June 9, 1999.

[206] *Congressional Quarterly,* July 26, 1997, p. 1765.

[207] Special Low-income Medicare Beneficiaries.

[208] *Health Care Policy Report,* July 28, 1997, p. 1167.

[209] Ibid., p. 1169. Earlier in July, President Clinton had sent a letter to Republicans laying out his tax priorities. *Congressional Quarterly,* July 26, 1997, p. 1766.

[210] Allowing those without health insurance between ages sixty-five and sixty-seven to "buy in" to the Medicare program.

[211] Also, it could get into the kind of trouble associated with the Medicare Catastrophic Coverage Act, under which affluent seniors were taxed more than the benefit was worth to them. Many of them lobbied strongly for its repeal.

[212] *Health Care Policy Report,* July 26, 1997, p. 1168.

[213] *Congressional Quarterly,* July 26, 1997, p. 1426.

[214] Ibid.

[215] *Health Care Policy Report,* July 28, 1997, p. 1165.

[216] *Congressional Quarterly,* August 2, 1997, p. 1997

[217] *Health Care Policy Report,* August 4, 1997, p. 1203.

[218] Ibid.

[219] Ibid., August 4, 1997, p. 1202–3.

[220] Ibid.

[221] *Congressional Quarterly,* August 2, 1997, p. 1832.

[222] Ibid., August 9, 1997, p. 1916.

[223] Chip Kahn, "The Era of Medicare+Choice," address to the National Congress on Medicare+Choice, sponsored by the Health Insurance Association of America, June 4, 1998.

[224] Ibid., p. 4.

[225] Q: How many economists does it take to change a light bulb? A: None. If the light bulb needed changing, the market would do it.

[226] Howard Cohen. Interview, June 6, 2000.

7

Implementation

This chapter has two main purposes. One is to give the reader a sense for what is entailed in the implementation of statutes of great scope and complexity, such as the Medicare and Medicaid acts of 1997. A second is to introduce the concept of implementation as an important element in understanding and evaluating the policy process.

One caveat is that implementation of BBA 97 was comprehensive in scope, involving over three hundred separate rules, new programs and provider entities, an array of prospective payment systems and revised payment mechanisms, and almost innumerable specific policy and technical adjustments. Keeping track of the tasks was, by itself, one of the major tasks. Time constraints were tight—in some instances, a few weeks after passage of the statute. For HCFA in particular, all had to be done while coping with a major reorganization, resignation of the administrator, and getting their data and information systems Y2K compliant. Many of the activities were routine, but some entailed bold adaptation, huge logistical problems, long hours under crisis conditions, and enormous individual and collective effort. For that reason, this particular episode loses some of its representative value as an instance of implementation. At the same time, it illustrates a wide range of behavior and gives a sense for the scope and complexity of Medicare and Medicaid implementation activities.

A chapter on implementation is included because it is part of the policy process and, for that matter, part of the politics of Medicare and Medicaid. In one sense, this states the obvious: that HCFA and the DHHS and other groups or agencies that review regulations or comment upon proposals are important in affecting how a statutory provision gets translated into a rule and is enforced. An additional point is that the Medicare and Medicaid programs—with our perennially divided government and the established access and effectiveness of the advocacy groups—are special cases approaching a kind of institutionalized syndicalism that threatens at times to overwhelm or paralyze implementation and invariably affects both the substance and process of policy.

Paying attention to implementation can help to get a sense for the possible, the prudent, and the cost-effective with respect to particular programs. A number of entities exercise oversight of Medicare and Medicaid programs, including the DHHS Inspector General, OMB, CBO, the GAO, MedPAC, and a dozen committees of Congress. Yet the administrators charged with the actual implementation are likely to have the best sense for what, in the context of a particular program, can be made to work in practice—at least, we hope they do. Bureaucrats, in the negative sense of that word, can take advantage of this asymmetry of information, especially in arcane fields like Medicare and Medicaid. Experience with or savvy about implementation, though, helps to separate authentic pleas of impossibility or necessity from bureaucratic dodges or stonewalling and, for that reason, is an important resource of the staff of congressional subcommittees and agencies such as MedPAC or the GAO.[1]

Both legally and politically, implementation procedures are important for accountability or assigning blame (cf. Mashaw 1996; see also Weaver 1987). For that reason, the implementation process is central to many of our current disputes about the future of Medicare and Medicaid and even the role of government in general. These are programs that occasion an enormous amount of blaming and especially blaming HCFA (or CMS) for whatever goes wrong: for delay in publishing rules, for onerous regulations or heavy-handed enforcement, for not adopting more private sector methods or pushing competitive bidding, and so forth.[2] Some of the complaints are appropriate; but sometimes they represent mainly blame shifting—behavior that is important to recognize. Often, for instance, it is Congress or OMB that is delaying the regulation. A perennial illustration is competitive bidding. Congress has long pushed HCFA to do competitive bidding demonstrations, but whenever HCFA has tried it, individual representatives have objected, importuned in turn by providers—especially HMOs—in their state or district who tout competition in the abstract but not as a real presence next door. Blaming HCFA or the "bureaucracy" can be both a way to shift blame and to cover over a significant reality.

Sometimes, too, it is important to have an account of undertakings that go well and are fulfilled creditably—both as an example of how to do it right and to give credit when deserved. Others learn from and are challenged by the example. Telling the story bestows honor upon a worthy achievement and may help restore some luster to the ideal of public service.

I. BACKGROUND

Implementing these statutes was mostly the work of HCFA, though a relatively small number of individuals within ASPE and the offices of the secretary, the general counsel, and the inspector general were important for reviewing regulations, for legal expertise, and for some issues of policy. HCFA also contracted for specific studies and services, worked closely on occasion with congressional staff and MedPAC, and consulted with the Department of Justice, the OMB, Treasury, and the IRS.

The HCFA (renamed CMS in 2001) is a small organization with about 4,500 employees that probably carries as much program responsibility per employee as any agency in the federal government. For FY 2000, the combined appropriation for Medicare and Medicaid was $313 billion, almost 12 percent of the entire U.S. federal budget. Not only is this a large amount of money, but it also funds a number of programs and activities remarkable for their range and complexity. Indeed, among the most common reasons given by HCFA officials for staying with the agency is that the work is interesting, challenging, and makes a difference.

One reason that the HCFA can cover so much with a relatively small staff is that it engages in little direct administration.[3] Among its activities are to supervise the carriers and fiscal intermediaries that pay the bills and the peer review organizations (PROs) and other entities that monitor compliance, and to work with state Medicaid agencies. The HCFA maintain a huge database, tracks developments, and provides information to beneficiaries, other agencies, and the Congress. It also supports research and demonstrations and helps devise new payment methodologies and service delivery models. One important task (and skill) is developing requests for proposals (RFPs) and writing and supervising the contracts that support these activities or purchase needed equipment and expertise. Most important, HCFA writes the policies, rules, manuals, and letters that implement payments and standards and that help maintain the integrity of the Medicare and Medicaid systems (for fuller account, see Appendix).

Despite this indirect mode of administration, HCFA is spread thin and increasingly so as its program responsibilities have grown. One reason is persistent underfunding. HCFA's administrative budget is a discretionary appropriation that Congress can more easily cut; and increasing HCFA's administrative funds is a hard sell politically. HCFA's staff, around 4,500, is roughly the same as it was in 1977 when the agency began—despite a tenfold growth in the budget, half again as many beneficiaries, and new and more complex responsibilities. In 1999, when collapse seemed imminent, a bipartisan group of health policy experts, including three former administrators, addressed an appeal to the Congress and the Clinton administration imploring them to do something about the impending management crisis. The malady has been chronic and is an important part of the background for 1997–98.

Programs that HCFA administers require—especially at the higher levels—people with talent, programmatic sophistication, and dedication. Another problem for HCFA has been a failure to renew this cadre as those who came in with earlier cohorts have retired or left.[4] The skills and capabilities of such people, along with their institutional memory and administrative expertise, were at a premium in implementing the Medicare and Medicaid amendments of 1997. This critical shortage of top-level staff was somewhat mitigated by the administration's opportunity—primarily through the reorganization of 1997—to recruit some able health policy veterans from the private sector, but for every major task, much was required of a few; and the implementation stretched a dwindling number of senior career executives to the limit.

By 1997, seven years had passed since HCFA had done a major reconciliation. This lapse of time meant that many of the staff had no experience with such a global effort and lacked some of the inventiveness and collaborative skills that grow from surviving such events.[5] Implementation of BBA 97 required HCFA to "go live" with some initiatives, such as the outpatient prospective payment systems, that were still in a developmental stage[6] and to design whole new systems, such as a consumer information program and the child health initiative. In practice, many of the HCFA staff had to learn as they went, teach others, and find new ways to collaborate across division lines.[7]

A major complication, some said "the worst," was the HCFA reorganization (see Appendix), which was getting seriously under way when BBA 97 was enacted on July 30, 1997. The reorganization process, which lasted well into the next year, involved an extensive restructuring of HCFA, including both administrative reassignment and physical relocation for most key personnel. Shortly thereafter, on September 12, Bruce Vladeck left.[8] With his departure, HCFA lost an experienced, effective, and highly regarded administrator as well as the guiding spirit behind the reorganization itself. People within HCFA disagree about the motives and the ultimate benefits of the reorganization, but most say that it was a traumatic process and that the timing was bad.

In the most obvious sense, the reorganization used up time and energy and added stress. It also, as Kathy Buto put it, "broke up many families" or workgroups, losing for some time a measure of their teamwork, institutional memory, and program expertise and requiring informal retraining in some instances.[9] This implementation effort especially demanded collaboration across division lines. But the reorganization, which may have facilitated this kind of cooperation in the long run, did not do so immediately. People were reassigned "notionally" but did not move physically, lacked updated telephone books, and often had no clear sense of what they should be doing or with whom they should be working or to whom reporting, so that the reorganization was not only a trauma and an aggravation but a physical impediment as well. Also, it came just before the biggest implementation task in HCFA's history.

At the time, HCFA was struggling with its Y2K problem. This was one of those problems that HCFA administrators had been conscious of, but not yet attentive to.[10] Troubles with their own Medicare Transaction System[11] had sharpened this consciousness for many; but implementing BBA 97 brought the real shock of awareness. For it was then they realized not only the magnitude of the Y2K project, but that it would be hard, or maybe impossible, to meet both the absolute Y2K deadline of midnight December 31, 1999, and the many other deadlines set by BBA 97.[12]

The Y2K problem[13] was exceptionally difficult because of two main factors: complexity and interdependence. The HCFA database is one of the largest, if not the largest, in the world. It is also unimaginably complex—because of the many programs and instructions involved, files by state, region, and carrier, and various instructions and modifiers added by technicians and researchers over the years. Moreover, much essential data is in the files of the intermediaries and contractors or the state Medicaid programs, so that these become, by extension, part of the Y2K problem as well. By way of comparison, the largest mainframe computers might operate with 50,000 lines of instruction. The Medicare data base has over 2,000,000 lines of instruction. The systems differ widely, and files are often tapped into for research or other purposes, and then returned with little, if any, indications of the instructions or modifiers that might have been added.[14] The other big factor is interdependence.[15] A failure in one line of instruction or information or an attempt to fix one part of the system can have serious and unpredictable consequences in distant reaches of this vast set of files. Because of this property, whole areas had to be walled off while data systems technicians worked to make them Y2K compliant. Meanwhile, people in program development and operations had to line up or queue for computer time or devise ways to work around the constraints imposed by the Y2K problem. For some people, this problem was minimal; for others it was huge and acquired maddening, Kafka-like properties.[16]

Altogether, the circumstances under which HCFA had to work were remarkably unfavorable. This is not to excuse any of the agency's failures in the implementation process, for there is little that needs to be excused. But it seems appropriate to comment that what they did was accomplished under conditions of great difficulty, with little complaint, and not much recognition from either Congress or the administration.

II. MEDICARE IMPLEMENTATION

Nancy-Ann deParle, the HCFA administrator who inherited the vast implementation project from her predecessor, Bruce Vladeck, recalled a meeting of the Executive Council that she attended with Vladeck to review a thirty-page draft from the Ways and Means Committee listing the various changes in the new legislation. As they worked down the list and she became aware of what the implementation tasks entailed, she grew increasingly uneasy and occasionally glanced at Vladeck. He seemed unperturbed and she was reassured.

When she later mentioned this episode to Vladeck he said that he was not worried because, as he put it, "I'm out of here." In other words, "It's your problem." Then, she said, she realized with full force the enormity of the task confronting her and the agency. However, she added, to tell the president they couldn't do it was not an option, especially knowing that he disliked the HCFA anyway.[17]

In fact, both she and the HCFA leadership were more prepared for the coming ordeal than this anecdote would suggest. Nancy-Ann deParle, a Rhodes Scholar with degrees from Harvard Law School and the Kennedy School of Government, had been a corporate litigator, commissioner of health services in Tennessee, and, as an associate director at OMB, deeply involved in federal health policy since the beginning of the Clinton administration. At her request, before formally taking over as administrator, she had "interned" as a deputy for three months, working closely with Bruce Vladeck, to get acquainted with the problems, routines, and agency directors. The Executive Council, a creation of the reorganization, had also been meeting to set priorities, to decide how tasks would be divided and aggregated, and to determine who would be the lead people on particular projects.

Planning at this juncture was difficult, in part, because the HCFA reorganization was in full course. The reorganization was time-consuming, created uncertainty about future responsibilities, and complicated the assignment of tasks. Until the end of July, moreover, the House-Senate conference was still in session and some of the language and numbers would not be worked out until July 28. Until then, HCFA staff literally did not know what some of the critical numbers and deadlines would be.

The new administrator, who was familiar with large organizations and programs, brought with her a strong sense of procedure. For this situation, it was important to have the priorities clear, limited in number, and effectively communicated. These priorities were (1) on-time implementation of the Medicare+Choice "mega-reg," (2) launching the Children's Health program; (3) completing implementation of the fraud and abuse legislation; and (4) getting ready for Y2K. Other activities, such as research and development, might suffer for a time, but so be it. With these priorities in mind, she began two-hour weekly sessions with the Executive Council to develop an implementation plan for Medicare+Choice. These sessions were supplemented by large, biweekly meetings with the implementation staff. During this phase, she also moved forward with plans to set up a comprehensive tracking system to coordinate tasks, keep up to schedule, and identify potential trouble spots.

Since HCFA was often blamed for whatever might go wrong, deParle recognized the importance of credibility in this venture. An early measure was to insist that staff inform her quickly and fully of any impending deadlines that would be missed or about glitches in the process so that she could be equally as forthcoming and well-covered in accounting to Congress or the president.[18]

She also used executive position authority established by the reorganization to appoint several individuals with strong program-related experience in addition to well-established reputations in the private sector. These included Bob Berenson, a physician and HMO executive, to head the new Center for Health Plans and Provider Operations; Carol Cronin, a consumer information and marketing activist and publisher, to head the Center for Beneficiary Services; and Mike Hash, a former staff aide to Rep. Henry Waxman and a health policy consultant, to work with Congress and the interest groups. Each of these added practical experience and expertise to HCFA. Individually and collectively they strengthened the administrator. They also had established relations and credibility with critically important outsiders, including providers, beneficiaries, and the Congress, who could help in getting through some of the political turbulence lying ahead.[19]

An early and critical set of decisions related to the management of this enormous project: how to prioritize and assign responsibilities, coordinate tasks, meet the scheduled deadlines, and monitor the results adequately. Much of the prioritizing and assignment of tasks was done through meetings of the Executive Council, the division heads, and special task forces, but BBA 97 was larger in scope and complexity than anything HCFA had dealt with before. It also required that many of the program changes—some of them entailing extensive development, data gathering, systems design, or training—be fully operational by specific deadlines. The deadlines were many and short. Altogether, management of the implementation project was, by itself, a major challenge.

HCFA's usual way of approaching this aspect of implementation was to do a "rack-up." This would typically be done within the (former) Bureau of Policy Development, by the division or task force with the major program responsibility. It involved analyzing the statute and defining the separate tasks; determining what each task would require by way of policy analysis, new development work, operations activities, and input from others within or outside DHHS; laying out critical paths and assigning time lines; establishing who takes "ownership" of the project; and specifying a "point" person for information or quick response. This method was informal, familiar, and good for planning work and assigning tasks, but it was less reliable for scheduling individual tasks, coordinating and monitoring progress, and assuring that all the parts were there on time and would work together.

Prudent administrative procedure for implementation tasks as complex as BBA 97 was to contract with outside consultants for various services ranging from advice, software, and systems design to the development and management of contracts or even the whole project. HCFA had done so, for instance, for the Medicare Transaction System, but in this instance, HCFA had contracted for a package program without an outside consultant to help manage and oversee development of the project.[20] It was an unhappy learning experience, and had led to three years of close and critical monitoring by the GAO, accompanied by complaints of poor management, failure to use approved techniques, and inadequate planning for a transition from the existing system of claims-processing to the new one (U.S. General Accounting Office 1997:2).

In the spring of 1997, there was an uneasy awareness within HCFA of what might lie ahead. In addition to troubles with the Medicare Transaction System, a gnawing concern about Y2K was beginning to develop. The HCFA reorganization—with its attendant disruption—was well under way. Bruce Vladeck was scheduled to leave early in September, and BBA 97 was expected soon, without, as yet, much knowledge of the details. With the future encroaching, a decision had to be made about management of the implementation process. At a Boston meeting late in the spring, HCFA administrators agreed in principle that they would contract with an outside source to develop a system of project management for implementing BBA 1997.[21] So began a tangled episode involving a troubled legacy from the past and a near-death experience for HCFA. It also illustrated the importance of redundant systems and the kind of administrative capabilities and experience that enable an organization to recover from a false start.

By July, a number of initiatives were under way. HCFA contracted with Coopers and Lybrand, a major accounting and management consulting firm, to help develop and operate a sophisticated project management system. For its part, HCFA undertook to develop its own matrix management capability that would serve as a foundation and counterpart to the project management system.[22] As an interim measure, Bruce Vladeck asked Barbara Cooper and the Office of Strategic Planning to do a traditional rack-up, which would serve to coordinate activities until the project management system became operational.[23] About that time, internal applications were solicited, and an experienced senior civil servant, Dan Waldo, was hand-picked to help arbitrate issues and coordinate the efforts of the policy staff with operations activities. According to Waldo,[24] one of his main qualifications, other than broad experience, was that he was seen as relatively neutral between policy and operations—an observation that touches upon HCFA's troubled legacy of the "two stove pipes."[25]

This expression refers to the historic division between the so-called bureau of policy development and the bureau of program operations. This division makes sense when viewed in the light of HCFA's basic mission, which is "to turn legislation into computer programs."[26] In other words, policy development translates the legislation into regulatory texts (with preambles) and operations manages the data files, creates the software, develops the manuals, and often provides the training to convert these rules into operating instructions for the carriers and fiscal intermediaries who pay the claims and, to some extent, monitor provider billing practices.

Over time, a troubling division developed between these two bureaus based in part upon attitude but also upon important differences in work style. People who write regulations tend to be like writers generally: they have a deadline and hope for insight and a "gestalt" to make the words flow as the deadline draws near. So they concentrate mostly on the big picture, not scheduling the steps. Operations people, on the other hand, have to think sequentially, about what needs to be in place before something else can happen. This kind of division in work style can, and did, lead to difficulties and even recriminations, especially when there were tight deadlines. The policy people, for instance, might meet their deadline but leave operations in the dark about important details for so long that they, in turn, would have to scramble hard to meet their own dates.[27] Operations people complained that policy would write a rule and "throw it over the wall," assuming that the matter was solved, with little awareness of what their prescription would entail for operations or whether it could be made to work at all. Policy people, for their part, objected that operations always wanted to know the details before the problem itself had been fully understood. There were attitudes that went with this division of work. Policy people were regarded as an elite but also as "long hairs," at times impractical or precious. Operations people were praised for their hard work and technical proficiency with inadequate equipment but viewed as "grunts," fit primarily to be instruments of another's will.[28]

Project planning could, in theory, make important contributions to the BBA 97 implementation. Most of the BBA deadlines involved not just writing a proposed or "interim final" rule, but program changes up and running by a certain date. In this situation, operations people especially needed an early view of tasks, sequences, and dates. They became strong supporters of project planning and of a concept of "management to completion," which would have research, policy, and operations working collaboratively from inception to final operational implementation.[29] This approach would not only help compensate for the "two stove pipes" division, it would largely do away with it.

Project planning with the aid of the Coopers and Lybrand consultants was less than a success. Some people in operations continued to like it and it was useful for getting support funds, but it seemed especially ill-suited for organizing the policy staff and regulation writers. "Like teaching pigs to dance," according to one observer.[30] In a more analytical vein, Kathy Buto commented that the consultants' version of project planning was more suitable for organizing tasks from the bottom up, like assembling the parts of a B-1 bomber, than for trying to coordinate a number of small regulation-writing cottage industries.[31] HCFA lacked the appropriate technical infrastructure and compatible computer programs, and there was a major problem with software licenses. HCFA managers had difficulty learning the new "org-speak" and resented being told what to do by Coopers and Lybrand "whiz-kids" fresh out of business school. Soon people began complaining that they were spending more time learning the new system than in getting useful work done. By February, the project planning initiative had almost ground to a halt.[32]

Fortunately, the standard rack-up was also being developed by the Office of

Legislation and the Office of Strategic Planning. This had originally been intended as a temporary substitute until project planning became fully operational, but Waldo and others were able to convert the rack-up into the primary planning device. Essentially, what they developed, working from the top down, was an animated spreadsheet. Through a series of iterations, lists would be sent out followed by telephone calls to sort the tasks, identify missing pieces and intermediate activities, and get names of project "owners" and point persons. This information would be made accessible on individual desktop computers—using Microsoft Excel, which was the agency standard—so that each person could know who was responsible for a specific task and how his or her own project stood. Each week, working from this common document, representatives from each division and each component would meet to report and talk through problems. Every two weeks the computerized spreadsheet would be updated with names, statutory completion dates, and red, yellow, and green markers to indicate project status.

This approach proved to be a successful adaptation, almost completely displacing the original Coopers and Lybrand method. The homegrown version could be done quickly, with familiar techniques and existing equipment. It established effective accountability and the administrator liked it. While it assumed collegiality and professionalism, it also built upon and enhanced these qualities. Also it worked well practically, coordinating efforts effectively, helping to identify additional tasks or problems,[33] and getting people to take ownership of them. Not least, it gave operations people advance notice and policy people their creative space.

Medicare+Choice Regulations

The Medicare+Choice (M+C) regulations dealt with an array of managed care plans that were either modified or created anew by BBA 97. "Traditional" Medicare—Part A and Part B, along with the outpatient prospective payment systems—was treated separately (cf. Appendix). The total number of regulations, their cumulative length, and their technical complexity—a testimonial in itself to the effort and achievement of HCFA and the DHHS staff—precludes any kind of comprehensive or even representative discussion. Their treatment here is necessarily selective, and restricted to some of the more important examples of implementation. These regulations dealt with new entities and posed novel challenges, In that respect they are atypical, but they illustrate a range of implementation activities and provide examples of the contributions that experienced civil servants can make.

"Mega-Reg."   The term "mega-reg" refers to the interim final regulation, published on June 26, 1998, that established the major outlines of the Medicare+Choice program. It was called mega-reg because it was the biggest

single job of the entire BBA 97 implementation. In the first draft, the regulation ran to over 800 triple-spaced pages. In the final edition, it filled 148 of the large, triple-column pages in the Federal Register, of which 52 pages were the regulation and almost 100 pages the preamble.

The deadline for this regulation was June 1, 1998, only ten months after passage of the BBA on July 28, 1997. The HCFA staff assigned to this task, although it had been given top priority, had doubts about meeting the schedule. Most difficult regulations, even with expedited procedures, typically take from eighteen months to two years. An earlier regulation of comparable scope had taken three years.[34]

For this rule, Congress had given HCFA authority to publish an "interim final rule." This is an expedited procedure that allows HCFA to issue what would otherwise be a "proposed rule" as "final" for the time being, without having gone through the initial "notice and comment" prescribed for typical informal rule-making. "Comment" by the affected private parties comes after the rule has been issued and typically leads to some amendment, but meanwhile the rule is in effect. In practical terms, this procedure drastically shortens the time required to get programs operational by transposing the comment phase and reducing it to one step.

In conferring this authority, Congress was reposing considerable trust in HCFA and in the clearance to which such rules are subjected by the department, OMB, and other administrative agencies. The professionalism and self-interest of the HCFA officials who developed the regulation enjoined them to be as faithful as possible to congressional intent and to be prudent and fair in interpreting the statute, filling in the gaps, and working out details. In this context, the part referred to as preamble is worth separate comment. HCFA preambles are typically lengthy accounts that explain in nonlegal language what particular provisions aim to accomplish, how they will be implemented or applied, what special duties they may entail, why a particular policy is desirable, and so forth. Their preambles are prepared with great care, to make them clear and accurate, consistent internally and with the regulatory text, and reliable as guides for action.[35] They represent an effort by HCFA to make regulations easier for intermediaries and providers to understand and to work with. And where an interim final regulation is involved, such prefaces are especially important in anticipating and allaying subsequent complaints by providers or beneficiaries, demonstrating a will to be responsive to Congress, and avoiding lawsuits or court injunctions.[36]

The mega-reg team was headed by Kathy Buto, an experienced senior civil servant much respected by the staff. To her we owe the project's informal title of "mega-reg." When the tasks were being sorted out she was assigned to chair the negotiated regulation for the PSO solvency standards. Later, when asked to lead the Medicare+Choice regulatory effort she made light of it, saying that since she was already "doing neg-reg," that she "might as well do mega-reg."[37]

She was a good choice for a number of reasons even though her experience was almost entirely with FFS Medicare, aside from a few managed care demonstrations. The former Office of Managed Care had almost no people experienced in regulation writing and Buto knew how to manage the development of regulations. In addition, a number of the Medicare+Choice regulations involved hybrid enterprises, such as PSOs and private FFS plans that would require sophistication with FFS regulations. Her lead associate for this task was Jean LeMasurier, director of policy development in the former Office of Managed Care, who organized and coordinated much of the ongoing work of the mega-reg task force.

The term mega-reg is somewhat misleading since it suggests that the size and complexity of a single regulation was the major problem. Taken as a whole, the task was huge, but for the most part it was broken into a number of team efforts, each of them characterized by its particular problems and differing demands for adaptive response. In some instances, the hardest part was the sheer scope and complexity of a new regulation; or it was the construction of new entities or dealing with unfamiliar expertise; or it involved moving farther into operations than before. Throughout, the HCFA reorganization and the Y2K problem were complicating factors, though how much so depended on the particular tasks. In any event, success in implementation owed much to adaptation as well as to dedication and effort.

The largest and most complex team effort was the managed care regulation. That was no surprise, since this regulation would affect the whole spectrum of managed care, all Medicare+Choice plans, private HMOs and health care providers, Medicaid, and state and local governments. The revised managed care payment formulas, the quality standards, and the consumer and provider protections added up to a huge amount of new regulation. New products such as provider sponsored organizations (PSOs), religious fraternal benefit societies (RFBs), and private FFS plans mixed risk-bearing and FFS payment mechanisms. They also involved complex issues of federal-state and public-private relations and the adapting of general standards of quality, solvency, or consumer protection to these hybrid entities.[38] With a deadline of January 1, 1999, to go operational, the time line was compressed, especially to get marketing and consumer information activities in place and operating. This meant working back in time from the deadline, so that the group had to be proactive, think ahead, and work closely with the operations staff.

To confront this array of tasks, the managed care group did for themselves what HCFA was doing collectively: they created their own steering group with representatives from policy and operations, quality and clinical standards, Medicaid, data and information systems, budget, and general counsel. This approach helped the group to respond quickly and adaptively to task needs and to monitor progress. Difficult issues needing a policy paper or higher level decision could be passed upward. In some instances, DHHS or

OMB representatives would be added or people from regional offices or the training staff included. In this manner, they were able to anticipate some difficulties, shorten the amount of time needed for administrative clearances, and gain lead time for operational activities.[39]

One of the most challenging problems for this group was lack of experience in developing regulations. Their background was managed care, working with health plans, the Adjusted Community Rate, risk, and solvency—not with glosses upon a statute and the fine-grained implementation of coverage policies or a fee schedule. Moreover, they had relatively little to work with. There were the original statute and a small number of managed care regulations, but much was in the form of operational policy letters and informal instructions.[40] In their small group of ten, left over from the Office of Managed Care, only one person had extensive experience with regulations. Others "didn't know what Sec. 1876 was," had never worked with regulations before, or did not write well enough to describe their policies to a regulatory staff or make regulatory texts clear to the operations staff.[41]

Given the circumstances, the task force members did what they could. As a first step, they set out to teach themselves, working in twenty or more subcommittees to inventory their existing managed care regulations, identify and try to think through the issues raised by the new statute, and to develop ideas and materials for their own regulations. They delegated much of the work on new entities and got the best people they could to take ownership of particular projects. They also borrowed key people, for instance, from the Office of General Counsel and the old Bureau of Policy Development.

The task force leaders readily acknowledged that the mega-reg suffered from the circumstances attending its creation. Jean LeMasurier said, for instance, that parts of the mega-reg that her staff worked upon directly were poorly written and did not include enough good "sermons" in the preamble.[42] Kathy Buto expressed a related concern, noting that for some of their regulations staff lacked the kind of experience gained from day-to-day dealings with the program specialists, and ceded too much to these specialists to the detriment of broader institutional and policy considerations. She mentioned particularly quality standards and the appeals procedures.[43]

Two of the mega-reg projects—Medical Savings Accounts (MSAs) and the quality regulations—exemplify the above points as well as illustrating the implementation process in more particular detail.

Medicare+Choice MSAs.   This task was larger and more difficult than it might seem. Private sector MSAs were familiar; but Medicare MSAs were another species. What the MSA task force had to do, in essence, was to devise a hybrid mechanism, adapt it for an alien environment, and have it ready for start-up in nine months. So time was critical. The scope of the task was such that they needed to deploy, on a lesser scale, their own version of the mega-reg: do the development work and write the regulation and marketing guidelines, but also work with the contractors to put the system together, with the computer people to generate a program for processing enrollment, and with the information people to develop an MSA guide and to mount an information campaign.[44] On a small scale, their project required "management to completion."

From the beginning, one of the biggest problems was statutory interpretation, important to get right since MSAs were a politically sensitive topic. The statutory provisions for the Medicare MSAs were highly prescriptive; but they left many issues open for interpretation and even independent decision. The most pervasive issue—not resolved by Congress—was inducements for insurance companies versus protections for the beneficiaries. Translating this into specifics, how much should the government contribute to the beneficiaries and how much should it pay to the insurance companies? Within the 300,000 global limit for MSAs, should there be any state or regional quotas? Does the statute require community rating? If so, what did community rating mean? Was it rated by government contribution or by beneficiary payment? Should coinsurance be considered? If so, who was responsible for balance billing, the insurer or the beneficiary? Did balance billing count toward the deductible? What did? Should there be a minimum deductible? If so, how high should it be? a token? leave it to the market? And so forth.[45]

The MSA task force members dealt with this problem of interpretation (or interpolation) in two ways. They tried to understand the underlying issues and principles involved, discussing these and aiding their efforts with short policy papers commissioned from the RAND corporation. They also sought to discover or infer what they could of the original legislative intent, searching in the conference report, consulting with their own lawyers and the Office of Legislation, and talking with committee staff.[46] Even so, legislative intent proved elusive.

In this situation, civil service "neutral competence" of a sort seemed both prudent and right. Aware that Democrats and the administration loathed MSAs and that MSAs could be detrimental both to the Medicare program and to beneficiaries, they saw no positive obligation to promote or market these MSAs aggressively. On the other hand, HCFA ought not to be seen as holding up this initiative. Therefore, they sought to discover intent where they could, stay neutral and be fair as between the parties, consult widely on how to make the system work, and give due weight to the underlying principles of the statute as a whole.

Although they were pressed for time, the regulations as such were not especially novel or difficult. Getting the policy right and assuring that it would seem right to potential critics was more of a challenge. To meet this challenge, they consulted widely. They questioned congressional staff about legislative intent. They worked closely with IRS attorneys and sought opinions from their own actuary. They met with insurance industry representatives over such issues as the deductible, quality standards, and minimum size of plans. They visited MSAs. They put application forms and procedures on the internet for comment. Some of these efforts, especially meetings with the industry, proved to be unenlightening, but they had made the effort.[47]

A critical and difficult part was reconciling this hybrid product with the principles of the main statute and the Medicare program. For this, they had to work out their own policies and send these on with instructions for writing the regulative text and preamble.[48] The preamble deals with this general problem in a number of different contexts, such as treatment of balance billing, quality standards, and consumer information. At many points it is apparent that there was little to rely upon to interpret the statute except general principles derived from the nature of MSAs, the M+C statute, and the Medicare program, so that it was a wise procedure for the task force members to begin with a study of these. Reading the preamble text on Medicare MSAs palpably demonstrates the importance of having a good writer to make the explanation clear and rhetorically persuasive.[49]

As they worked toward a conclusion, this task force, like a number of others, encountered its own version of the Y2K problem. They needed computer time and assistance to develop a system for processing and monitoring enrollment, keeping track of plan membership, who the insurers and depositories were, and so forth. Initially, the task force members were put off because their job was too small—because the big tasks of Y2K compliance or managed care payments could not be sidetracked to deal some MSA affair "involving 80 people in Chattanooga."[50]

Eventually they got their computer time and, working at home and on weekends, were able to finish within their deadline. Shortly after the MSA regulations were published, the task force members held a special meeting with insurers to explain the system. After that, they began going through the comments coming in that would be a part of the "final-final" iteration of mega-reg.

QISMC and the quality regulation.   QISMC, which applied to Medicare, came about in a rather unexpected way. In 1993, HCFA developed a contract with the National Academy of State Health Policy and began working under Section 1115 waivers with state Medicaid bureaus and with managed care plans and their medical directors on a Quality Assurance Reform Initiative (QARI), a two-year project to develop better state quality measures. These were published in 1995. HCFA then moved on to develop a Medicaid version of HEDIS and add process and outcome indicators.[52] The Medicare program—with its 1985 quality indicators inadequate and out of date—built on these efforts to develop a state of the art version of its own, with common standards, performance and outcome measures, and continuous quality improvement.[53] So, in effect, Medicaid led the way for Medicare—an unusual provenance with at least one significant side-effect.

At the time QISMC was being developed, the quality movement was both strong and growing. Business groups were touting private sector efforts such as HEDIS and FAcct. Both the JCAHO and NCQA subscribed enthusiastically and somewhat uncritically to outcome measures and continuous quality improvement. Much to the point, quality of care, especially as applied to HMOs, was getting a lot of attention in Congress and from the administration: to improve care, but also as a way to include access standards and patients' rights, and as a political tactic to focus discontent on HMOs.

One consequence was that persuading Congress was easy. Few representatives or their staff were interested in the technicalities of quality assurance—in contrast, for example, to a so-called patient's bills of rights. From a congressional, and especially Republican, point of view, quality without legislative or bureaucratic micromanagement made sense. Approaches such as QARI and QISMC, which emphasized outcome measures rather than process variables, suited them and appealed to the health plans as well. So, Congress largely accepted the HCFA approach,[54] with the statute prescribing both outcome measures and continuous quality improvement (CQI). Politically, QISMC and QARI were the best games in town.

What the mega-reg did was to incorporate QISMC, with some appropriate modifications and rhetoric. However, QISMC came with some biases it had incorporated, and DHHS and the administration had their agendas as well. The result could be described as an instance of " overregulation," illustrating the kind of concern expressed by Kathy Buto about too much influence from specialists and special groups.

The problem began with the development of QISMC itself. As explained by the project director, Jeffrey Kang, both QARI and QISMC had the same technical advisory group, made up of one-third each of providers, consumers, and health plans. This distribution tended to underrepresent the real stake of the health plans, and it also overrepresented staff-model HMOs—a distinct minority among Medicare plans—in relation to the less structured network models. Thus, QISMC itself was based on a false assumption that HMOs had more control over their own structure and procedures than they did in reality.

A mobilization strategy that accompanied QISMC was also important. Quality assurance and improvement is often described as a "movement," and movements are largely impelled by their aspirations. For a movement, it is important to aim high—for morale, to carry others along, and to reach a desired level of achievement. Jeffrey Kang said, for instance, that in developing the regulation they sought more than they expected so as to reach at least a level of the NCQA standards. In this movement, HCFA was also hoping to engage the "flagship" plans and HMO leadership to bring others along in the process. For that matter, one school of thought within HCFA saw raising these standards as a way to get rid of some of the lower quality and more opportunistic Medicare health plans.[55]

In keeping with the spirit of the quality movement, the preamble stressed aspiration and moving toward national performance standards, leaving their number and the pace of movement unstated. The tenor of the preamble, though, conveyed a sense that the standards would be numerous and the pace brisk. This forthright approach sounded alarms among the Medicare HMOs, especially the network models, many of them lacking the data and protocols to develop such standards. For that matter, Kaiser-Permanente, the biggest staff-model HMO in the country, did not keep encounter data at all. When HCFA later asked for seven such standards as a beginning installment, the health plans mounted a political offensive that brought about a radical reduction to one or two per plan.

The department and the White House also had their managed care priorities, a number of which found expression in the regulation. These included items from the president's Consumer Bill of Rights and Responsibilities;[56] civil rights issues pressed by the secretary, emergency services and poststabilization care; and access and provider protection standards. Some of these were not necessarily quality issues though they could be, arguably, subsumed under a quality rubric or associated with it. In any event, they were pushed from above with little awareness of the specialized problems of health plans. Meanwhile, HCFA officials were seeking to moderate or remove such provisions where they could.[57] Whether this quality theme was carried too far remains to be seen, but heavy regulation and regulatory costs have been one factor—probably less important than reduced payments—in motivating an increasing number of HMOs to withdraw from Medicare participation.

In this instance, those associated with QISMC were trying to moderate political pressures and protect the integrity of their programmatic initiative. Yet the episode illustrates and supports Kathy Buto's concern about the need to counter programmatic particularism. Professional enthusiasms, like the quality movement, are liable to overreach realistic objectives or be used by others for ulterior purposes, so that they are especially in need of critical review—which in this situation was hard to provide because of the ongoing HCFA reorganization and the administration's political agenda.

Creating a final product. A first step in the review process was to have something coherent to review, i.e., a complete version of the mega-reg. For this, the drafts resulting from the various task assignments were assembled, with instructions, and sent to the regulation writers to develop both regulatory text and preamble. They produced an 850-page, triple-spaced document. This step also provided an initial opportunity to smooth writing styles and check for glitches in policy, inconsistencies between regulatory texts and preambles, and problems needing more thorough solutions. Because of time constraints, this mega-reg iteration was written while some policy drafts were not yet complete and many conflicts in policy remained to be resolved. As a consequence, the review process was both delayed and protracted while option papers were produced and discussed and erupting policy issues appealed or, in many instances, resolved by means of ad hoc improvisations.[58] To review this document, HCFA set up thirteen committees, each with its own specialized expertise and responsibility. In addition, the agency staged an early "roll-out" in February inviting comment from representatives of providers and other stakeholders, six hundred of whom came to Baltimore for the occasion.[59] This first iteration produced 604 comments, filling 242 single-spaced, typewritten pages, according to Donald Kosin, an OGC attorney who read them all. That was the bad news. The good news was that a second iteration got only 144 comments; and a third one very few at all.[60]

"Never before or since" in his eighteen years as a DHHS attorney, said Kosin, had he seen anything like the mega-reg review. He expected it to last two weeks and it lasted six. He recalls reading comments twelve and thirteen hours at a stretch, separating them into piles for action or no-action; working until 2:00 or 3:00 in the morning, on week-ends until 5:00 or 6:00 in the afternoon, driving from Washington to Baltimore through traffic; leaving his speaker phone open for hours at a time; trying to figure which committee needed him the most; whether they could lawfully do this or that; asking ASPE, OMB, Hill staff, and Ed Grossman about the meaning of a word and coming up dry; then thinking "really hard" about how to implement some provision where the intent was not clear.[61]

Within HCFA, there were two additional levels of review. One was a steering committee, made up of chairs from the thirteen initial review committees, which coordinated tasks and sorted out issues for appeal to a higher level. At this next level, seven or eight of the major project leaders attempted to resolve remaining policy issues. Meanwhile, regulatory text and preamble writers worked together to put language into a finished state, ready for submission to Bob Berenson and Kathy Buto, the director and associate director of CHPP.[62]

At the department level, there was an additional stage of review that was both comprehensive and detailed. This review began in April and worked through several iterations, down to the final publication on June 26, 1998. The group of seven or eight primarily involved were experienced senior civil servants from the office of the secretary. Included were specialists in managed care and representatives from Planning and Evaluation (ASPE), Management and Budget (ASMB), and Legislation (ASL)

This level of review was conducted by written comment, faxes and telephones, and conference calls between this group and HCFA representatives.[63] Mostly the review involved this group and HCFA staff, but a number of issues would be referred to other administrations or services—such as the Health Resources and Services Administration (HRSA) or the Public Health Service

(PHS) There was a final appeal to Kevin Thurm, the DHHS chief of staff and, on a few occasions, to the secretary, Donna Shalala.

The department-level review of the HCFA draft proceeded from comments to an agreement in principle, to proposal of a recommended text, and to a final resolution. The topics addressed in some of the comments suggest the particularity of the concerns as well as the importance and complexity of the policy issues: beneficiary rights in cases of disenrollment for disruptive behavior; counting privately contracted services toward MSA deductibility; antigag rule language; poststabilization guidelines; and enforcing submission of health plan encounter data. The comments themselves bring to mind the lawyer's advice about always preparing the opponent's brief. They also illustrate the importance of virtues attributed to senior civil servants, such as institutional memory, expertise, and professionalism.

The policy review was most important, but there were still other stages. A departmental review for regulatory impact and paperwork reduction occasioned no delay, and HCFA felt it had met its deadline of June 1. However, OMB held up final clearance for three weeks to allow the Department of Justice time to complete its review of the fraud and abuse provisions.[64] Even so, the 833-page document—earlier estimated at 600 pages—was made available for inspection on June 18 and finally issued on June 19. It was published in the *Federal Register* on June 26, less than eleven months from the enactment of the Balanced Budget Act—a record for a regulation of this scope.

PSO Solvency Standards and Negotiated Rulemaking. The mega-reg was only an element—though the largest single one—in an array of Medicare+Choice implementation regulations and activities, which included technical and complex topics, such as the solvency standards and private FFS plans, and major operational activities, such as the consumer information program. Two examples described below—the solvency standards and the consumer information program—further illustrate the range of activities and the adaptations required for developing individual rules and for putting them into practice.

Provider-sponsored organizations (PSOs) were a controversial initiative that was included in the Medicare+Choice legislation. Under that heading, solvency standards were a particularly difficult problem. Since PSOs would be risk-bearing entities, it was important that they be "solvent," i.e., that they be able to provide or pay for the services in the contract, immediately and for the long term. Yet to hold them to the kind of capital and reserve requirements set for insurance companies would shut out most prospective PSOs, and especially the more enterprising and experimental entities that this new option was intended to encourage. More established managed care plans, though, were wary of "quick-buck" artists who might rush in, reap quick benefits, and then disappear, and so the solvency standards were a high-stakes issue, politically sensitive, and clouded by particularistic interests and ideology.

These standards also involved technical issues of risk, actuarial soundness, and what should count as working capital and reserves. Resolving these matters in Congress, either at the staff level or in subcommittee, would inevitably prove difficult, time-consuming, and probably unsatisfactory. So a committee staff suggestion[65] was adopted to delegate the matter to HCFA, with a directive to employ a rarely used though increasingly popular technique known as negotiated rulemaking or, in the parlance, "neg-reg."

Negotiated rulemaking, as its name might suggest, grew out of the American labor tradition of collective bargaining (Kerwin 1999:179) and mixes bargaining and conciliation with some of the legal requirements for administrative rulemaking. It is thought to save time, promote consensus, and reduce future litigation, though opinions differ with respect to each of these putative benefits (ibid.). This and closely related variants have been used in labor, environmental, educational, and civil aviation rulemaking. Negotiated rulemaking was looked upon with favor by the Clinton administration and strongly supported as part of Vice-President Gore's "reinventing government" campaign.

At the same time, neg-reg was new to HCFA, which had "never done anything like that before."[66] Achieving a consensus among a group of provider and beneficiary representatives on an issue as technical and divisive as solvency did not seem as though it would be easy. Going in, HCFA staff thought there was less than a 50 percent chance of success.[67] And the stakes were fairly high. The secretary (practically speaking, HCFA) could abort the process and write the regulation in the usual manner, but that would be time-consuming and unpleasant. It would also be seen as a HCFA failure.

Given these circumstances, HCFA staff tried to make good use of the resources available to them. The DHHS office of hearings had done a number of negotiated regulations and was able to give the HCFA staff advice on procedures and the pitfalls to avoid.[68] From the department appeals board, HCFA got assigned an experienced arbitrator, Judy Ballard, to act as facilitator—acquainted with the procedures, but not sitting as a judge for this proceeding. Kathy Buto, the deputy director of CHPP was detailed as the sole HCFA representative, in part because of her experience and credibility; also because FFS expertise would be essential. In addition, HCFA created its own committee, to provide staff support for the HCFA representative, develop position papers, and monitor the process.[69]

A first difficult decision confronting HCFA was who should participate. Except to say that the negotiating committee should be named within forty-five days after its passage, the statute was silent. It mentioned the National Association of Insurance Commissioners, the American Academy of Actuaries, and "organizations representative of medicare beneficiaries and other interested parties" as groups to be consulted about publishing a notice, but not necessarily appointed to the committee. Some of the appointments—the

AMA, AHA, NAIC, AAA, AARP, and BC/BS—were both obvious and politically prudent selections. Beyond that, the list was not easy. Several beneficiary representatives in addition to AARP were also included. To keep the group manageable, the size was restricted to fifteen, which left a number still urgently seeking to be appointed. The group as finally constituted was broadly representative of the affected interests but composed mostly of lawyers, CPAs, and a few vice-presidents—technicians or people skilled in negotiation, which was probably important for eventual success.

Doctrine on negotiated rulemaking generally holds that time should be strictly limited, especially because of the temptation to leverage the process by stalling (Kerwin 1999). Time was certainly limited in this instance, though probably more for political reasons than doctrinal ones. The statute, passed on August 5, called for the negotiating committee—which would be appointed by mid-September—to report to the secretary by January 1 on whether "a consensus is likely to occur," no later than one month before the final publication date of April 1, 1998. Practically speaking, this schedule meant that the committee, assembling in October, would have little more than two months to educate itself on solvency, sort out and discuss the issues, and decide by Christmas whether it could reach a consensus. As it happened, the committee selected Christmas as the "point of no return,"[70] which at least had a positive symbolism as compared with the April 1st deadline. Effectively, the working time from beginning to end would be seven and one-half months, about a quarter of the time required for most HCFA rules.

The HCFA steering committee moved expeditiously, quickly selecting the committee so that meetings could begin on October 1. Most of the group were specialists in one discipline or another, but not in the law and economics of solvency, so that much of the time from October until December was spent in getting the group as a whole up to speed and operating with some common understandings of insurance principles, solvency requirements, the economics of managed care, and current HCFA regulations and policy.[71]

As this learning phase progressed, the group began to confront tough and complex issues, such as how to define "sweat equity" and how much it should count; how much liquidity to require how to treat risk-based capital where a parent organization provided the assets; and what guarantees should be required.

These questions were obviously difficult in a technical sense. They also went to the core of the controversy over PSOs—essentially a question of how much the insurance and managed care rules should be adjusted to enable physicians and hospitals to go into this business for themselves. This issue combined professional passions and ideology, deep conflicts of interest, intricate technicalities, and the political clout of powerful organizations with much at stake.

Some standard dispute resolution techniques were adopted and were probably useful. Each of the committee members was given training in alternative dispute resolution and interest-based negotiation.[72] Outside experts were brought in and HCFA policy papers developed. The group met several times over lunch or dinner; and Kathy Buto held six or seven three-day meetings.[73] The facilitator, Judy Ballard, also broke the committee apart into working groups that cut across divisions between HMOs, providers, and beneficiaries.[74]

Even so progress was slow, especially before Christmas. A HCFA staff person recalls his own sense of panic over the approaching deadline. One member of the committee could not take the stress and resigned. As the deadline approached, members wished strongly to continue, and resolved to go ahead, but without any great assurance that they would be able to reach a consensus.

After the holidays, with the group committed to reaching a decision, the pace quickened, but a final resolution did not come easily. Work on a definition of PSOs dragged along, even though the committee had an early draft by February. The committee continued to wrestle with stubborn core issues such as how much liquidity to require and how to count "sweat equity" and "going concern" value. Late in March, it was not clear that a consensus could be reached.

The final meeting was dramatic. Philip Doerr, a principal HCFA staff person, recalls the meeting vividly. The group met in the DHHS penthouse, resolved to make this their last meeting. They broke into smaller groups, with the facilitator switching them from group to group, keeping them going nonstop, allowing no one to sit down until they finished.[75] The meeting lasted for twelve hours, but the group reached consensus and finished within the deadline. After other clearances, the regulation was published on May 7.

In this instance, negotiated rulemaking was a notable success. The neg-reg group achieved a consensus on difficult, multiparty issues. Because of their agreements on substantive policy the regulation almost "wrote itself," cutting the time for completion in half.[76] Subsequent comments on the regulation were also drastically reduced. The participants worked together, got to know each other, and left with good feelings. Among reasons mentioned for the success were the deadline and the knowledge that DHSS would do the regulation its way if the panel defaulted; the joint learning experience and the bonding; good staff support; the skill of the facilitator, Judy Ballard; and the adroitness of Kathy Buto in leveraging her position as HCFA representative. One participant, asked if he would do it again, said "in a heartbeat."[77]

Consumer Information and Medicare+Choice.   One of the biggest operational tasks associated with the implementation of Medicare+Choice was the expansion of the consumer information activities to match the new program. This particular example is of special interest because it illustrates some of the range of activities involved in operations, as opposed to regulation writing, as well as some of the issues that might be controversial about this kind of enterprise.

To keep matters in perspective, one should be aware that the total HCFA M+C operational effort was enormous, involving writing new contracts for each of the plans, continuing and intensive outreach and consultation with individual plans, getting the HCFA regional offices up to speed, creating and testing a web-site, developing data systems and software and getting them to run properly, training people in their use, approving applications and marketing materials, and monitoring plan compliance.[78]

Consumer information was a sensitive topic, in part, because of some recent history. In 1995, the Republican Congress had proposed "two HCFAs" with separate agencies to administer the FFS program and the managed care plans (see p. 103) At that time, the Institute of Medicine had unintentionally rubbed salt in the wounds with a draft report suggesting that HCFA might do well to delegate the consumer operation to some private entity that would be more adaptable and experienced with consumer information techniques. Since 1995, the IOM had published a second report that was less "directive" and Congress had retreated from its two HCFAs recommendation, but the underlying sensitivities were still there.[79]

Apart from the issue of HCFA's capabilities, the consumer information program and who administered it bore pretty directly on the future of Medicare+ Choice and how public or private that system would be. For example, if consumer information were to be spun off, then a system modeled on the FEHBP might seem a plausible next step. However, an FEHBP model would be rather anomalous if consumer information remained an integral part of HCFA. Indeed, this kind of consideration was a major reason for HCFA's unhappiness with the first IOM report.

Another sensitive issue was what consumer information should include. For example, consumer information might comprise nothing more than the kind of spreadsheet with comments issued by several then-current private sector consumer reports (e.g., Check List, Health Pages). Both Congress and HCFA were aware, though, that more was needed for the Medicare population and, especially, to reach rural areas, cultural and linguistic minorities, the blind, and the illiterate. Moreover, HCFA and many of the consumer information advocates wanted the Medicare beneficiary to be more than a passive recipient of information—to become a knowledgeable consumer and even a self-directing "navigator" through the health care system.[80] But to educate the consumer to this point, the information system would need, at a minimum, to be interactive and ideally to have some entity with "a pulse and an address" at the other end of the line.[81] If we go this far, why not a local office and agents similar to the local Social Security representative? If the local representative provides information and counseling, why not case work and advocacy, especially for the frail elderly or Medicaid recipients? These agents might even be useful informants about some of the abuses of managed care plans and other providers. These examples are, of course, hypothetical extensions of the program, and were not being contemplated at the time. They serve to illustrate how implementation can be a way of "institutionalizing the future" and why the issue of who administers consumer information is controversial.[82]

Like the 1995 statute, BBA 97 contemplated a broad and inclusive program of consumer information with an enormous responsibility settled upon "the Secretary"—i.e., HCFA—and a demanding time schedule.[83] In fact, a major "information campaign" to acquaint Medicare beneficiaries with the new program was mandated for November 1998, only thirteen months after the passage of BBA 97. According to one official, they were "naively aware of what was coming" on August 5, but there was not much they could do in advance, and no one comprehended "how big it was."[84]

Essentially, HCFA's charge was to create the infrastructure and materials for a national Medicare+Choice educational program and have it up and running, full bore, before November 1999. That, by itself, was a tough assignment. But a year before that, HCFA had to stage a trial run, on a smaller scale, with essentially the same working parts. As prescribed in the statute and as HCFA interpreted its responsibility, this included: a new toll-free hot line and a website; a revised Medicare handbook; collecting, assembling, and reviewing the materials needed for the annual information fair including health plan comparative data; developing a strategy to reach special populations and work with regional and state and local consumer information groups; and, generally, providing whatever additional information would assist beneficiaries in choosing their plans.

Two observations are helpful for understanding the operations aspect of implementation. One is that for systems to operate elements have to be in sequence—something is always preceded by something else. The other is that HCFA itself does very little of the actual operating. Instead, the operations and systems people issue instructions, purchase, or contract. These activities, of course, require lead time and planning—for instance, to consult on what the Spanish edition of the handbook should say to beneficiaries, to get that written, to pretest and amend it, and to get it printed and mailed. All of these steps require planning, coordination, developing protocols, writing the contracts or purchasing the services, and evaluating the product before going public.

For the Center for Beneficiary Services (CBS), there was both a policy and an operations aspect. Their primary responsibility was operations, to use the older terminology. There were regulations to be written, dealing especially with definitions of new entities, such as PSOs, PPOs, and MSAs, and with eligibility, the enrollment process, marketing guidelines, and beneficiary protections, for which they shared a responsibility with the Center for Health Plans and Provider Operations (CHPP). For these, CBS participated in the policy or regulation writing team led by CHPP, to provide its perspective and to assure that the text and preamble fit with what could be done and what the health plans were being told about the changes being made.[85]

The statute provided for national, comprehensive, "annual, coordinated elections" with "Medicare+Choice information fairs" beginning with November 1999. This would allow over two years to plan and develop a full-scale election program. The legislation also ordered a dress rehearsal—an initial "special education and publicity campaign" to take place November 1998. This separation carved out time for longer term planning and development, but it left a year or less to settle on a strategy, get organized, do the policy work, write specifications, negotiate contracts, and have the component parts operational for the early preview.

The statutory language allowed HCFA wide discretion with respect to the initial information campaign. Except that HCFA should inform the beneficiaries about the M+C options and the selection process, no specific requirements were included, so that HCFA's initial campaign could have been minimal. In retrospect, HCFA made a wise choice to begin phasing in most of the elements of a full-scale model, a step that meant that the first iteration might be rough and missing some parts, but would be valuable for developing the finished product. The main elements of this campaign included:

- completing, printing, and mailing a new Medicare handbook to 5.5 million beneficiaries in five states with a condensed version to all other beneficiaries;
- phasing in a toll-free telephone line beginning with five pilot states;
- creating an Internet site that included the handbook and detailed plan comparisons;
- organizing a National Medicare Education Program to "partner" with agencies;
- training seven hundred individuals from these agencies to be leaders for others.[86]

As was common—and recommended—for projects of this size, CBS contracted with an outside consultant, Arthur Anderson, for project integration services. From these consultants, CBS got several kinds of technical expertise, including help in working through a plan, developing critical paths and time lines, strategies to acquire information from health plans, expertise on particular technologies, and the development and management of contracts. The HCFA staff still had to winnow this technical input, understand the options, and make the final choices. For this, they were on a "very fast learning curve," with little room for mistakes.[87]

The Medicare Handbook was not mandated as such, though the statute directed that new enrollees receive various kinds of information about both the FFS and the M+C programs that added up to a pretty substantial packet. Moreover, from the HCFA perspective, the handbook was both traditional and seemed, as its title indicated, something that every beneficiary should have at hand, especially for a new and potentially confusing array of programs.

The handbook project was not so much technically difficult as simply huge. A text had to be written incorporating the changes and explaining a complex new reality clearly and in language "easily understandable by Medicare beneficiaries." To meet the needs of the various regions and cultural and linguistic groups, twenty-seven different versions, with plan data as timely as possible, were developed and reviewed. Because of its political sensitivity, some of the language dealing with MSAs, had to be cleared with Congress.[88] To print the handbook and arrange for simultaneous distribution by the U.S. Postal Service required three months, which added to the time pressure for many other activities.

The hotline presented its own particular problems. HCFA had some experience with hotlines, but not of this sort. The Arthur Anderson consultants supplied some specialized expertise on hot line operation and resources. Eventually, CBS used a "simplified acquisitions process" and ran a competition to choose the operating company. However, to write contract specifications CBS still had to decide, in general, how the hot line should be adapted for the M+C program and for Medicare beneficiaries. Would the number of calls be more like private health plans (medicine) or like Social Security (elderly)? Would the questions be complex and probing or short and simple? What kind of interactive protocols would be most helpful? For many such questions, CBS had no experience—so they had staff and other handy helpers, such as mothers-in-law, call in from five different regions. The system worked; but they had to go live with one month of testing and leave many of the changes for a second iteration. As the CBS director later observed, "the shakedown was rough."[89]

Reports from the field and CBS's own monitoring confirmed the wisdom of beginning the phase-in early and using an iterative process. CBS learned, for instance, that the first handbook was comprehensive and informative but also intimidating and not much consulted by beneficiaries. The hotline was used infrequently, mostly by less educated beneficiaries, to ask short and simple questions about benefits and enrollment. The web-site was mostly consulted by college graduates, especially to seek information useful to someone else, such as a parent or spouse. The most common source of information, particularly for picking a plan, was the health plans themselves.[90] Feedback like this was useful not just for designing the next handbook and supplementary bulletins or for tweaking the hotline and web-site menus, but also for redirecting CBS's own efforts, for instance, toward more informative and sophisticated plan comparison information.

One of the biggest challenges in preparing for the future, especially the

November 1999 health fair, was to develop Medicare Compare, a database that could be fed into the Internet site and would enable consumers to comparison shop for health plans. In general terms, this would involve assembling, for each plan, information on premium costs and services provided, plan-specific quality performance measures and consumer satisfaction ratings; and then designing a user-friendly web-site. Operationally, the tasks included talking with beneficiary groups to find out the principal reasons for selecting a plan; reviewing the Consumer Assessment of Health Plans Survey (CAHPS) and the Health Plan Data and Information Set (HEDIS) to decide which comparison measures to use and testing them for usefulness and accuracy;[91] translating these indicators into workable reporting requirements for the health plans; developing protocols with the health plans about data to be submitted through the ACR annual process;[92] and deciding upon and developing the necessary software to store and process all these data, and interact in a user-friendly way with the beneficiary, relative, or friend seeking information; and, finally, pretesting and making the final modifications before going fully operational.[93]

Outreach was another important element of the national education campaign. This outreach served two main purposes: to get meaningful feedback from group leaders with a stake in consumer information and to encourage local health information efforts. Among the activities were bimonthly meetings in Washington with leaders of advocacy groups and "partnering" agencies engaged in health information activities; contracts with ten PROs in different regions to investigate and develop methods for reaching local populations; and administering a small program ($250 million) of grants to local state health information programs (SHIPs) and community health insurance counseling projects.[94]

Outreach activities of the sort described were helpful in finding out which information activities were working and which were not. Among important discoveries—as reported at one of the Washington meetings—was how little beneficiaries knew about Medicare; how much misinformation there was; and the average beneficiary's limited information horizon and capacity to understand the implication of decisions.[95] HCFA reported plans to conduct focus groups on these and related topics. From the conference participants came suggestions about the need for a personal contact, for counseling, and even for an ombudsman, all of which makes a fairly obvious point that HCFA's National Medicare Education Program was, almost inevitably, an exercise in constituency building that could lead to mission creep and politically controversial program enhancements.

CBS staged an ambitious information campaign in November 1998 and began phasing in the various systems. There were glitches in the first iteration—the overly compendious handbook, 60,000 Spanish language versions sent to random addresses, misjudging the type of hot-line questions and the

usage patterns of the various information resources. This was also a first iteration of a new kind of activity. In the opinion of several outside observers, CBS
moved promptly and effectively to adjust the system, and was "doing as well
as could be expected" with a delegated responsibility of this size and a statute
as prescriptive as BBA 97.[96]

FFS Medicare: Hospital and Physician Payment; Outpatient PPSs

As with the treatment of Medicare+Choice, the aim with respect to amendments of the "traditional" FFS program is not to provide a comprehensive
account of implementation but to deal selectively with a few topics and
episodes that illustrate characteristic activities and problems encountered. A
brief inspection of the table of contents (see Appendix A) for Medicare and
Medicaid is useful to get a lively sense of the size and complexity of the statute
itself and to suggest the amount and variety of activities needed to implement
and administer these subtitles, chapters, and sections of BBA 97.

The two selections that follow illustrate different parts of the policy process
as well as two kinds of challenges. The hospital and physician payments
were exercises in regulation writing under almost crushing circumstances
of time compression, number and complexity of tasks, and Y2K obstacles.
The outpatient prospective payments systems provide an example of inade-
quately developed technical foundations for the regulations that had to be
written.

Hospital and Physician Payment.   In most years, implementing the hospital
and physician payment changes would be, for HCFA, a familiar exercise.
Many of the changes were formula-driven or involved small percentage
increases or decreases in the existing payment provisions. Wage, case mix, and
other indices had to be recalculated. Congress would usually tinker with some
parts of the system, for example, changing the hospital capital reimbursement, imposing a copay or a global cap, or even adding a simple fee schedule—most of these with lengthy consideration and recommendations from
ProPAC and PPRC (now MedPAC). All of this was fairly routine. The former
Bureau of Program Development had a computer program for the annual
update that allowed much of the regulation to be developed by filling in the
blanks, and there were often previous rules or antecedent policy amendments
to serve as templates for implementing the more substantive legislative
changes. For that matter, one of the concerns in 1997 was that HCFA had not
done a major reconciliation in seven years and lacked that particular and
unique kind of learning experience.[97]

Implementing BBA 97 was different, though, much as a tempest differs
from a gentle summer rain. What transpired was familiar in some ways, but

it came quickly, in great volume, and with unexpected twists. In addition to the sheer number of amendments, many of them were accompanied by aggravating factors: changes that required additional data and technical work; drastic time compression; the HCFA reorganization and Y2K problems; and not enough experienced personnel or hours of sleep.

The deadline for hospital payments was one of the harshest constraints. The regulations and payment rates for both PPS and TEFRA[98] hospitals had to be ready for the September 1, 1997, Federal Register. It helped that physician payments were not due until November; but they were the smaller and easier task. September 1 meant publication on that date, so that time for clearances and printing had to be allowed.[99] Some of the most important decisions on hospital payments were made in conference and became known in detail only with these reports, so that there was almost no lead time on important parts of the legislation.[100] The statute was enacted on August 5. Practically speaking, that left about two weeks of working time to deal with a number of important amendments and finish the regulation.[101]

One dimension was the sheer volume of regulations—$40 billion worth— in the first-year payment changes alone for PPS and PPS-exempt hospitals. These involved, of course, the regular update, with the hospital marketbasket, the various indexes, and alternatives in modifiers or in methods of calculation. Changes in outlier payments were especially difficult since these had to be budget neutral, requiring meticulous, iterative calculations. There were a large number of adjustments for special categories of hospitals: rural, Medicare-dependent, cancer, and long-term care. More basically, a number of payments were terminated, capped, or restructured, such as Medicare DSH payments, capital reimbursement, discharge payments, the DME/IME formulas, the TEFRA hospital caps, and the outpatient prospective payment systems.

The scope and complexity of the regulatory task meant that an intense and coordinated effort had to be mobilized quickly. Meanwhile, HCFA was in the midst of a comprehensive reorganization, with regulation writers being reassigned, divisional responsibilities altered, and telephone numbers changed. Fortunately for this particular effort, many of the physical changes had not yet taken place, so that policy people and regulation writers could still work closely together even if no longer in the same organizational box.[102] At the same time, prioritizing and coordinating were difficult because responsibilities had changed and people were packing offices and moving. Getting the work done under these conditions required heavy reliance on personal loyalties, the willingness of individuals to take ownership of projects, and the "super-dedication" of key individuals.[103]

Another important dimension was complexity. Some of these changes required development and/or data, policy analysis, and writing a regulation— all to be done within the compressed time-frame. The transfer regulation—which dealt with how to split payments for early hospital discharges involving ten DRGs—required analytic work to select the DRGs, calculations of payments, introduction of new codes, and creation of a regulatory framework.[104] To cite another example, payment ceilings for TEFRA hospitals were set at 75 percent of the target amount for FY 1996. That sounds simple enough. But to get those target rates all the intermediaries had to be surveyed. For yet another example, changing the IME was a simple matter of a formula, but the GME—the direct payments for educating residents—involved definitions, calculating "full time equivalents" (not an easy task with medical schools), "rolling averages," and—if the secretary thought fit to prescribe rules—aggregating the numbers for an entire institution. Writing a rule for this kind of situation, involving individual histories of 125 or so medical schools, was a challenging activity. It also required learning to "think like a medical school administrator" to know what to anticipate and guard against.[105]

The Y2K problem, difficult for most programs, posed special hardships for this group. Changes in the payment formulas, especially developing the various outpatient PPSs and other modifications, typically involved the vast HCFA and intermediary data files, but these files were the biggest part of the Y2K problem, and a number of them were closed or partially blocked while the data management experts worked to get the files and the computer systems compliant.

One example of the sort of difficulty occasioned by Y2K was the DME "carve-out." Under this provision Medicare general medical education (GME) payments that had been made to managed care plans for treating Medicare patients were to be "carved out" and paid directly to the medical schools and teaching hospitals. To do this, the secretary was to estimate the amount paid to the plans and transfer that amount directly to the teaching hospitals that had provided the care. That, in turn, however, required that HCFA get into the managed care files and work with the encounter data—much of which was fragmentary and varied from plan to plan—in order to estimate the level of historic payments.

Another example was the $1,500 cap for services under the new prospective payment system for rehabilitation. Under the statute, payment would be based upon the existing fee schedule, including balance billing limits, but with a different rate for hospital-based facilities. Special provisions were made for outpatient occupational and physical therapy that was furnished incident to a physician's professional services. A global cap of $1,500 was set for 1999, 2000, and 2001. Congress also asked for a report on the functioning of this new system, not later than January 2, 2001. On its face, this mandate would seem simple. Obviously, though, Congress intended for HCFA to enforce this global cap and monitor its effects. Therefore, a separate system had to be created to keep track of the billing, check for errors, establish provider screens, and assess the impact. This relatively simple global cap required a large amount of development work and extensive access to the existing files—for data that might or might not be available.

The impact of Y2K has to be viewed against a background of an enormous collective effort in which the individual work groups were processing huge files through multiple iterations that might take days or weeks to run. The first-year October 1 payments had top priority. Many other programs that were Y2K sensitive did not. These took meetings and negotiation to see what was available, centrally and locally, and to get resources and time committed. Typically, individuals or groups had to arrange access to the needed file, then queue for a limited slot of computer time—often late at night or early in the morning. They lost their place and had to queue again if the task was aborted or interrupted. Barbara Wynn estimated that her deputy spent 80 percent of his time for two weeks in meetings, mostly dealing with Y2K problems. Work went on after hours, over the weekends, and past midnight, not infrequently running into computer instructions stating that some operation "may not be made." At times a quick permission could be gotten from the data systems people. Often, the expedient step was to devise a way to trick the computer and work around the barrier.[106] At best, the work was demanding, frustrating, tense, and physically exhausting. As Wynn said, "It was Y2K that told me it was time to leave."

Outpatient Prospective Payment Systems. A remarkable feature of the Medicare legislation of 1997 was the wholesale adoption of prospective payment systems, almost as though invoking the formula "PPS" was by itself a major step toward cost containment, appropriate resource utilization, and fair payment. Prospective payment systems were prescribed for rehabilitation hospitals and services, long-term care hospitals, outpatient department services, skilled-nursing facilities, and home health services.[107] Budget savings and CBO scoring were factors in some instances for the choice made. HCFA was concerned about the time schedule and the work that still needed to be done on these systems, but also wanted the mandate.[108] Despite forewarning and some misgivings, Congress endorsed the approach. The results have been mixed and serve as reminders that prospective payment systems take time and persuasion and, even when developed, work no special magic.

Development of outpatient prospective payments systems began in the early 1970s, predating the formation of HCFA itself, with R&D on ambulatory payment groups (APGs). Since then, demonstrations had been supported in various areas, including home health care, outpatient services, rehabilitation hospitals and services, and mental health.[109] However, HCFA's budget for research and demonstrations during the 1980s was limited. It was especially difficult to get money for low-profile items.[110] Moreover, the agency had no power to compel submission of data, so demonstrations had to be on a voluntary basis.[111] In retrospect, it is easy to say the agency should have anticipated the future, but grave concern about outpatient cost containment only began in the 1990s; and not until 1997 would many people have bet that Congress would order every PPS on the menu.

One problem for those charged with implementing the various outpatient PPSs was that these systems were still in process and needed development before they could become operational.[112] Each one of these was technically difficult. Also, in addition to the PPSs, a number of complex demonstrations such as competitive bidding, PACE, and the S/HMOs needed specifications developed, contracts written, and sites arranged.[113] One PPS would have been a challenging assignment; doing all at once with severe time constraints was almost overwhelming.[114]

HCFA reorganization and the Y2K turmoil also cut across the development effort. The existing Office of Research and Demonstrations had been split up, with demonstrations and policy development for the outpatient PPSs going to the Center for Health Plans and Providers. This dispersion left behind in ORD several experienced leaders with a small cohort of research people to work on implementation. More disruptive, though, was Y2K, since development and demonstrations were critically dependent upon access to data files, many of which had to be sealed off while HCFA worked to get its own internal computer systems Y2K compliant, along with those of its contractors and intermediaries.[115] This constraint meant, practically speaking, that additional development on the outpatient PPSs, unless of a routine sort, was hard or impossible to do; and that much of this work would have to wait until the Y2K problem was resolved. It was in this context that the administrator, Nancy-Ann deParle, acknowledged in July 1998 that HCFA was falling behind in its work schedule. She requested delays in some of the statutory deadlines, including outpatient services and home health care.[116] At the time, Chairman Thomas, of the Ways and Means Health Subcommittee, deplored this delay in "the two prospective payment systems . . . originally proposed by the administration." Blaming the delay on the lagging Y2K efforts of the contractors, Pete Stark, the ranking Democrat, introduced the Medicare Contracting Flexibility Act, to give HCFA more authority to compel the contractors to make year 2000 corrections.[117] Neither approach helped to move the process forward.

Skilled nursing facilities (SNFs).   Since the mid-1980s, HCFA had centered its efforts to develop a PPS for skilled-nursing facilities on "resource utilization groups" or RUGs, a concept that was now in its third iteration (RUG-III). Based upon information in "minimum data sets" submitted by the facilities, this approach used activities of daily living scores and measures of nursing and rehabilitation time to create twenty-six different RUGs and to classify patients into four different categories—one that required rehabilitation services and three that did not. SNFs would then be paid a single per diem rate that covered routine, ancillary, and capital costs as well as Part B charges during the stay, with the RUGs serving as a case mix adjuster (Medicare Payment Advisory Commission 2000:59).

Although HCFA had been refining this approach for over a decade, there were some difficulties with it, especially as perceived by MedPAC and its staff. One persistent concern was that a per diem payment would encourage SNFs to "game" the system: lengthening stays to gain on end-of-stay low-intensity days and underserving patients by scanting on rehabilitation services and ancillaries, especially if not adequately compensated for them (Medicare Payment Advisory Commission 1998:94–95). A second problem, noted by MedPAC, was that RUGs did not adequately account for increases in the case mix intensity of contemporary SNFs. Although the RUG-III system distinguished categories of patients and included a "rehabilitation" hierarchy, it was based historically on amounts of staff time, which did not take account of shifts in patient population and SNF practice. Therefore, RUGs would tend to overpay SNFs that provided little rehabilitation or therapy and underpay those that provided more—neither a desirable consequence (Medicare Payment Advisory Commission 1999:88–89).

Mindful of these problems, MedPAC had urged HCFA, early in 1998, to explore a "discharge based" PPS as "most appropriate" for SNFs. It recommended a system, used for rehabilitation hospitals, that was based on "function related groups" ["Functional Independent Measure-Function Related Groups (FIM-FRGs)"; Medicare Payment Advisory Commission 1998:95–97]. This system, which had been shown to work well for rehabilitation patients, used twenty-one diagnostic categories, such as stroke, spinal cord injuries, and cardiac conditions, along with age and the patient's functional and cognitive abilities, to create some seventy FRGs that would predict length of stay and resource use. MedPAC recommended that the HCFA staff continue working to refine its RUG-III rehabilitation category, but that they use FRGs.

From a policy perspective, the FRG solution might have seemed the elegant one. But within HCFA, a more pragmatic view prevailed. For Tom Hoyer, director of chronic care, and his deputy, Janice Flaherty, FRGs were a "black box" and probably easy to game. In dealing with something as tricky as a new outpatient PPS, they preferred to start with the familiar and let experience build up for a time. Moreover, RUGs and FRGs were two different payment methods—a per diem and a per discharge—and would be difficult to meld within one system, requiring intricate cross-walks and other adaptations. Beside that, their Division had a July 1, 1998, deadline, which they expected to meet. As Hoyer explained, there was time to do one system or the other, but not both. Given that choice, the RUG-III approach was the best single system, so that was the way they went. HCFA met the deadline.

No one supposed that was the end of the story; and it was not. HCFA worked on further refinement of RUG III. MedPAC continued to express its concerns about the system, and Congress included several provisions in the Balanced Budget Refinement Act of 1999,[118] enacted at the end of November. Colloquially known as the "give-back" act, this legislation—among its many other provisions—addressed the RUG issue both generally and in particular, increasing the SNF market basket and temporarily raising the rates for a number of individual RUGs in the "medically complex" category while awaiting HCFA's next refinement. In May 2000, HCFA issued a proposed rule, with final publication promised for October of that year.

The iterative process just described has characterized the development and implementation of prospective payment systems, though at times "process" seems a more appropriate term than "system." It also illustrates a tension between further technical refinement in the payment mechanism of a sort often pushed by MedPAC or its predecessors and pragmatic experiment and incremental adjustment favored, in this instance, by HCFA. There may be no elegant solution to this kind of dilemma; but divided government or partisanship can surely be calculated to make it worse.

Home health care.   Home health care is one of those problem areas that provides useful reminders of why health policy is unexpectedly difficult, given American institutions and attitudes. A series of decisions by Congress, the courts, and HCFA beginning in the 1980s had transformed the home health benefit from a restricted coverage for posthospital care into a widely available kind of in-home subacute or long-term care. Modifying or undoing these concessions proved difficult—because of differences in the types of care being given, regional variations in utilization, divisions within the industry, technical problems of devising a case mix adjuster, and the fact neither Congress nor the administration had the political will for more direct solutions.

Experts in the field have long said that Congress and HCFA needed to say more clearly what they will pay for and what establishes eligibility—for instance, to define "intermediate care" or say what qualifies as "homebound." Why not? One answer is that Congress and HCFA have tried that, and it did not work. At one point, a definition of "homebound" was to have been included in BBA 97, but that project was abandoned and HCFA was told to study the topic, even though the agency already had a definition in its provider manual.[119] As one experienced administrator put it, there are aspects of the concept you just "don't want to consider," such as whether the beneficiary lives alone or has in-house caregivers.[120] Even winning on the issue is probably not worth the moral anguish you or the political price.

Another kind of direct approach would be to discourage utilization by instituting a copay, with $5 usually suggested. This was rejected by Congress in part because both the industry and the administration had strong objections in principle to a HHC copay. Opponents of the copay added that visits often totaled more than two hundred a year, so that even a $5 copay could be burdensome for poor beneficiaries, and difficult to collect.[121] BBA 97 did provide for a surety bond of $50,000, which was seen in considerable measure as a way of screening out some of the opportunistic or dishonest agencies. The $50,000 bond was decried as burdensome for small rural agencies and deserving Visiting Nurse Associations. Within weeks after its publication, it was suspended on the initiative of a bipartisan group of senators from rural states.[122]

The main emphasis of the legislation was upon a per episode PPS with a case mix adjuster and outlier payments. This was an approach strongly favored by industry leaders and backed especially by the for-profit chains, that were even then pushing a version they had developed.[123] HCFA had grave misgivings. One concern was how to prevent gaming and risk selection—which a per episode system would invite, especially without a reliable and discriminating case mix index. Some analysts, both within and outside HCFA, doubted that it could be done.[124] Another major problem was that HCFA had no database with which to work—a prerequisite for designing a competent case mix index. Since CBO did not score promises or even prospective designs, it was incumbent upon HCFA to come up with an alternative. That was the origin of the Interim Payment System (IPS)—a temporary method of reducing payments sufficiently to meet the deficit reduction target.[125]

The IPS was to go into effect on October 1, 1997 and last until Ocober 1, 1999, when the prospective payment system would begin. Under the IPS, providers would get the lesser of: (1) 105 percent of a national median; (2) a blended rate of 75 percent of agency costs and 25 percent of a regional average; or (3) the per visit cost limits. The payments were for an episode of care set at 120 days, with 1994 selected as the base year.[126]

With an implementation date of October 1, 1997, the home care industry, led by the NAHC, developed an impressive campaign aimed especially at the IPS and the surety bond. As for the IPS, industry representatives objected that the rates were too low and would drive a number of agencies out of business. They challenged figures about how widespread abuses were. In their view, the combination of per visit and aggregate limits would hurt both the acute, service-intensive and the longer term chronic cases patients—so that the neediest would suffer. They were particularly distressed when Congress postponed the deadline for the prospective payment system to October 2000, extending the IPS another full year.

The home health campaign was effective. The surety bond was suspended in July, less than a month after publication of the regulation. In mid-October, barely two weeks after implementation, modifications of the IPS were passed as part of the omnibus appropriations bill. At a cost of $1.7 billion this legislation eased payment limits and postponed a 15 percent overall reduction until October 1, 2000.[127] Though not perceived that way at the time, this was the first of a number of Medicare "give-backs" from the budget savings achieved by BBA 97.

One of the biggest obstacles to the development of a home health PPS was the lack of adequate data. Home health care agencies varied greatly in size, professionalism, and practice patterns. So did their definitions of services provided, procedure codes (if they used them), and billing practices (Medicare Payment Advisory Commission 1998:93). HCFA's way of working around this lack of data was to adopt a standard assessment instrument, widely accepted in the industry, and make it a requirement for home health agencies participating in the Medicare program. The Outcomes and Assessment Information Set (OASIS) had been used by larger home care agencies, primarily for patient assessment and to develop treatment plans. Early in 1997, before BBA 97 was passed, HCFA issued a proposed regulation that would have required all home health agencies to use OASIS for patient assessment, but the final rule was never published. Then BBA 97 was enacted, mandating the development of a case mix–adjusted PPS. OASIS became much more important. Employing this tool, HCFA could get a flow of standardized data without needing to work from unreliable billing files.

Following a usual practice, HCFA got some ninety home health agencies in eight states to agree to submit OASIS data and work with them to develop a database. HCFA also engaged ABT Associates to provide technical assistance. Their primary purpose was to collect data; but in pursuit of this objective, they discovered that OASIS could itself serve as a good case mix indicator, and provide the foundation for the payment system.

The essential elements of the PPS were made public on March 18, 1999, by Tom Hoyer, HCFA's director of chronic care and insurance policy. The system would be based upon episodes of care lasting sixty days, use of OASIS for patient assessment, and a case mix adjuster with patient groups determined by clinical data, functional status, and utilization factors. October 1, 2000, was set as the implementation date.

The sixty-day period deserves separate comment. Setting the length of the episode of care was critical for the home health PPS: too long invited gaming and overpaid long stays, and too short was costly and burdensome. Skeptics about a home health PPS doubted, in fact, that any case mix adjuster could be effective over the current 120-day episode of care and recommended, at a minimum, some system of postepisode cost reporting and auditing.[128] The sixty-day period was a compromise that improved the performance of the case mix adjuster and provided additional occasions for patient assessment—upon entry, each sixty days, and then upon discharge. More frequent episodes would also help monitor costs and quality, especially when linked to a powerful data-collecting instrument like OASIS.

To get this system operational, HCFA needed a wide and representative data flow for a number of months—in other words, OASIS reports coming in from around the country and from a large and representative sample of 10,000 home health agencies. Keenly aware of time constraints, HCFA sought emergency clearance from OMB on paperwork requirements for an April rule mandating home health agencies to use OASIS in their reporting.[129]

Since BBA 97 says explicitly that, beginning with October 1, 1997, "the Secretary" could require "all home agencies" to submit "information needed to develop a case mix system," one might have thought that HCFA could do as it chose in this matter. From the provider perceptions, though, OASIS was an elaborate data set that was expensive and required large amounts of professional time to administer. It could be an onerous requirement for small or rural agencies to develop this capability and pay for the computers, software, and training that would be required.[130] The government made no offer of compensation for these expenses. Moreover, using such data in-house for patient assessment or quality enhancement is one thing. Giving patient information to an outside government agency is another and raises questions about confidentiality and privacy. OASIS, which started as a protocol for patient assessment, was beginning to seem like a much larger affair.

Again, the home health agencies lobbied Congress and the administration to good effect, especially on the privacy issue. Members of Congress complained that the data to be collected were extremely personal and they were concerned that it would be included in a national data bank.[131] Vice-President Al Gore requested a comprehensive review of the privacy issue, and OMB held up the paperwork clearance. Rather quickly, the implementation deadline moved from April to June 19, with transmission of data to HCFA to begin August 25, 1999. HCFA also published a "notice" indicating a number of steps it would take to protect privacy and reduce the reporting requirements, though insisting that agencies would still have to report data essential to determine appropriate payments and assure quality.[132]

So far, the score card would seem to read NAHC, 3; HCFA, 0. The surety bond was suspended in June 1998, less than three weeks after publication of the rule. Legislation amending the Interim Payment System and increasing payments was signed into law November 1998. Home health agencies continued to push for additional changes. In March 1999 reporting requirements for the PPS were stalled and were later substantially modified.

This could be seen as one more example of providers exploiting their access and lobbying skills to profit at the expense of the public, but home health agencies had some equities on their side. The Interim Payment System, for instance, was an expedient to gain time while a proper PPS was developed. It was also a harsh deficit reduction measure devised with little regard for the industry. A major factor in the financial distress of home health agencies, which was genuine, was a CBO miscalculation—use of a behavioral offset of two-thirds, which tripled the budget reduction from $16 billion to $47 billion and forced hundreds of closures in some states.[133] The $50,000 surety bond was part of a general section dealing with disclosure and surety bonds (Section 4313) and seemed not unreasonable to Congress, but then HCFA added "or 15 percent" of Medicare or Medicaid payments, "whichever is greater," and required that the bond be posted annually, making the provision much more onerous.[134] The OASIS reporting requirement was costly, especially difficult for small agencies to meet, and raised serious issues of privacy and confidentiality.

As was often the case, there was blame to go around. There was a history of abuses by the home health industry. On the other side, Congress and the administration made mistakes and overstepped. One merit of our pluralistic system is that it facilitates redress. On such occasions, especially with an election in prospect, local areas and interest groups may do especially well for themselves.

Hospital outpatient prospective payment system.   Revising the nonsystem of hospital outpatient payments was both a challenge and an instructive experience, especially considering some of the contemporary trends in health care. For many years, hospitals had been moving services, procedures, and diagnostic tests to outpatient sites. The establishment of an inpatient PPS in 1984 provided impetus to this movement, as did patient preferences and technological developments. Outpatient activities grew from 7 percent of hospital business in 1983 to 20 percent in 1997, in dollar volume an increase of about 14 percent a year.[135] This rate of increase was one of the problems, since more and more activity was falling outside the purview of effective regulation. In addition, hospital outpatient activities, with their multiple sites, mix of payment systems, and rates of technological and practice innovation, invited a good bit of entrepreneurial site-shifting based on payment differentials. Another motivation behind the development of a PPS was to remove or diminish incentives for this kind of gaming. This same pluralism and dynamism made regulation especially difficult, it was also important not to discourage the shift to outpatient sites since this was, overall, a good thing. Beside that, for providers the stake was enormous and many of them liked the situation the way it was. The efforts by Congress and the administration to confront this complex reality and deal with the interests and issues at stake provide a good illustration of interaction between legislative policy and administrative implementation. They also show why implementation sometimes takes unexpected amounts of time.

Developing a PPS was not the only important problem. At the time, methods of payment for hospital outpatient services included cost reimbursement, charges, fee schedules, and a blended rate. Moreover, not all of the outpatient services and procedures would be included in the PPS. Some changes could and should be made in the interim, while the PPS was being developed. One of these was the so-called formula-driven overpayment.

The formula-driven overpayment came about because of a curious anachronism that allowed hospitals to bill patients for outpatient services and procedures according to their charges rather than their costs. Since many of these charges were not under a payment limit and were higher than costs, beneficiaries paid more—in some instances more than half again of the total charges because of copays and balance billing. Because of blended formulas the full amount of the copays typically would not get deducted by the intermediaries from their payments, so that there would be a "formula-driven" overpayment.[136] Providers took further advantage of this situation by raising their charges, so that not only did patients and the government lose money but the payment methodology was itself an invitation to further gaming.

Following the House proposal, the statute dealt with this issue rather neatly—requiring that all provider copays would be deducted at the end of the reimbursement process so that, effectively, Medicare payments would be correspondingly reduced—thereby removing the formula-driven aspect and the incentives to continue raising charges. It was a neat solution, but this one line of text in the statute meant that HCFA had to develop the software program to track, edit, and check these copays for the individual providers and the particular services and procedures—a time-consuming process that also involved access to carrier and intermediary files and Y2K complications.[137]

HCFA planned to use Ambulatory Payment Classification (APC) groups for the outpatient PPS, an approach that had been under development for at least fifteen years.[138] An earlier version, known as Ambulatory Patient Groups (APGs) was one of the first technically sophisticated attempts to deal with the outpatient payment problem (Smith 1992:115–16). Basically APC groups were a bundling or packaging device that grouped together services and procedures that were clinically related and required comparable use of resources, then paid for these groups on the basis of established codes (HCPCS). The primary rationale for such an approach is fairly obvious—substituting a *prix fixe* method of pricing for an *a la carte* one and thereby reducing the incentives to proliferate and upcode individual services and procedures.

From the hospital perspective, there are a number of reasons to be concerned about devices like the APC groups, but they usually come down to what is included in the bundle and how "coherent" the groups are. As to size, how much is included under the one payment—for instance, a related procedure or ancillaries such as drugs and devices—is a vital concern. If the bundle includes a number of high-cost along with low-cost elements, then the hospital could be at considerable risk should it get the wrong patient mix, for instance, by developing an unfortunate reputation for good treatment of high-cost patients. Hospitals are also leery of such devices because they make them increasingly responsible for physician decisions that they cannot control. So they are likely to insist strongly that APC groups be as coherent as possible, and for that reason smaller and more numerous. That moves the PPS back in the direction of an ordinary fee schedule and makes it prone to similar inflationary pressures, such as code proliferation and volume increases.[139] No matter which way this tug-of-war turns out, it is fundamentally about shifting costs and risks.

In the legislation, Congress addressed these concerns of the hospitals specifically and with a sophisticated awareness of the kinds of problems likely to arise in the course of developing and implementing such a system. Rather than attempting to take a large amount of money out of hospital outpatient payments, Congress provided that the new system should be "budget neutral" with respect to the old—in other words, set payments so that outpatient departments in the aggregate neither gained nor lost by moving to the new system.[140] In recognition of the fundamental issue of shifting risk, the legislation provided that services classified within each group should be "comparable clinically and with respect to the use of resources" (Section 4532). Mindful of what this implied, Congress directed the secretary to "develop a method" to control increases in volume with an authorization to reduce the update for subsequent years to offset volume increases, much as had been done under the physician fee schedule (Section 4532).

A proposed rule for an outpatient PPS was published on September 8, 1998, only five weeks after the rule for skilled-nursing facilities. At the time of publication, HCFA delayed the implementation date—which had been set for January 1, 1999—until early 2000, citing Y2K problems.[141]

Y2K was especially important for several reasons. One was that the most central task, to refine and adjust the APC groups, required extensive work with the data files and the intermediaries. This activity was slowed because of Y2K complications. An immediate delay, according to a HCFA official, was a corrupted data file and an earlier computer program that proved to be faulty.[142] Remedying this required a protracted effort to review and clean the data files and rebuild much of the program.[143] Seemingly minor items in the legislation made their own unique contributions. For instance, the statute provided that beneficiary copays should be frozen until they reached 20 percent of the outpatient department's fee schedule amount. This simple formula required a system for monitoring the payments collected and, therefore, use of the existing files to develop the software. Congress also directed that payments under the outpatient PPS should be budget neutral with respect to the payments outpatient departments would have received under the existing system. Implementing this provision was both conceptually difficult and required the development of complicated cross-walks. It also involved activity that was Y2K-sensitive . All of these tasks took time, but Y2K made the tasks more difficult and protracted.

From the hospital perspective, there were a number of problems with the HCFA proposal, including the variance associated with and the distributive effects of particular APC groups, whether ancillaries would be included, exemptions for particular hospitals and pass-throughs for drugs and new technology, payment levels, and transition rules. HCFA was responsive to some of these concerns. They sought and have continued working to improve the performance of APC groups and to reduce their distributive effects. They did not attempt to include ancillaries. HCFA also increased the number of groups from 346 in the proposed rule to 451 in the final version, and did not implement a volume control.

The hospitals wanted more than incremental adjustments, however, and for these they took a legislative route.

The amendments sought by the hospitals were part of a general campaign, planned in advance and begun in January 1999, that eventually culminated in the Medicare Balanced Budget Refinement Act of 1999 (BBRA). For their part, hospitals hoped both to make a preemptive strike against additional payment cuts and to lessen the size of the scheduled BBA 97 reductions. One attempt that failed was to persuade Congress to revoke or modify the hospital transfer provision. The hospitals' other major regulatory priority was to amend the "flawed"[144] outpatient PPS. Efforts on this front succeeded dramatically.

Passed in November 1999, BBRA was remarkable for the explicit "marching orders" given to HCFA. Congress also displayed great solicitude for providers, perhaps with the future election of November 2000 in mind. The major outpatient provisions fell under six headings:

- Rural and cancer hospitals were exempted from the PPS, with a proviso that the secretary study the matter.
- Cost reimbursement pass-throughs were legislated for drugs, biologicals, and new technologies, in some instances with specific pricing formulas.
- Outlier payments were mandated for high-cost cases.
- Special "corridors" were established to phase in payment reductions over a three-year transitional period.
- No service included in a APC group could have a mean or median cost more than two times the mean or median for the lowest cost item.
- Payment groups would be reviewed annually and updated as necessary.

The specific outpatient amendments were developed initially by the majority staff of the Ways and Means Subcommittee on Health. Some of the changes added little to the existing regulatory tasks of HCFA, but the pass-throughs and the transition corridors were troublesome. Pass-throughs were especially difficult because they created exemptions and stirred up intense lobbying efforts by scores of manufacturers of drugs or devices. In addition, HCFA had to define devices and develop application procedures for new and existing drugs and devices, determine the "average wholesale price" for drugs (often when the industry had none), impute their contribution to specific procedures, and meanwhile deal with the pleas and complaints of the lobbyists.[145] The transition corridors were not complex, but they made a substantial contribution to costs. Under the earlier proposed rule, outpatient payments would have been reduced by 3.8 percent. With BBRA, according to HCFA calculations, hospital payments for the coming year would be increased 4 percent over the current cost-based system and would be more than 10 percent higher than the earlier proposed regulation,[146] not counting the indirect costs of pass-throughs and exemptions.

HCFA published its regulation—over seven hundred pages—on March 31, 2000, after departmental and OMB clearances. That was by no means the end of the story. HCFA delayed final implementation from July 1 to August 1, citing software and other technical problems. The hospitals then sought an additional two-month delay, saying that they were not challenging the rule itself—which would increase their outpatient payments by $800 million in the first year—but that neither they nor the intermediaries were adequately prepared to start operating under the new program.[147] Their reasons for requesting the postponement illustrate some of the final steps and additional occasions for delay in the operational aspects of implementation:

- a two-month delay in issuing the processing format for a line-item change in claims,
- unavailability of outpatient code editor and PRICER software,
- additional time needed for testing prior to August 1 implementation,
- intermediaries' lack of adequate plan for contingency payments should the PPS malfunction,
- lack of adequate training, especially where final instructions were not issued or all elements of billing and payment were not yet in place.

One objective of implementation, especially for most Medicare programs, is to take the legislation, turn it into regulations, and then into computer software. As these hospital concerns about the outpatient PPS regulation would indicate, another important aspect is getting operational in the fuller sense: issuing the manuals, operational policy letters, and new forms; instructing and negotiating with the intermediaries; and working with the providers to assure that the system will function in practical, everyday situations—all of which takes time.

HCFA began operating under the new outpatient PPS on August 1, 2000, without acceding to the hospital's request for a delay. The agency continued to work on outlier payments and a volume control device and to reduce the variance in APC groups, and provider groups continued to lobby for further concessions in a second BBRA, and beyond that.

Much of the delay of the outpatient PPS seems rightly attributed to the complicating factor of Y2K. It should also be clear that developing such a payment system is, at best, a labor-intensive and time-consuming task freighted with a large burden of persuasion. The new payment system can hardly fail to be an improvement over the irrational nonsystem that preceded it, though it may not save much money. In any event, this example helps illustrate one point: prospective payment systems can be oversold, especially as a quick or easy route to cost containment.

Midcourse Corrections: The Balanced Budget
Refinement Act; Medicare+Choice

An important part of program implementation is "midcourse" corrections. As with BBA 97, these are often occasioned by an awareness that the original legislation or a subsequent regulation "overreached" or did not go far enough; by changing circumstances or "unforeseen consequences," actual or alleged; or by the continuing pursuit of an existing policy agenda. Barring unusual circumstances, major programmatic changes are unlikely, but the American system of government provides numerous opportunities for incremental amendments to ease hardships and make significant improvements in a program. These changes can amount, cumulatively, to billions of dollars and substantially delay or alter the thrust of a particular program. At the same time, incremental amendments alone may not be enough to avert a major calamity. The Balanced Budget Refinement Act illustrates the first of these statements, and Medicare+Choice the second.

The Balanced Budget Refinement Act of 1999. As for midcourse corrections, 1998 was not a year in which much happened. For an item, relatively little of BBA 97 had been implemented. It was an election year, which meant that the legislative cycle would be short and that much of health politics would consist of position-taking and partisan bombast. In addition, Congress was distracted by the Monica Lewinsky scandal and the impeachment process had raised partisanship to a level that made constructive legislation difficult. As previously noted, the home health agencies got the surety bond suspended, the interim payment system modified, and a 15 percent reduction postponed. The AAHP, along with the HIAA, sought modifications in the managed care payment formulas and an easing of the regulatory burden. The AMA initiated a lawsuit to block implementation of HCFA's resource-based fee schedule for physician practice expenses.[148] Aside from more vigorous prosecution of Medicare fraud and abuse, though, Congress showed little interest in amending BBA 97.

With the election of 1998, the political scene changed. Democrats saw in the election some vindication and an endorsement of their domestic policies, which encouraged them to push health care reform more aggressively. Republicans, lacking a working majority in the House, discerned a message that bipartisan collaboration would be prudent and probably essential to get any significant domestic legislation passed. In similar circumstances, Congress had passed both HIPAA and BBA 97, so that significant progress on substantive issues might have seemed likely. Because of important confounding factors, however, the most important health care legislation of the year was the modest, low-profile Balanced Budget Refinement Act of 1999—and even that was almost overwhelmed by larger initiatives.

One circumstance favoring minor BBA amendments was the poor prospect for major health care legislation negotiated at the leadership level. With the third speaker in as many weeks, the House Republicans were in disarray. Facing the Senate was the trial of an impeached president. In both houses, partisan rancor was high, making negotiated deals unlikely, and most of the major health care issues—a patients' bill of rights and HMO reform, the Bipartisan Commission and Medicare Reform, and a Medicare pharmaceutical benefit—were already caught up in the political campaigning for the November election of 2000. These initiatives involved political and strategic issues that could not be resolved at the committee level, and higher level leadership was in no fit state to resolve them either. Therefore, the legislative agenda was relatively open for a traditional, incremental kind of "fix" for BBA 97 to be developed at the committee and subcommittee level.

At this point in time, Congress was just beginning to get used to a politics of budget surplus, as opposed to the perennial struggle with deficit reduction. This was the first year for which a surplus was predicted; but later projections through the year opened an expanding vista of surpluses as far as the eye could see. By midyear, CBO made the prospect yet grander, adding $10 billion to a surplus already estimated to reach $120 billion. Over ten years, CBO projected a truly impressive $2.9 trillion surplus.[149] Another important midyear datum was that Medicare spending for the year would actually drop by $1 billion in overall expenditures.[150] Economists and health policy experts did on various occasions point out that such numbers could not simply be taken at face value—but many people did, and the numbers supported arguments that Congress might well have been too hard on providers and that money was available for some relief.

Meanwhile, several levels of budget surplus politics affected Medicare policy directly and indirectly. At the highest and most global level, there was a debate over tax cuts versus deficit reduction or using some percentage of the surplus—with 15 percent most frequently mentioned—to extend the solvency of the Social Security and/or Medicare trust funds or to add a pharmaceutical benefit to the Medicare entitlement. Some of these considerations had important spillover effects for the BBRA amendments. For instance, a major objection to using the surplus to shore up the trust fund was that it would remove the impetus for long-term reform of Medicare and for moving quickly to address the forthcoming recommendations of the Bipartisan Commission. Either of these major initiatives could have crowded out BBA reform. As it was, two impending and potentially distracting issues tended to cancel each other. President Clinton was backing his own version of Medicare reform, which involved a pharmaceutical benefit and additional spending. This spending would have been paid for in part by additional provider cuts totaling $39 billion over ten years.[151] The administration also proposed its version of BBA amendments, putting $7.5 billion on the table as a "quality assurance fund" to help with provider relief.[152] The intention was to include the BBA amendments with the Medicare reforms. This move would have gained political support for the administration's Medicare reforms but, since there was little chance for these to be enacted in 1999, joining the two might doom the BBA relief package for that year. Representative Thomas was seeking to restore considerably more to providers but hoped to include this relief in a Medicare reform bill next year, that would be based on the proposals of the Bipartisan Commission.[153] Meanwhile, both the provider lobby and many individual House and Senate members wanted tangible results in the current year. Happily for them, failure of the two larger initiatives left an opening in the legislative agenda.

Major provider groups that saw themselves as unfairly or harshly treated by BBA 97 began developing their campaigns for relief in January 1999. Initially, the predictions were that they would face stiff resistance and that Congress might even come back for additional budget reductions. As home health agencies went bankrupt and HMOs withdrew from Medicare, provider complaints began to seem more credible. The debate took a new turn, with CBO projections of huge budget surpluses and the astonishing $1 billion decline in Medicare spending for 1999. Providers could argue not only that they and their patients were being subjected to needless injury by specific BBA cuts but that Congress had misjudged and taken more out of Medicare payments than needed to meet the savings targets. Republicans in Congress pushed this theme, at the same time blaming HCFA for not helping them to identify BBA "fixes" or taking administrative action to ease the afflictions of providers.[154]

While providers were making their case, others expressed doubts about their claims of hardship and interpretations of the data. MedPAC, for instance, said in May that the hospital industry had overstated the effects of BBA and that Medicare margins would continue to be positive for the life of the statute.[155] HCFA and the GAO attributed provider distress to factors other than BBA, such as bad business decisions, enforcement of fraud and abuse legislation, and slowness of various payments.[156] As one small footnote to history, the $1 billion decline in Medicare spending resulted in large measure not from BBA expenditure reductions but from a drop in hospital case mix and a lag in home health care payments, cost factors that would end in July. HCFA, MedPAC, and individual committee members noted as well the lack of any credible evidence of harm to beneficiaries. A panel that included HCFA, the GAO, and MedPAC testified before the Senate Finance Committee against any general "give-back," though the panel members did say that some targeted relief might be justified, particularly for skilled-nursing facilities, home health agencies, and hospital outpatient departments.[157]

Targeted relief was something that Congress and the lobbyists understood quite well, and it seemed to them both right and plausible to expand the list of targets. Managed care was an obvious candidate since HMOs were, without doubt, an instance where Congress had underestimated the BBA impact.[158] Both the House and Senate moved quickly to include physicians and hospitals and add creative adjustments for SNFs and hospital outpatient departments. The Senate bill, which provided some relief for almost every provider group seeking it, totaled $9.7 billion over five years or $15.2 billion over ten years. The House bill would cost $9.4 billion over five years to which Chairman Thomas planned to add the $5.6 billion in administrative adjustments that the president had already put on the table.[159] An explanation given by Representative Thomas was that the administration contributions would reduce the amount of relief that Congress would need to provide. However, that was largely an "add-on," not an "instead of."

The final legislation—passed as part of an omnibus appropriations act— gave Medicare providers $16 billion over five years, $27 billion over ten years. The House rejected a Democratic proposal to add $2.7 billion to benefit mostly poor or severely ill patients and the providers treating them.[160] Republicans promised to return to the issue of Medicare reform in the coming year, and providers said that they regarded the bill as a good beginning, but only that.

This whole episode falls somewhere between a genuine midcourse correction and a thinly disguised give-back. It seems clear that there were some instances of severe hardship (home health agencies) and of drastic unintended consequences (managed care). On the other hand, there was little, if any, credible evidence of harm to beneficiaries. Moreover, hospitals and medical schools made out the most handsomely, with enormous political clout but without evidence that they had suffered proportionately from BBA stringency. Deficit reduction techniques were adapted effectively to target relief for providers but without the discipline of an overall total limit or following the standards of proof suggested, at various points, by MedPAC and the GAO. As a result, this process lacked the elements of objectivity and the appearance of policy-driven decisions that often characterized the collaborative efforts of Congress and staff agencies such as ProPAC and PPRC. The fact that the common name given to this process was "give-back" should provoke some reflection about the behavior to expect with a budget surplus or, for that matter, with credible symptoms of provider distress. The correlation between political power and the amount of relief suggests that we have moved uncomfortably in the direction of old-fashioned budgetary incrementalism and perhaps as well toward a growing capacity of the regulated, under a system of administered pricing, to determine the ultimate payment.

The year 2000 generated an even bigger giveback: $35.3 billion over five years compared to $16 billion in the BBRA. The Medicare/Medicaid and SCHIP Benefits Improvement and Protection Act (BIPA), passed as part of an omnibus appropriations bill on December 15,[161] cleared the way for Congress to adjourn. Hospitals were the biggest winners this time, with $13 billion, followed by health plans, with $10.3 billion. Beneficiaries were third with $5.7 billion.[162]

The second time around, there were more indications that BBA 97 was hurting providers: declining margins for hospitals and HMO losses or service withdrawals. Still, there was little to assure that the remedies prescribed were proportional to the injuries, and "correcting" BBA 97 seemed so attractive an enterprise that it raises a concern, as Justice Stephen J. Field once put it, that "the medicine of the Constitution [would] become its daily bread."[163]

In 2001, providers geared up for another round, but Congress showed little interest, and even some reaction to past give-backs. In the House, Thomas and Stark joined in a bipartisan denunciation of MedPAC as an "organized forum for the voice of self-interested lobbying." Gail Wilensky, the chairperson, was replaced by Glenn Hackbarth, in part, according to rumor, because of her support for doubling the hospital update recommended by Congress.[164] The Bush administration also opposed additional give-backs.[165] There the matter rested—no general relief bill was considered. Even specific efforts to increase managed care payments failed, despite continuing plan withdrawals.

Medicare+Choice. Implementation of the Medicare+Choice program furnishes us with a cautionary tale for our time. The BBA provisions with respect to managed care were, at best, a precarious compromise with a number of tensions unresolved, and a good many unforeseen consequences, both fiscally and administratively. In addition, managed care remained a politically and ideologically charged issue from 1998 through 2001, caught up in both partisan conflict within Congress and policy differences between the administration and Congress. These historic factors may or may not have contributed to the waves of HMO withdrawals from Medicare, but they helped to create a sense of crisis about the future of managed care in the Medicare program and had a potentially significant impact upon national health policy as a whole.

An important part of the background is that Congress, especially the Republicans, seemed to have greatly overestimated the attractiveness of a number of the new M+C options for either producers or providers. In the first round, for instance, HCFA got only three applications, two for provider-sponsored organizations, one for a preferred-provider organization. No applications were received for Medicare MSAs or for the private FFS option.[166] Late publication of the regulation and hard times financially for managed care organizations were some of the factors mentioned. HCFA was blamed in some measure: for requiring MSAs to employ a community rate and for setting the "substantial proportion" of health care that a PSO had to provide at 70 percent (60 percent for rural). Whatever the causes, the fact remains that, outside Congress, there was little clamor for these new options.

The new payment system established by BBA 97 proved especially disappointing, if not onerous, for the MCOs. This system was intended to achieve several objectives. One was to establish a floor or minimum payment to encourage HMOs to move into areas with historically low rates and enrollment. Another was gradually to sever the connection between HMO payments and the historic and inequitable AAPCCs. To do this, Congress based HMO payments on a new national per capita Medicare growth rate that would be the basis for annual increments. County rates would then be a blend of national and local, with the national rate being phased in, gradually reducing the disparity in rates. Annual updates would be based on the rate of increase in the national Medicare growth rate. Because capitation rates were generally regarded as too high, percentage reductions in the update were also scheduled for the next five years, amounting to a total of 2.8 percent; but no plan was to receive less than a 2 percent increase in any year.

A large number of simulations had been done on this formula, indicating that it should work effectively and fairly to promote these several objectives. However, the scheme was budget neutral and tied to the traditional FFS Medicare rate of increase. For a variety of reasons, including the effects of BBA 97, the rate of increase in FFS Medicare spending was dropping and would turn negative in FY 99.[167] This decline, of course, would ratchet down the national capitation rate. In addition, there were the annual percentage reductions in the update. CBO estimated that these payment changes would reduce budget outlays for managed care by $23 billion over five years. Most of this diminished annual increment was taken by the two floor payments, with the practical effect that the lowest payment counties got their minimum—for them a substantial raise—and the rest got 2 percent. Blending occurred for the first time in 2000, and was not expected to apply for 2001, so that little progress toward equalization could be made.[168] With medical costs generally expected to increase from 6 to 12 percent in 1999 and 2000,[169] a 2 percent update seemed inadequate, almost confiscatory.

There were additional exactions. One of them, small in size but seen by the managed care plans as unjust and irritating, was a user fee imposed on managed care organizations to finance the beneficiary education program for M+C, which would be administered by HCFA. This levy would amount to $95 million per year, or $475 million over five years. Much more substantial was the "carve-out" of medical education payments, allotting the MCO share of these funds directly to the hospitals. This was an additional $4 billion over five years.

Congress had also directed the secretary to develop a risk adjustment methodology that would help to account for the variations in costs per beneficiary experienced by the health plans. BBA did not specify whether the risk adjuster was to be budget neutral, but HCFA intended to reduce much of the favorable selection that MCOs allegedly enjoyed under Medicare and planned for savings on the order of $11 billion between 2000 and 2004.[170] This was not an inconsiderable sum of money, regarded either by itself or as an addition to the other BBA payment reductions. Moreover, the development of a risk adjuster would add an element of uncertainty for HMOs in their fiscal calculations and planning, and a major burden of providing the encounter data needed to develop the risk adjuster.[171]

At the time, a number of developments within the managed care industry began to make the Medicare market seem relatively less attractive. By 1997, managed care plans were abandoning their strategies of increasing market shares—typically by adding benefits and keeping premiums low—and recognizing a need to raise premiums and generate profits or surpluses.[172] For several years, increasing Medicare enrollments had seemed an attractive way to offset some of these losses, especially by reaping the benefits from moving beneficiaries into managed care plans, many of them with high capitation rates because of local AAPCCs. Then came BBA, with its harsh payment reductions. In effect, MCOs faced a private market that was bad enough, requiring premium rises—projected for 1999, for instance, at 8.3 percent.[173] Medicare, rather than offsetting some of these losses, now made the situation worse. Furthermore, much of the attractiveness of HMOs for Medicare beneficiaries was add-ons such as medical devices, new therapies, and a pharmaceutical benefit, all of which were becoming increasingly expensive. At that time, it was pretty much received doctrine within the industry that these add-ons could not be abandoned—especially not the drug coverage—since they were the main reason Medicare beneficiaries chose HMOs. Because of considerations like these, for-profit HMOs were being advised to drop or curtail their Medicare participation; and health plans generally began reconsidering their relationship with Medicare.

For various reasons, the managed care industry had difficulty getting a favorable hearing. One was the belief that HMOs were already overpaid by Medicare—with subsidies for medical education (removed by BBA), payments based upon historically high AAPCC rates, and a favorable selection that gave them a disproportionate share of the younger and/or healthier beneficiaries.[174] Another alleged overpayment, amounting to $1.9 billion in 1996, according to the DHHS Office of the Inspector General,[175] resulted from a faulty method of calculating MCO administrative costs. Pete Stark, ranking member of the Ways and Means Health Subcommittee, pointed to additional losses from a failure to recompute the 1997 baseline and from a one-year delay of the risk adjuster.[176] Aside from "overpayment," others remained unconvinced that managed care plans had demonstrated need or made a case for increased payments. MedPAC, for instance, recommended no change in HCFA payment formulas,[177] and Interstudy, a widely respected foundation, saw indications that a three-year decline in HMO profitability might be ending, in part because of successes in controlling medical costs.[178] In addition, 1998 and 1999 were years in which both parties in Congress and the administration were advocating Patient's Bills of Rights and in which "HMO bashing" was rife, so that sympathy for managed care plans was neither wide nor deep.

By mid-1998, Medicare health plans began to complain more urgently and persistently not just about payment levels but about their regulatory burdens, especially those attending implementation of BBA 97. Health plans, which both insure and provide medical care, were already closely regulated at the state level and by HCFA. While they welcomed some elements of the Medicare+Choice regulation, other parts were regarded with fear and loathing, because of the compliance costs, data requirements, and intrusive micromanagement they would entail.

There are numerous illustrations that could be adduced (cf. Fried and Ziegler 2000) but QISMC was a particularly sore point about this time. This program set an ambitious goal of transforming traditional quality assurance methods into an advanced version of systemic quality improvement replete with performance measures and national outcome indicators. Health plans were concerned about a "one size fits all" approach, the hardships of adapting existing quality assurance methodologies, the data reporting requirements, and the aggressive implementation schedule. One HCFA operational policy letter, for instance, set a schedule of sixty days to submit a detailed work plan (suggesting one hundred pages or more for guidance) indicating how they would comply with M+C regulations—this followed by another letter requiring a plan of similar scope on compliance with QISMC (ibid.:12). Then the MCOs received notification that a goal for the first year would be seven new outcome standards. For most plans, getting QISMC in place and completing one such standard would be difficult and, for some, impossible. Seven seemed not only difficult, but gratuitously onerous—and the plans said so. HCFA officials readily conceded the point and reduced the standards to two, one of which had already been developed in the private sector.[179] This was one quickly remedied example of overreaching. But other instances—such as HCFA micro-management of plan marketing and the projected requirements for encounter data needed to develop a risk adjuster—along with the steady accumulation of operational policy letters and other HCFA directives—gave HMOs an additional disincentive for Medicare participation (Fried and Ziegler 2000:12).

Another early implementation mishap came about because of a shift in the date for filing the adjusted community rate (ACR) proposals with HCFA. Previously, that filing date had been November 15. However, BBA 97 provided for a special education and publicity program to inform beneficiaries and eligible parties about the new program and the available choices. Accordingly, Congress had moved up the submission deadline to May 1 in order to provide time for HCFA to include plan descriptions in the Medicare manual and make other materials available for consumers. The plans were unhappy about this radically compressed schedule in part because it left them little time for planning and decisions about their offerings. They complained especially because they would have to file their ACR proposals before the managed care regulation—which would affect their costs, payments, and operating environment—was scheduled to be published on June 1.[180]

The plans asked for a delay of the filing date or, if not that, to be allowed to amend their rates after inspecting the managed care regulation. HCFA officials refused, since from their perspective either alternative would have entailed major disruption at a time when they were still plagued with Y2K difficulties and working around the clock to get the Medicare+Choice program operational.

Fortunately, the filing date predicament was a one-time occurrence. In the following year, the date was moved back two months from May 1 to July 1.[181] Still, the episode was illustrative of a third major complaint of the health plans—that doing business with HCFA was often irksome and costly. Even thoughtful and sympathetic plan representatives complained about regulations and data requirements that were expensive, time-consuming, and unduly constraining.[182] Plan managers, especially those of network models and for-profit entities, found that HCFA's frequent changes of policy and payments made planning and administration difficult. The uncertainty and modifications could and did on occasion significantly affect the stock market valuations of for-profit health plans that were calculated by reports of quarterly earnings (Hurley and McCue 1998:15). As this example illustrates, the problem may have been primarily one of different cultures and operational requirements; but it was not being effectively addressed.

During the summer of 1998, both Medicare and Medicaid plans were thinking about their future prospects. The exodus of health plans began with withdrawals from Medicaid—soon to be followed by Medicare HMOs.[183] In August, Aetna U.S. Healthcare, a major participant, announced that it would stop offering Medicare HMOs in nine states and the District of Columbia.[184] That same month, Karen Ignagni, speaking for the American Association of Health Plans, warned that further defections would ensue if health plans were not given additional time and the opportunity to amend their filings. The AAHP joined with the Health Insurance Association of America to urge amendments that would address concerns expressed by managed care plans with the recently published Medicare+Choice regulation. These included—in addition to payment rates—quality standards and "over-regulation" generally, transition measures, and risk adjustment.[185] The complaints and testimonials gained additional credibility, early in November, when forty-two health plans elected to withdraw from Medicare and another fifty-three announced that they would cut back on their services.[186] Cumulatively, these decisions would affect over 400,000 beneficiaries, or about 7 percent of the total enrolled in managed care plans—a dramatic change from a few years ago when Medicare enrollment in managed care plans was growing by as much as 28 percent in a single year.

The bad news continued. With the July 1 filing of 1999, another fifty-eight plans withdrew, affecting 327,000 enrollees or about 5 percent of the Medicare HMO membership. An additional 900,000 beneficiaries faced premium increases of $20 or more per month.[187] In July 2000, HCFA's own estimates were that over 900,000 enrollees would be affected by plan withdrawals in that year. As plans were withdrawing, new ones were entering; and, in fact, Medicare managed care enrollment grew slightly in 1999, but in 2000, for the first time, total managed care enrollments were not expected to increase at all during the year.[188]

In response to the economic threats posed by BBA 97 as well as the political opportunities such numbers represented, the AAHP, joined by the HIAA, began in the fall of 1998 to organize a large-scale public relations and lobbying effort[189] that continued over the next two years, culminating in major legislative victories in both 1999 and 2000. It would be an understatement to say that the campaign was well-organized. It had everything, including a website, research and policy papers, expert testimony and stacks of impact data, elders demonstrating on the Capitol lawn accompanied by their local representatives, "grass-tops" organizations in fifty states, and articles and research papers in local newspapers and journals.[190] One theme of the campaign was that HMOs were underpaid and overregulated, but its most telling thrust was the vivid portrayals of elders dropped by their HMOs, paying higher premiums, or losing their drug coverage because of BBA 97.

The major premise of the campaign—that BBA underpayment was the prime explanation for the health plans' behavior—did not go unchallenged. The GAO and the DHSS Office of Inspector General, along with Congressman Pete Stark, continued to insist that HMOs were still overpaid, especially relative to FFS Medicare.[191] Early in 1999, MedPAC refused to recommend changes in managed care payments, despite the defections, though it did urge HCFA to phase in the risk adjuster gradually and administer some provisions more flexibly.[192] HCFA, the GAO, and others that tracked the withdrawals argued that, mostly, these were plans in low-AAPCC areas or plans that were doing poorly for other reasons, or had made "business decisions" to withdraw related more to their own experience or market conditions than to BBA payment reductions. As was often the case, the countering message lacked volume and got less attention.

The AAHP campaign has been an ongoing success. In 1999, AAHP took the lead in pressing for the Balanced Budget Refinement Act, from which managed care plans netted the largest gains, after the hospitals. Also in 1999, HCFA made several concessions, moving the filing date to July 1, appointing new advisory panels, publishing a "mini-final rule," and dropping a number of specific requirements. In 2000, a presidential election year, AAHP efforts helped to promote over a dozen bills in the House and Senate coming to the aid of Medicare HMOs. The Benefits Improvement and Protection Act of 2000 (BIPA), the second give-back, was much more helpful to HMOs than the first, with a relief package scored at $10.3 billion, rises in the national floor and the minimum rates for urban and rural HMOs, and a ten-year phase in for the risk adjuster.[193]

The gains made through the AAHP campaign could have some significant long-term effects. The increase in unity, purpose, and political clout of the managed care coalition may, for instance, moderate the populistic and some-times mindless HMO bashing that has, on occasion, substituted for serious policy. It might lead to a more sustained effort to bridge the cultural differ-ence between HCFA and the managed care industry. Health plans also showed a robust capacity, both on their own behalf and that of the plan members, to get increases in plan payments despite weighty opinion that they were not needed.

Health plans have not flocked back to Medicare despite the inducements. On the eve of taking office as the new HCFA (CMS) administrator, Tom Scully observed ruefully that the number of Medicare beneficiaries in managed care plans had declined by 1.6 million members over the last two years, and that the plan share of Medicare enrollees—projected by CBO to reach 25 percent in 2000—stood at 15 percent and was declining. By December 2001, another 536,000 seniors were expected to be dropped (Pear 2001a). Plans were also less accessible geographically, especially in rural areas, "no matter how much money we throw in them." Even fewer were offering zero premiums without copays or drug benefits, features especially attractive to seniors. All of this despite serious efforts by Congress and the administration to induce plans to stay or return. The episode leaves behind a disturbing question of whether HMOs can be a major and reliable source of cost-saving for the Medicare program.

III. MEDICAID AND SCHIP

Medicaid and the State Child Health Insurance Program (SCHIP),[194] like Medicare, were also dealt with comprehensively by BBA 97. Medicaid was recast and amended in detail, and the child health program was created new. For several reasons, the implementation phase of these two programs will be dealt with less extensively than Medicare.

One reason for a briefer treatment is that much has already been said about implementation. A central purpose of this chapter is to illustrate different aspects and problems of implementation, especially rule making, rather than covering in detail the more than three hundred identifiable tasks and projects involved in implementing BBA 97. The particular episodes and activities that relate to Medicaid and SCHIP were chosen primarily because they illustrate aspects of the implementation process in an instructive way.

Implementing the Medicaid amendments and setting up the child health program involved, in the initial phase, tasks of less scope and complexity than required for the Medicare amendments. In part that was because of differences in the programs and, therefore, in implementation itself. Medicaid and SCHIP are, in a word, more cooperative and less regulative. Rather than regulating (or instructing intermediaries) in prolix detail, for Medicaid and SCHIP, HCFA seeks to establish cooperative working relationships with the states, which, in turn, do most of the regulating. An important procedural detail, for instance, is that the Medicaid program does not first issue a proposed rule and then ask for comments. Instead, letters to state directors are sent out and proposed rules are based in part on the responses HCFA receives.[195] In other words, the Medicaid program relies considerably more upon letters and manuals both before and after the issuance of a rule—so that rule making as such plays less of a role, is less technical, and is generally less legalistic.

Most of the major implementation projects for Medicaid either involved traditional rule making of a nontechnical sort or were shared with Medicare. For Medicaid, the biggest elements were the managed care regulation, the PACE program, fraud and abuse, and protections for the disabled.[196] In addition, there was a host of minor regulations and payment amendments dealing with eligibility, enrollment, and beneficiary protections. PACE and fraud and abuse were shared concerns with Medicare, which carried much of the regulation writing responsibility for those projects. The Medicaid managed care regulation was in a category by itself; but most of the other and smaller amendments involved regulation writing of a fairly routine sort. SCHIP required extensive program design, outreach and consultation, the development of a model state plan, and a monitoring device. Neither for Medicaid nor for SCHIP was there extensive technical "development" of the kind required for Medicare programs such as the outpatient prospective payment systems or the "health fair" and consumer information program.

Because there was a relatively small amount of technical development required, the Medicaid and SCHIP task forces suffered little of the Y2K aggravation that so bedeviled Medicare. For Medicaid the biggest problem was that the states and Medicaid managed care providers needed to achieve Y2K compliance in order to continue participating in the program; and for that HCFA had to "jawbone" laggards to the very end of 1999. But needing little technical development, the Medicaid and CHIP task forces had no major Y2K problems themselves—which spared them one major hardship.

None of these introductory comments are intended to make light of the efforts and accomplishments of the Medicaid and SCHIP task forces—only to put in context the particular examples of implementation activities selected. Like their colleagues in the Medicare program, these people worked evenings and weekends for long months. They took pride in doing the best they could under the circumstances—in meeting the deadlines and faithfully interpreting their mandates. In part, these examples of implementation—establishing SCHIP and the Medicaid managed care regulation—are chosen because they illustrate political appointees and civil servants operating with considerable discretion, in situations requiring imaginative and yet responsible interpretations of their mandates.

Establishing the State Children's Health Insurance Program

As background to the legislative implementation and initial establishment of SCHIP it is important to recall some history. Child health might seem a relatively uncontroversial, nonpartisan issue. In fact, it revived a number of sharp differences over block grants and entitlements, added a new issue of increased access to health care for adults as well as children, provided some easy money, and raised the political stakes for the administration and both parties in Congress. There was the deceptive quiet of a storm center about this particular initiative.

The child health initiative began in a significant way with a Kennedy-Kerry proposal (see p. 214) in 1996 to expand the Maternal and Child Health Block Grant to cover uninsured children. This initiative failed, but in 1997, the Kassebaum-Kennedy bill (HIPAA) did pass—important as a bipartisan effort to increase access to health care for employed workers. Early in 1997, President Clinton's budget message strongly supported efforts to increase insurance coverage for children and uninsured workers. Building upon this initiative, another bipartisan proposal, the Hatch-Kennedy bill, would have used money from an increased tobacco tax to provide insurance for children in low-income families or to support coverage provided by employers. After that, congressional partisans on both sides weighed in with health care liberals generally advocating Medicaid expansion and conservatives pushing for a block grant.

As noted earlier, BBA 97 combined both approaches, institutionalizing the conflict and keeping the political stakes still fairly high. For HCFA officials confronted with implementing the SCHIP legislation, there were several important priorities. One was to maintain a steady and true course roughly midway between Medicaid and a block grant. At the same time, SCHIP had strong presidential backing and historic rhetoric about insuring five million children. The administration was also pushing for stronger quality standards and patient protections for both Medicare and Medicaid. On the other side, there was a Republican Congress, especially the House Commerce and the Senate Finance committees, with their own views about the statute, and fifty states, the District of Columbia, and the Territories, that needed to be sold on the merits of these new options. There was also was a big, new appropriation of $24 billion funded by tobacco taxes, a lowered CBO baseline, and an already promised appropriation—money that seemed to be burning holes in the pockets of legislators and the administrative officials and that cried out for programmatic employment. For HCFA and DHHS it was important to move carefully but also to implement the program quickly and effectively.

Two specifics of the legislation—expressing congressional exuberance about SCHIP—were especially important in determining how HCFA officials would approach the establishment of this new program. One was the unexpectedly large authorization of $24 billion over five years. As recalled by Judy Moore, then deputy director, HCFA officials had been working with $4 billion as a figure when $24 billion unexpectedly came through, much of it from a last-minute decision by the conference committee. That action changed the nature of the task from one of incremental amendments, largely to existing programs, to the creation of whole new structures.[197] In addition, SCHIP had to begin almost immediately. On August 5, 1997, the BBA became law. It provided SCHIP funds beginning in October of that year—less than two months away. That meant HCFA officials would have to begin reading and approving state plans even as they were developing policy and structuring the program.[198] Generally, it is not regarded as prudent to design an airplane while in flight; but that, metaphorically, was what they had to do.

A first step, much as with the development of the managed care "mega-reg," was to organize a steering committee. This committee was chaired by Debbie Chang, from the HCFA Office of Legislation, and by Earl Fox, director of the Health Resources and Services Administration. HRSA was included because of its jurisdiction over the Title IV Maternal and Child Health Block Grant. The "HHS CHIP Steering Committee" as it was officially known, was huge, with a hundred members representing over forty organizations within DHHS. The steering committee met twice a week, often for hours at a time, over the next year and a half.[199] It was highly successful in setting priorities, resolving policy differences, getting people to take ownership of particular tasks, and monitoring progress.[200]

Much of the success of the steering committee should be credited to the strategy guiding its organization. Two key elements were inclusiveness of representation and bringing together program development and administrative clearance. Accordingly, the steering committee included program chiefs or their deputies from every significantly involved program or staff agency within DHHS and representatives from OMB, the Department of Justice, and the White House. As the steering committee had to combine both planning and development, inclusiveness helped to resolve issues as they emerged, since the affected parties were there or represented by deputies and could often reach agreement quickly. With representatives from the key staff agencies, clearance issues could be largely settled in advance, drastically reducing the time needed to develop and gain approval for final drafts.[201]

Almost immediately, state plans began trickling in, without as yet program guidelines in existence to serve as criteria for approval. As a result, much of the substantive policy was developed like case law, from ad hoc approvals. Each state plan had, within HCFA, a point person in charge and a review team with representatives from the steering committee, OMB, and the White House. From reviewing these state plans, wider policy questions and additional task priorities would emerge, to be dealt with as the occasion demanded—in some instances, through forming a small task force or working party and getting someone to take ownership of the project; or when in disagreement by developing alternatives with policy papers and deciding upon one of the options. Failing that, there was a final appeal to Kevin Thurm, the DHSS chief of staff. By mutual agreement, issues once settled were not reopened except under exceptional circumstances.[202]

The steering committee recast its emerging policies, with comment, into a series of "Questions and Answers," and made these available in print and on the internet for the guidance of regional and state officials, providers, and other interested parties.[203] Published in installments, the list eventually grew to one hundred questions and answers,[204] dealing comprehensively and in minute detail with aspects of the program. As they learned more about program and issues through this iterative process, the members of the committee formulated policy guidelines and communicated them to the states in "Dear State Director" letters, three of which were of major scope.[205] Using "Questions and Answers," members of the steering committee collaborated with the National Academy for State Health Policy to develop a model template for SCHIP state plans.[206] Working from these materials, in collaboration with the regulation writers in Baltimore, a small task force developed most of the proposed regulation. As a rather elegant addition, HCFA officials, in cooperation with a number of states and the National Association of State Health Plans, created a monitoring tool, which could be adopted by states, on a voluntary basis, if they chose to do so.[207]

As the steering committee progressed in its work, other important activities were going forward. Task forces were formed to work on early guidelines; to develop recommendations on waiver policy, on "crowd out," cost sharing, and the 10 percent limit on non-health-related expenditures; and to collaborate in the development of a monitoring instrument.[208] Data collection, especially getting figures on eligibility and enrollment, was a difficult but essential task. HCFA regional offices had to be instructed and readied for their role in assisting and monitoring the development of the new SCHIP state agencies.[209] Communication with and outreach to the states was a major, ongoing activity: answering questions from more than fifty jurisdictions; preparing letters, explanatory material, and action kits; and briefings and conferences with state officials.[210]

The steering committee approach was especially useful for working with the states. State SCHIP officials knew the composition of their HCFA review teams and were in frequent communication with them. HCFA also allowed states to file "placeholder" state plans[211] and would help them to achieve full approval. For some technically difficult or controversial issues—such as enrollment procedures, maintenance of effort, or crowding out—close involvement with individual state plans helped identify some unacceptable practices and to appreciate the nicety required to achieve acceptable solutions.[212]

As intended, the steering committee strategy saved a significant amount of time. First, this approach proved to be a successful technique for resolving differences, especially when backed with the strong presumption that issues once decided were taken as settled. In addition, most of the difficult questions of design and procedure were dealt with along the way, in the process of reviewing state plans and developing policy guidelines. As a result, the regulation was largely a codification of this experience, and, as several HCFA officials said, almost "wrote itself." The preclearance process also largely obviated one of the most time-consuming procedures of all in the development of regulations. The steering committee was able to finish its work in just over a year with a full "roll-out" and OMB clearance. The proposed rule was published on November 9, 1998, only fourteen months after the passage of BBA 97.

It could be argued that the steering committee's methods contributed significantly to the success of the program—in expediting approvals, quickly sending out letters and policy guidelines, and getting the program fully operational. The major complaint with SCHIP implementation has been the numbers enrolled—considerably short of the five million goal set by the president. However, five million was mostly campaign rhetoric and with two million enrolled in the first two years of full operation, SCHIP did well by CBO's more realistic projection (Moore 2000). Program officials have also been pleased with the energetic and innovative response of many of the states. It would be hard to estimate how much the pragmatic, case-sensitive approach of the steering committee contributed to that outcome, but it certainly did not hurt.

The Medicaid Managed Care Regulation

The Medicaid amendments in BBA 97 were strong and clear in their underlying philosophy, which was to balance flexibility for the states with protections for Medicaid beneficiaries, but the legislation provided little guidance in deciding how to weight flexibility as against beneficiary protections, especially for the disabled and other dual eligibles. House and Senate versions had disagreed on that particular topic, with the Senate Finance Committee coming down more strongly for beneficiary protection and House Commerce for flexibility. Among the Medicaid constituency and within HCFA itself there were divisions over how flexible or protective to be in writing the regulation. The White House also had more than a routine interest in this issue because of its stand on patients' rights and Executive Order 13040, which mandated the Consumer Bill of Rights and Responsibilities for federal health agencies.[213]

The managed care regulation was embroiled in this conflict of values and objectives. A major reason states wanted more flexibility was to have greater freedom to utilize and to negotiate terms with managed care plans. Freedom would be increased by no longer requiring waivers for MCOs and by allowing states to make enrollment in them a condition of receiving benefits. Other concessions to managed care plans abolished the 75/25 restriction on Medicaid dominant plans and allowed greater freedom to impose cost-sharing requirements. At the same time, it was understood by both political parties in Congress that—in addition to existing managed care regulations—special attention would be given to quality improvement and to protections for vulnerable populations. But how far should this protective philosophy go, and how should it be applied? Should states with waivers continue as before? Should QISMC standards be pushed for Medicaid as well as for Medicare? How should the at-risk populations be defined, identified, and protected? What provisions of the Quality Commission's "bill of rights" should be included? And what provisions should be made for enforcement, for instance, with respect to providers contracting with the states?

An additional complexity was added by past history, in particular, the way in which legislation and implementation interact in the Medicaid program. Medicaid legislation is complex, dealing with the different needs of fifty states, the territories, and special populations as these needs have been historically addressed with layer upon layer of legislative amendments and administrative regulations, accumulated over thirty-five years. A common practice in developing legislation was for HCFA staff to prenegotiate textual language with congressional subcommittees so that the legislation being drafted would make appropriate allowance for the complexities of the situation being addressed.[214] Legislation would build upon existing regulations and would, in effect, endorse and provide legal foundations for administrative practices, though often without making clear the extent of that endorsement. Then would come more legislation, such as the BBA 97, which added new provisions in areas never previously addressed by the department, with little or no guidance about what to do when old practices and new legislation were in conflict or when, between them, they did not cover the situation for which a regulation was being written (Rosenbaum and Darnall 1998:12).

Unlike Medicare, the Medicaid program is, of course, a federal-state program, a difference that substitutes one kind of complexity for another. Medicare regulations have to be written with an eye especially to their immediate impact upon providers, the health care industry, and the beneficiaries or "consumers" of the services. For Medicaid, the regulations are written, in the first place, for the state agencies, each with its own local history and immediate problems, and at a second remove, they address the contracts between these agencies and the providers, leaving up to the states themselves the details of regulation. The ultimate federal relation either to providers or Medicaid recipients is mediated and remote. As a consequence, Medicaid regulations require a special kind of judgment about how much to say and how specific to be in dealing with a particular situation. Institutional memory, local experience, and a trained intuition play an important part in this kind of activity.

Work on the managed care regulation was similar to SCHIP in scope of effort and in some of the activities involved. It did not, however, require the creation of a whole new program; nor was there the same imperative for a quick start. On the other hand, it was fully as difficult. The central task was to put together a major regulation, smaller in scope but similar to the Medicare mega-reg, that would deal effectively with a relatively new regulative domain, be adapted to the layered complexities of the Medicaid program, meet legal constraints, both clear and unclear, and be acceptable to the Congress, the states, and the Medicaid constituency.

Like SCHIP, those working on the managed care regulation had their own steering committee. This steering committee had a previous incarnation, having been used in developing regulations for welfare reform. In that capacity, it had been successful enough to commend itself as a model, and was adapted both for the managed care regulation and for SCHIP. The chair was Judy Moore, then director of the Medicaid Bureau. Her deputy for this assignment was David Cade, an attorney with a depth of experience in health care, including Medicaid and Medicare. As with SCHIP, this steering committee had departmentwide representation, following a similar strategy of inclusive consultation and administrative preclearance. Since its task was narrower in scope, this steering committee was somewhat smaller; but it worked the same long hours and followed similar procedures.

In contrast to SCHIP, the managed care regulation was more like a traditional rule. As state plans and requests for waivers were submitted to the committee, some would be quickly approved, but not with the intention of using them to develop the content of the regulation. For that, the steering committee broke the statute into a list of provisions. For each one, a staff person would take ownership and work with a task force on the particular assignment. For controversial issues policy papers were developed with a number of options. These were then discussed by the steering committee and if they could agree, approval was sought from Nancy-Ann deParle. Failing agreement, an appeal could be taken to Kevin Thurm, the HHS chief of staff. Upon approval, a "Dear Director" letter was sent to the states for comment.

One of the earliest issues to arise was also one of the most important: what to do about waivers, either existing ones or new requests? BBA 97 exempted existing Section 1115 and 1915 demonstration waivers from the new standards. Since half of the states were operating under one kind of waiver or another, to take such a blanket exemption at face value would have rendered the new beneficiary protections—the standards and exclusions—without much effect within those states. The larger purpose of the legislation, though, was to protect beneficiaries under a managed care regime, even though no language in the statute provided explicit guidance. Faced with this situation, the steering committee took a common sense approach and applied a lawyerlike distinction between general and specific preemption. In simpler terms, *existing* waivers would not be exempted generally, but where the terms of the waiver set forth a specific exemption that conflicted with one of the new standards—for instance, requiring managed care enrollment where only one plan existed—that provision could be exempted until the date for the waiver renewal came around, at which point all BBA restrictions would apply. *New or amended* Section 1115 waivers would be permitted only if the state agency could demonstrate that the beneficiary protections and quality standards provided for the proposed demonstration would equal or exceed the BBA requirements (ibid.:14, 15).

The waiver dilemma was one of those situations where there seemed to be no discernable congressional intent. As previously noted, the House Commerce Committee was probably on one side and Senate Finance on the other. Even though the HCFA interpretation was common sense and seemed implicit in the statute, it is difficult to say how or where that interpretation was to be found. Moreover, the distinction was not clean or simple in its application, for with it came perplexities over how to interpret a "specific" waiver, especially as to how much "understood" agency policy it included or excluded.[215] Deciding what was exempted still took a lot of sorting and judgment and especially close work with legal counsel. The decision itself, though, would seem to be one of those instances where policy had to be uppermost or, as a judge might say, where law could not be entirely "found," with some of it needing to be "made."

A similar kind of dilemma arose with the Consumer Bill of Rights and Responsibilities, which the president had mandated for federal health agencies, including Medicare and Medicaid. The statute itself was influenced by an anti-HMO patients' bill of rights philosophy and contained a number of similar provisions, but not the same ones nor using the same terminology. For the steering committee, there was a clear presidential mandate, and there was some sentiment that it was fair game to get back through an executive order part of what had been lost in the legislative process. There was also a belief that the law was the law, and a concern about the hammering that HCFA might get from Congress if their interpretations were too creative.

The steering committee's approach to the bill of rights acknowledged the realities of divided government in a way that was both principled and prudent. In general, they sought to implement the executive order fully, even though at times it was not their preferred option and they knew that the states would not like it. On some points, for instance emergency medical care, the statute and the Consumer Bill of Rights and Responsibilities said much the same thing. Where the statute said nothing, the steering committee did not take the view that silence was license. They sought to "find support" in related provisions or "ground themselves" in the statute, and, failing that, would omit the provision. In this respect, their position was not unlike that of a judge in an administrative law case deciding whether there was "law to apply." It was an approach that successfully rationalized the inclusion of a large part of the consumer bill of rights and would be reasonable and defensible if caught between the president and the Congress. Little objection was raised either by the Congress or the administration. However, Judy Moore reported that she was "booed" at a meeting of state Medicaid managers in June 1998—the only similar occasion being when HCFA reported on implementation of the Boren Amendment repeal.[216]

Some of the most important beneficiary protections occasioned relatively little work for the steering committee. The information requirements and the enrollment and disenrollment guarantees, for instance, were delineated in the statute in enough detail that developing regulatory text and preamble for these was comparatively straightforward. The quality standards could have been an enormous undertaking, but were not because of the years spent working on QARI with the state Medicaid agencies.

An issue that, in retrospect, turned out to be important was the general treatment of the quality standards: how much emphasis they should receive, and whether the Medicaid standards should be nudged closer in philosophy and requirements to the Medicare QISMC standards. The statute said little about the general philosophy that should inform Section 4705. But it assigned special importance to quality, requiring each state to adopt a broad quality assessment and improvement strategy and including appropriateness of care, access standards, grievance procedures, and marketing and information under the general rubric of "quality assurance standards." Also, QARI and QISMC had developed together and shared much of the same basic philosophy and approach. Some assimilation of the two would be relatively easy and in keeping with the a broadly shared goal of bringing Medicaid closer to Medicaid and more into the mainstream of American medicine. Yet, the statute did not authorize this; and QISMC standards were a reach, even for Medicare HMOs.

The approach taken by the steering committee seemed reasonable in general and prudent under the circumstances. The preamble text dealing with quality contained an introductory "sermon" on the importance of QISMC, data collection, and the quality movement in general. This step signaled that HCFA might be heading that way in the future, but the actual prescriptions for the quality "strategy" stopped short, largely implementing the approach contained in the House bill, which stressed the quality improvement process and projects rather than uniform standards and outcome measures.

This moderation of the steering committee with respect to QISMC standards did not mean that quality assessment and improvement as a strategy was any less central. In fact, restraint with respect to standard setting was matched by an increased commitment to quality as a pragmatic and inclusive strategy. A sentence from the proposed regulation captures the thought underlying this approach:

> We believe that the Quality Assurance and Performance Improvement strategy developed by each State agency should be used as a tool to assure that contracts with MCO's are effective in delivering quality health care services.[217]

The open character of the phrase "used as a tool to assure" is worthy of note, especially with respect to how broad and aggressive the strategy should be.

One way in which this commitment was expressed was to come down hard on the concept of "access" and make it a vehicle for extending quality care more broadly to categories and individuals.[218] Access to care included, for instance, assuring services for children, pregnant women, and persons with special needs or complex and difficult conditions. Access covered the information beneficiaries needed to make initial plan selections—supplied as need be in "specified prevalent languages"—and to participate in medical decisions and have their complaints addressed, with the aid of translators, sign language, or Braille interpretations. Access meant not just available staff, but state certification of credentials and appropriate staffing ratios. It included an initial assessment of health status within ninety days of enrollment, and shorter periods for pregnant women and people with "complex or serious conditions." It incorporated provisions from the Consumers' Bill of Rights and Responsibilities, such as access to specialists in women's medicine, emergency medicine and poststabilization care, and respect for the privacy and dignity of beneficiaries.

The other major emphasis of this overall quality strategy was to require that state agencies themselves or through their provider contracts assure that HMOs or other "managed care entities" fulfill their obligations—contractual and otherwise—to provide quality care. In this respect, the proposed rule was broadly prescriptive in laying out, often in detail, what state plans must do with respect to structural standards and marketing and enrollment; what provider contracts should contain; and how plan performance would be monitored, evaluated, and corrected. In addition, state plans had to include a strategy for employing intermediate sanctions and civil monetary penalties, conferred by Congress in BBA 97 to help states discipline the Medicaid health plans.

The regulatory strategy underlying the proposed rule seemed both soundly conceived and well executed. The conflation of quality and access provided a

persuasive rationale for the inclusion of a number of needed protections for
Medicaid beneficiaries. It is not difficult to make a case that each of these
applications of the concept of access, especially when tied to quality, addresses
the condition and needs of Medicaid recipients. The close association of quality and access in the statute supports this interpretation. Moreover, with
mandatory enrollment in HMOs permissible without a waiver, quality assurance and beneficiary protection are much more important. It is arguable,
though, that an approach developed in the House bill was adapted in a way
that favored Senate and administration priorities and that could seem like
micromanagement by proxy to many states. Mentors can say too much, even
though they may be right.

Knotty and legally difficult questions arose in deciding when and how
these standards would apply to some providers. For instance, rural managed
care plans were treated differently. There were new statutory definitions of
"managed care entity" and "primary care case manager." The "prepaid health
plan" did not appear in the legislation, but had been a creation, an artifact of
past regulations, that was well established as a program entity and needed to
be accommodated. Getting definitions that worked and specifying how far
enrollment protections, solvency requirements, nondiscrimination rules and
provider protections, and access and quality standards applied to these entities required a considerable amount of work as well as overall programmatic
knowledge and specialized legal expertise

A tough individual issue was who should be exempt from state mandatory
enrollment in managed care plans. Protections for the handicapped, dual eligibles, and "special needs" children against being "dumped" into Medicaid
HMOs or other "managed care entities" had been important in the committee deliberations and the legislation, and BBA 97 specified clearly under several titles that children could qualify for this exemption, but without defining
"special needs." That left the definition up to HCFA.

"Children with special needs" (under Title V) was a term well established
in state child health programs, but states varied in their interpretations. With
this important statutory language left open, advocates for children with cere-
bral palsy, Downs syndrome, and a variety of other special conditions lobbied
HCFA intensely for broad interpretations. HCFA struggled with the problem,
but definitions in such matters are hard, tending either to include or to
exclude too much. There was the related issue of the assurances to require
from states to protect these beneficiaries from being improperly enrolled in
managed care plans. Depending on the regulatory text, the provision could be
quite onerous, requiring states to identify such individuals, keep separate
records, and track the cases through the system.[219] One concern of the steering committee was that states might be discouraged from trying useful experiments with managed care because of this kind of administrative burden.
Moreover, if HCFA could not define the concept, there might be both practical and legal problems with regulating the relevant behavior.

The steering committee resolved this particular issue by leaving the determination up to the states, specifying that eligibility for Title V children could
be "defined by the state in terms of either program participation or special
health care needs."[220] In other words, delegate the matter, but with a proviso
that the treatment of such children under a waiver would be judged according to "a growing body of State experience and best practices." As explained
by Moore, on issues of this sort, a primary need is to get terminology that will
work and still allow states room to experiment. Specific corrective action can
be taken *ex post,* as needed, through the Medicaid manual, letters to directors,
or review of state plans.

In addition to approving and reviewing state plans, HCFA exercises some
oversight of the contracts between states and the providers as a way to monitor service and compliance with state plans and federal requirements. HCFA
also sets forth provisions that such contracts must contain: for instance, spec-
ification of benefits and details of coverage and authorization of services; the
actuarial basis for premiums; and methods the plan will use to assure that
marketing plans and materials "do not mislead, confuse, or defraud the recipients or the state agency."[221]

An important contract requirement was the assurance of adequate capacity
and services. This assurance required documentation showing that the health
plan offered an appropriate range of services including access to preventive
services, primary care, and specialties and a provider network adequate in
"number, mix, and geographic distribution" to meet the needs of the
enrollees. Plans also had to demonstrate that they could meet state standards
for urgent care.

Since this requirement put the burden on plans to show adequacy, it would
give states powerful leverage to exclude marginal providers or bargain for concessions. It would also provide HCFA with an effective and nonintrusive
method to monitor the adequacy of services. At the same time, members of
the steering committee had misgivings, with this and similar requirements,
about problems of notice and due process and other legal consequences of
making many private activities into public functions or state activity. Nor did
they think that HCFA should be specifying services and staffing ratios for
physicians and other personnel. Aside from the objectionable measure of
micromanagement involved, HCFA itself lacked the staff to enforce such a
requirement.[222]

The path ultimately taken was to require health plans, every two years, to
forward their documentation both to the state agency and to HCFA. The
states would certify plans as having met the requirement, but the materials
would also be available for HCFA to review. New documentation would be
required whenever a plan renewed or entered into a new contract or the state
determined that there has been a significant change in the delivery system or
the plan enrollees (Rosenbaum and Darnall 1998:35). This resolution would
have the states deal with the adequacy issue in the first instance and allow

HCFA to intervene but not require the agency's involvement. There would still be opportunities to flag a serious problem.

This example of assuring capacity illustrates one of the generic problems of indirect regulation that frequently confronted the steering committee. The 1997 Medicaid amendments were both comprehensive and ameliorative. Congress wanted Medicaid managed care improved as well as regulated and wrote in substantial and detailed sections on increased beneficiary protection, quality assurance standards, and fraud and abuse. Congress and the states were also concerned about oppressive mandates and micromanagement. For the steering committee, the challenge was to craft a provision that would strike an appropriate balance between beneficiary protection and state flexibility, enable and motivate the states to control and improve the behavior of MCOs, and allow HCFA to monitor results with some capacity to encourage compliance.

The same example also illustrates the difficulty of enforcing compliance with federal mandates. HCFA (CMS) can delay or condition approval of state plans or waivers. It can query provider contracts. In extreme cases, it has the legal authority to exclude plans, terminate contracts, withhold payments, take over the management of plans, and/or impose civil monetary penalties. However, the political clout of governors and the congressional state delegations and the importance of good working relations with state agencies and Medicaid directors make these sanctions, practically speaking, almost worthless. On a few occasions, HCFA has taken over the management of an MCO. According to the GAO, HCFA has never withheld payments from a Medicaid MCO.[223] Serious and continued misbehavior has generally been dealt by the courts or Congress rather than administratively.

One way in which Congress sought to strengthen enforcement was by extending to Medicaid and requiring the states to implement a number of intermediate sanctions of the sort already legislated for Medicare.[224] The proposed regulation required state plans to include provisions for applying these new sanctions, adding some particulars of administrative process. In the light of past history, it will be interesting to see what the states do with these new powers.

Developing the proposal for a grievance system was an exercise that called for creative efforts, putting the steering committee in peril of doing too little or of doing too much. The statute provided only that MCOs had to establish "an internal grievance procedure"—nothing was said about a "grievance *system*" or an external review.[225] Treated in a minimalist way, the statutory requirement would have accomplished very little. Moreover, both thought and practice had moved beyond this point: for instance, with respect to appeals from Medicaid MCO decisions, review by external bodies, and the right to a "fair hearing." On the other hand, to create a fully developed grievance system would require building a large edifice on a small foundation with the use of some dubious materials.

According to the preamble, the grievance system must include, at a minimum, (1) a designated office within the MCO for inquiries, (2) "two tracks for MCO review (the complaint process and the grievance process)," and (3) access to the state fair hearing system.[226]

A strategically important step, in developing the regulation, was to make a distinction was between a "complaint" and a "grievance." The statute makes no such distinction, using only the term "grievance," but both terms had been adopted by many states, supported in the "Model Grievance Act" of the National Association of Insurance Commissioners, and seemed a practical necessity given the realities to which it applied. A complaint, according to the regulation, dealt with "any aspect of an MCO's or provider's operations" and could be either oral or written. A grievance was a written communication "explicitly addressing dissatisfaction with(the availability, delivery, or quality, payment, treatment, or reimbursement of claims for services, or issues unresolved through the complaint process."[227] Grievances, as illustrated by the definition, dealt with medical care, quality, and payment—involving weighty and technical matters of legal and professional obligation, evidence and proof, for which the formal requisites of notice and hearing and a courtlike adjudication would be appropriate.

This distinction was strategically important in several ways. It supported an argument for a more structured and formalized grievance system than required by the statute. It tied in with quality improvement and sanctions, especially by identifying availability, delivery, and quality of care as actionable. MCOs were also required to maintain a log of complaints and grievances and their disposition that would be subject to inspection (within some limits) by state agencies, so that there was ongoing oversight. The distinction also established an important link to the state "fair hearing" requirement.

The requirement of a fair hearing was critically important for the managed care regulation. For Medicare+Choice, the statute provided, in detail, for appeals from MCO coverage decisions to an "outside entity" and for a hearing before "the Secretary." The Medicaid legislation made no provision for an external appeal, but there was a long history of the fair hearing requirement originally established for AFDC in the Social Security Act of 1935, extended to Medicaid in 1965, and given constitutional status by the Supreme Court in 1970.[228] There was no question about a Medicaid right to an external appeal. The question was whether and how it could be applied to Medicaid MCOs.[229]

This matter was not without difficulty. Historically, the fair hearing had been used for public agency denials of eligibility and benefits in welfare and disability. cases. Within the states, courts and legislatures had taken some small and halting steps, but were slow to extend this right to prospective acts of private agencies (HMOs) and their judgmental decisions about medical care. Nevertheless, the fair hearing was a legally important doctrine. HCFA had been receptive to Medicaid and MCO appeals. A number of states were moving this way—though some were not. Moreover, Medicare+Choice included elaborate statutory provisions for appeals with a hearing "before the Secretary," and judicial review of final decisions.[230] From these sources, the steering committee found support for an external appeal for Medicaid MCO grievances.[231]

In addition to providing "multiple avenues of recourse"[232] the grievance system was intended to be one that MCO enrollees could use effectively. These beneficiaries often have special problems: unable to read or speak English, suffering from mental disabilities, ignorant of their rights and how to proceed, severely ill and unable to secure medical care while waiting for a resolution. On this account, the regulation was both prescriptive and sensitive to beneficiary needs: directing MCOs to make available user-friendly materials and staff an office to help beneficiaries file complaints or grievances; setting forth elaborate notice requirements that included information about beneficiary rights and how to proceed; requiring expedited procedures for protection of beneficiary rights and continuation of benefits during grievance or fair hearing appeals.

The grievance system provision, which was elaborate and perhaps too prescriptive, illustrates a subtle aspect of Medicaid implementation. Old hands in Congress and the Medicaid administration understand the importance of trying to accommodate fifty states and leave "wiggle room" for state agencies to administer their programs at the same time that they defend federal priorities. One of their most important contributions is to develop accommodations between legislative text, administrative priorities, and the needs and desires of the states. Yet, when the statute says only "internal grievance procedure" without more, it opens the way for particular enthusiasms, such as patients' rights or quality improvement. It can also leave those who seek to develop a more balanced version without the statutory authority with which to ward off these or other importunings.

The actual writing of the regulation—getting from the option papers and policy decisions to the regulatory texts—was a hard task for the steering committee.[233] Medicaid specialists knew their own program; and they had the benefit of experienced and specialized legal counsel. But as Gertrude Stein once said, "Remarks are not literature." Knowing what they wanted to say, they still struggled with the task of saying it right and producing a coherent whole. Within HCFA, most of the preamble and text writers were occupied with Medicare. Those regulation writers detailed to Medicaid had experience primarily with Medicare, not Medicaid. Institutional memory and program expertise substituted in some measure for experience in writing regulations, but it was a difficult phase.

The managed care regulation was completed within its deadline. There was even time for a comprehensive roll out, with Hill briefings, meetings with providers, and conference calls with Medicaid state directors. The proposed

385-page regulation was published in the *Federal Register* on September 29, 1998. The final regulation was withdrawn in January 2001 at the request of the Bush administration and never went into force.

Medicaid and the Bush Administration: First Year.   Medicaid did not figure significantly in the presidential election campaign of 2000; and the Bush administration did not take office with a particular Medicaid agenda.

The new president, as governor of Texas, had not been a strong supporter of Medicaid. Furthermore, he appointed Wisconsin governor Tommy Thompson—a leader in the attempt to block-grant Medicaid in 1995—as his secretary of DHHS. Historic background and some of the early developments in the new administration, though not conclusive, may be significant as a portent of the future and as a test of the bipartisan consensus on Medicaid that was reached in 1997.

Two early developments will be discussed briefly: (1) the suspension and replacement of the Medicaid managed care final rule, and (2) the National Governors' Association proposal, early in 2001, to restructure Medicaid, together with the Health Insurance Flexibility and Accountability (HIFA) demonstration initiative, a response by the Bush administration to the governors' proposal. These episodes illustrate both contingent nature of the Medicaid bipartisan compromise in 1997 as well as some of its latent staying power.

The Medicaid managed care rule.   One of the first acts of the Bush administration on January 20, within hours of the inauguration, was to delay any final rules not then in effect—which included the managed care regulation. After review by OMB, the effective date of the regulation was moved from April 19 to June 18, a delay of sixty days.[236] At the end of this period, the date was again moved, this time to August 17.

During these months, quite a bit of controversy was stirred up over the regulation. It was denounced by the National Governors' Association, which called for review of this, other regulations, and Medicaid directors' letters that "undermine state flexibility." In his address to the NGA February meeting in Washington, D.C., Secretary Thompson told the governors that he would "work with them" to make DHHS more responsive to states and assured them that they had "a friend in the White House."[237] At the request of the Bush administration, the Medicaid directors sent a fourteen-page letter, criticizing almost every aspect of the regulation, but singling out especially the quality provisions and the grievance procedures as "too detailed and prescriptive" and "over the top."[238] In July and August, an NGA campaign for a major restructuring of Medicaid was going forward, with support form the administration. Because of Senator Jeffords's defection, Republicans no longer controlled the Senate; but this loss increased the incentive for the new administration to gain what it could while it could by administrative action. In this kind of political environment, supporters of the managed care regulation waited with apprehension, afraid of what this political agenda might produce and expecting, at the least, that the regulation would be drastically modified.

On August 17, as the third sixty-day postponement expired, CMS published an interim final rule with comment that delayed the effective date for the regulation one year, until August 16, 2002. Then, on August 20, a new proposed regulation was published, modifying the January final rule. This procedure raised some eyebrows, since interim final rules are usually authorized by Congress when there is an emergency or, at least, an urgent need for haste. But the sense of it, in this situation, was that it extended consideration of the managed care rule for a year, but only for that period, to allow a fuller consideration of the comments and the regulation. Some officials, experienced with rule making, said at the time that they doubted that a year would be enough.

The amended rule of August 20 was surprisingly moderate, considering the partisan atmosphere of the time. Mostly, it followed the preamble and text of the earlier final rule. To a considerable extent, it was the same sermon, but with modified rhetoric. It took out or tempered references to the Consumer Bill of Rights and Responsibilities, QISMC, and taking Medicare as the model.[239] It eased the pinch for the states and providers, extending time periods, reducing data requirements, leaving more details to states, using words like "adequate," and emphasizing collaborative approaches. It changed the quality requirements to make them less like Medicare and the grievance system to make it more like Medicare.[240] Generally, as the earlier final rule of January 18 seemed to tilt moderately toward beneficiary protectiveness, so the proposed amendments of August 20 moved back, moderately, toward provider protectiveness and state flexibility.

What the future may hold is another matter. CMS lacked time to consider a fundamental revision of the final rule; and the proposed regulation of August 20 may be no more than a "placeholder," dealing with minor, relatively uncontroversial issues and providing a delay for more drastic amendments to be considered. However, HCFA final rules often track proposed ones closely, differing incrementally rather than in basic principle. Creating preambles and regulations is a craft—taking time and skill, requiring the reconciliation of differing views, and the production of a consistent and compelling text. Of course, major amendments can be made by changing a definition, adding a modifier, or "transposing a 'not.'" Like a statute, though, a regulation, or an amendment, faces a critical "audience" of stakeholders and the courts, adept at finding loopholes, inconsistencies, weak arguments, or policy glitches.[241] With such thoughts in mind, comparing the "final final" rule with the "final" rule should be an instructive exercise, to see what evidences there may be, if any, of constraints the rulemaking process imposes upon political agendas and stakeholder claims.

The governors' proposal and HIFA.   Rising Medicaid costs and other economic factors help explain this emergence of a major restructuring proposal so soon after BBA 97. In a word, states were being financially squeezed or, if not presently in distress, saw trouble ahead. Medicaid costs have usually grown faster than state per capita incomes or tax revenues; and this disparity seemed to be increasing even as states were losing some of their capacity to close the gap (Holahan 2001:17–18). Rising prescription drug costs, growing numbers of elderly and disabled, and federal mandates (ibid.) increased costs. States had meanwhile lost DSH money and seen lucrative loopholes closed. Savings from managed care declined. Raising taxes was hard because of such factors as interstate competition, a slowing economy, and a regressive tax base. These were powerful and relentless realities that tended to upset earlier deals and make a strong case for more money or fewer constraints—maybe both.

The plan reflected the agendas of two groups within the NGA. One of these, represented by the Democratic co-chair, Howard Dean of Vermont, wanted more money and greater flexibility to enroll the uninsured. The other, led by the Republican co-chair, Donald Sundquist of Tennessee, wanted more freedom to alter benefits and to reduce the existing Medicaid requirements. In effect, both groups wanted more money and more freedom.

The prescription was comparatively simple: add some money and alter the structure and state obligations to make the Medicaid program more like SCHIP. Three broad categories would be established. In Category I would be current "mandatory" populations—those required by the Medicaid statute to be covered. These would receive current mandatory benefits, with no cost sharing; but could be subjected, with a few exceptions, to cost sharing on optional benefits. For this group, states would be paid the regular Medicaid matching percentage for the mandatory benefits but would get a 30 percent reduction in their matching requirements for optional benefits—the match prescribed for SCHIP. A second category included both optional populations (such as the "medically needy" or children above the FPL) and optional benefits (such as dental care or prosthetic devices). For optional populations, states could provide a reduced benefit package, such as that prescribed for SCHIP or an actuarial equivalent. And for optional services, states could charge premiums, copays, and deductibles, up to 5 percent of family income. For optional populations, including optional benefits, the states would get the 30 percent reduction in their match. Category III would allow states to target specific categories, define the benefit package, and set the cost sharing with no restrictions. For this, they would receive the regular federal match.

The logic of this scheme was compelling. By extending the SCHIP concept to adults, states could reach a large uninsured adult population. The 30 percent reduction in state match would provide an attractive incentive to reach out to this population, expand benefits for Medicaid beneficiaries, help pay for the high-cost and long-term care population, and ease the fiscal pinch for the states. Flexibility with respect to the optional benefit packages and Category III would, in addition, enable the states to manage more efficiently and to experiment with new programs.

As always, there was another side. The scheme could help the states, but with a major shift of costs to the federal government and a downside risk of reducing protection and services for Medicaid beneficiaries. For instance, states would get a higher match for enrolling the near-poor than they would for the poor or traditional Medicaid beneficiary. They could save at the expense of the optional category by offering minimal benefits and imposing cost-sharing requirements. Since most Medicaid benefits are optional anyway, states would be paid handsomely for services they were already providing, with no assurance they would use the freed money to cover the uninsured or improve benefits for the severely ill or those in long-term care. Also Category III, with no "strings," could be used for almost any related health purpose and possibly even find its way, as in the past, to football stadiums and highways (Holahan 2001). Like many a scheme contrived by those expecting to benefit from it, the NGA scheme had little in it to protect against its abuse.

The most dramatic aspect of the governors' plan was the shifting of costs to the federal government. With no change in coverage or benefits, according to John Holahan of the Urban Institute, states would save $16.5 billion, because of the enhanced match. At 200 percent of the FPL, coverage for children and all adults would cost the federal government $39 billion. The states could still save $6.5 billion, One simulation by Holahan showed that states, by imposing some cost sharing and reducing optional benefits 40 percent for the optional category and 10 percent for the mandatory group could increase savings to $18.1 billion, or 21.3 percent of their current program costs. Of this amount, only $2.4 billion would come from "flexibility" savings; $15.7 billion or 87 percent would be from increased federal support.[244] Two important points illustrated by this simulation are that the states would have a considerable incentive to game the system; and that the federal government would foot most of the bill.

This proposal, if successful, would have been an astonishing coup. It would have accomplished much of what the NGA sought in 1995 in flexibility gains and would have shifted the fiscal burden of increased coverage to the federal government. (see pp. 47–48) At 200 percent of FPL, this initiative could add as many as fourteen million new beneficiaries, making a major contribution to coverage for the uninsured and working poor. Even before the surplus vanished, though, informed observers. including the NGA, realized that the prospect Congress would enact such changes and set aside this kind of money with minimal safeguards was remote.[245] But there was another way to gain some of the same objectives.

Restructuring Medicaid was only one topic. The NGA policy paper of February 2001 expressed a focused discontent with several aspects of Medicaid administration: relations with HCFA, the review and administration of state plans, and waiver approval. Pointing out that the new administration had delayed the managed care regulation, the governors said that they hoped for a "more collegial and cooperative mindset," and looked forward to "working with this administration . . . in developing solutions."[246] With respect to state plans, waivers, and Medicaid director letters, they wanted, generally, quicker approval, more limited review, greater flexibility with respect to management, reimbursement and cost sharing, and a relaxation of the "budget neutrality" requirement.[247]

Tommy Thompson had more than a general sympathy for the governors' plight and for their proposal. He had been one of the key Republican governors working through the NGA in 1995 to block-grant Medicaid. While still governor of Wisconsin he had worked over the summer of 2000 to develop the February NGA proposal. When appointed secretary, he began putting into effect the administrative component of the scheme, by dramatically expediting waivers and by initiating the Health Insurance Flexibility and Accountability Demonstration Waiver (HIFA).

HIFA was formally announced on August 4, 2001. Ostensibly, it was a Section 1115 waiver[248] demonstration, but its aim was to transform the Medicaid program in line with the governors' proposal. The basic conception was simple: states could apply for a Section 1115 waiver to increase health insurance coverage for low-income individuals and receive, in turn, programmatic flexibility to modify existing benefit packages and impose cost sharing. The waiver specifications tracked the governors' plan closely, though they did not permit modification of the Medicaid benefit package contained in existing state plans. HCFA (CMS) promised to give priority review to state applications falling within the project guidelines. The same day, it also published an "application template" that drastically simplified the application process and the information required.

HIFA differed from the governors' plan in two other important ways. It did not provide for an enhanced match, which would require congressional action.[249] The NGA proposal also sought a relaxation of the budget neutrality requirement, so that states could apply savings across all federal programs or, failing that, offset from any program falling under the Social Security Act. The NGA addressed these changes in a three-pronged effort aimed at Congress, DHHS and OMB, and continued to lobby their proposal in all these venues.[250] With a vanished budget surplus, a recession, and the international crisis over terrorism, thought, additional money for a new Medicaid initiative or relaxing the budget neutrality requirement was not forthcoming.

Meanwhile, the DHHS continues to implement the HIFA initiative, creating an unusual situation in which a demonstration authority is being used directly in an attempt to transform a major statutory program without even a blessing from Congress. For this initiative, the agenda of an advocacy group was adopted with no countering voice being heard. The Clinton administration's efforts to implement the Consumer Bill of Rights and Responsibilities could be cited as a similar example of partisan overreaching, but that was at least more openly avowed. The comparison is instructive, though, because some procedural checks were important in each instance. For the CBRR, it was the Bush administration's sixty-day hold on new regulations. For the NGA and HIFA initiatives, it was the need for an authorization and appropriation and the OMB budget neutrality requirement. Still, it is discouraging to observe the speed with which the Medicaid bipartisan consensus of 1997 was abandoned following the election of 2000.

IV. DESIGN AND CONSTRUCTION

As noted earlier in this chapter, there are a number of reasons for studying implementation, such as widening the consideration of policy, learning about the practical and the prudent, and assigning blame. Another reason is to see how initiatives turn out: what was or was not accomplished and why. In this respect, the implementation of BBA 97, including the various midcourse corrections, provides useful materials for analysis and reflection.

Of the initial goals sought for Medicare in BBA 97, the greatest successes were in saving money and assuring more than ten years of hospital trust fund solvency. As noted (see pp. 192, 221) , most of these successes came from traditional methods of cost containment, from the decline of Medicaid and Medicare baselines, and the growth of the economy. This success was also uneven and offset in part by undesirable consequences. The new prospective payment systems required years of additional development, involving delayed implementation, intervention by MedPAC, the GAO, and Congress, and a series of "give-back" packages (Medicare Payment Advisory Commission 2001:Chs. 2, 3). Use of the "sustainable growth rate" to limit physician payment now appears simplistic, and the managed care payment rates were a major factor in plan withdrawals, a continuing disaster for the Medicare+Choice program.

The most dismal failure was the centerpiece, Medicare+Choice. This program was to have introduced new models and more choice for beneficiaries, promoted managed care participation and competition, increased efficiency and provided more benefits, mitigated regional inequities and attracted more rural plans. As Thomas Scully, the new administrator of CMS observed in May 2001, BBA 97 may have increased beneficiary information, but in almost every other dimension, except for reduced payments, the legislation has been a failure: almost zero new models in service and decline in rural plans; smaller percentages of beneficiaries with access to one or more MCOs, fewer with zero-premium plans or pharmaceutical benefits; and 1.6 million nonrenewals in the first two years (Council on Economic Impact of Health System Change 2001; Gold 2001). In mid-September of 2001, the Bush administration announced that it expected MCOs to drop an additional 500,000 Medicare enrollees in the coming year.

With Medicaid and SCHIP, the distance between expectation and outcome was less, in part because the changes were of a more traditional kind and/or less technical than Medicare, especially Medicare+Choice. SCHIP enrollments have been fewer than hoped, but reached the level of realistic estimates. Some states gamed the system by enrolling Medicaid eligibles in SCHIP, but that was expected, and steps were taken to counter such behavior. For Medicaid, the withdrawal of the managed care regulation represented the defeat of an implementation effort—or its correction, depending on the point of view. The governors' plan and HIFA were major challenges to the accommodation reached in the BBA 97 Medicaid legislation. However, the first of these has been laid to rest—temporarily, at least, and, so far, HIFA has not met with much of a response.

For interpreting these developments, a useful distinction is that between design and construction, with legislation thought of as design, and implementation as construction. Reality is not that simple: the administration gets into design and Congress into the details of construction. The terminology is deliberately chosen for some of its normative implications: that Medicare and Medicaid need to be designed, not just stuck together; and that construction is a craft with technical constraints and elements of gildlike custom. Like the "policy-administration" distinction, a major purpose of these terms is to help with analysis.

Applying the distinction, the major failure with the Medicare legislation was design. The cost-saving provisions were, variously, poorly coordinated, too drastic or procrustean, and/or politically unsustainable. Several of the new plans offered in the broadened spectrum of "choice" were ideologically driven or concessions to advocacy groups with little or no foundation in experience, research, or demonstrations. It should occasion little surprise that they have found few takers. Even the outpatient and postacute prospective payment systems were in part a failure of design to the extent that Congress accepted HCFA's assurances that they were doable.[251]

The overselling of HCFA's capabilities with respect to the prospective payment systems can also be seen as a failure on the construction side. One serious consequence was that it left administered pricing in this area more politicized and less effective than it might have been. HCFA administrators do not see themselves as blameless in this matter, admitting that they wanted the mandates. They did the best they could under circumstances that they helped to create.

A less ambiguous example was the quality standards and QISMC. This was an instance of constructing more than agreed upon or of overregulation that

contributed in some measure to subsequent plan withdrawals. HCFA specialists seemed caught up in the quality movement and bent upon improving the
Medicare program with national standards and quality improvement exercises. It was also true that HCFA officials resisted pressure from ASPE, the secretary, and the White House to go farther with respect to QISMC standards,
the CBRR, and various civil rights. They pushed for quality, but also defended
the integrity of the program as they saw it and argued for more recognition of
the realities of managed care. When it became clear that they had overreached
they were quick to pull back, especially on QISMC standards.

Medicaid was simpler: smaller and with fewer moving parts. As for creating a design that balanced flexibility and beneficiary rights, the Congress—
with some assistance from the administration—seemed to have gotten it
about right. Arguably, the Senate went too far in its zeal to protect Medicaid
beneficiaries, especially vulnerable populations, from various abuses; but it
remains to be seen if they *can* be protected sufficiently with a number of safeguards weakened, as they have been, in the current revision of the managed
care regulation.

The governors' plan and the HIFA demonstration initiative were efforts to
undo the bipartisan compromise on Medicaid reached in 1997. Time will tell
how durable that compromise proves to be. In any event, the design was good,
even though advocacy groups or partisans may choose to change it.

As noted earlier, the final Medicaid managed care regulation of January
2001 arguably went beyond the legislative mandate—or interpreted that
mandate in a one-sided way—with respect to level of prescriptiveness, overall
quality strategy, information requirements, and its protectiveness of beneficiaries, including an elaborate grievance system and imports from the Consumer
Bill of Rights and Responsibilities, and the secretary's "special needs report"
(Department of Health and Human Services 2000). As with Medicare,
though, there were two schools of thought within HCFA, and much of the
putative overreaching came at the insistence of the secretary's office and the
White House.[252] In other words, the faults in construction—if they were
faults—could be ascribed in large measure to the intervention of a second
principal.

One conclusion from this chapter is that design is much more of a problem
in the amending of Medicare or Medicaid than construction or the implementation of a design. For that matter, the worst failures in construction often
came from efforts by advocacy groups, the Congress, or the administration to
continue or reopen the design phase. The study of implementation provides
evidence that design matters and often why and how it does. From a larger
perspective, divided government, partisanship, the campaign style of legislation, and the constraints of the reconciliation process work against good
design. So does haste, inadequate staffing, the failure to develop and consider
policy alternatives, and the substitution of ideology for evidence. Fortunately,

our system of government has checks and balances and staff agencies that warn and advise, though preventing mistakes does not create the imaginative, workable designs needed to improve Medicare or Medicaid.

NOTES

[1] James Bentley, senior vice-president of the American Hospital Association, said of attempts by Congress to direct HCFA that you "can't push a wet noodle." In other words, Congress had the power to stop the administration, but directing it requires more understanding and finesse. Interview, November 18, 1998.

[2] Adapting Ambrose Bierce's definition of a cat: a furry object "to be kicked when things go wrong" (cf. *The Devils Dictionary*).

[3] Marketing and consumer information for Medicare+Choice was an exception; but this exception also generated a large amount of controversy.

[4] Probable reasons would seem to be parsimonious authorizations; attractiveness of alternative opportunities in the private sector or on the Hill; and lack of big events that bring new recruits, such as passage of Medicare/Medicaid and attempts at health care reform.

[5] Nancy-Ann deParle, Kennedy School of Government; formerly, HCFA administrator. Interview, March 8, 1999.

[6] Barbara Cooper, Institute for Medicare Practice, Mount Sinai School of Medicine. Formerly, director, Office of Strategic Planning, HCFA. Alphonse Esposito, deputy director, Office of Strategic Planning. Interview, April 20, 1999.

[7] As the medical residents' saying goes, "See one; do one; teach one."

[8] He had announced his intention to resign early in February.

[9] Informal organization was important for division of labor and sharing tasks, for consultation, and as a source of valuable institutional memory. Some positions were apportioned: for instance, 60 percent in coverage and 40 percent payment. With reorganization, a part of that person's institutional memory would be lost. Kathy Buto, Congressional Budget Office; formerly, director, Center for Health Plans and Providers. Interview, April 15, 1999.

[10] Judy Moore, National Health Policy Forum. Formerly, Medicaid director, HCFA. October 15, 1998.

[11] A failed project to create a megasystem for Medicare data and computerized transactions.

[12] Nancy-Ann deParle, interview, March 8, 1999. Gary Christoph, director of information services, HCFA. Interview, May 5, 1999.

[13] So called because of the dating problem that would arise on January 1, 2000, at 12:00 A.M., because most computers and computer programs had only two spaces for the year date. In this situation, not only would dates be missing but programs could begin "crashing"—failing in part or entirely—with unpredictable and even catastrophic results.

[14] Gary Christoph. Interview, May 5, 1999. Christoph compared the system to "grandma's quilt," also to a "Model T Ford with a Cadillac engine."

[15] Christoph used the concept of "propinquity," illustrated with an example of a steel bridge. A weakness in the bridge is usually characterized by propinquity—which means that if a bolt is missing or a crack appears in the frame, the fracture is likely to be near in space to the visible defect. Computer programs are not like that: a failure in some tiny, remote part of the program can bring the whole edifice crashing down. He also likened these programs to a plate of spaghetti: you pull on one strand but you cannot predict what it may affect.

[16] Kathy Buto. Interview, April 15, 1999. Barbara Wynn, RAND. Formerly, director, Plan and Provider Purchasing Policy Group, HCFA. Interview, May 13, 1999.

[17] Nancy-Ann deParle. Interview, March 8, 1999. Clinton had been governor of Arkansas and, like many other governors, saw HCFA as a nuisance.

[18] Interview, March 8, 1999.

[19] A similar appointee, though not one with previous HCFA experience, was Gary Christoph as director of the new Office of Information Services. Christoph had an impressive scientific background, had worked in the laboratory of Linus Pauling, and had spent fifteen years managing Cray computers at the Los Alamos laboratory.

[20] Peter Bouxsein, Institute of Medicine. Formerly, deputy director, Office of Managed Care, HCFA. Interview, February 16, 2000.

[21] Dan Waldo, director, Strategic Planning Office; earlier, Office of the Actuary, HCFA. Interview, April 14, 1999.

[22] Dan Waldo. Interview, April 12, 2001. Steve Pelovitz, director, Survey and Certification Group, Center for Medicaid and State Operations, HCFA. Interview, April 12, 1999.

[23] Barbara Cooper. Interview, April 20, 1999.

[24] Dan Waldo. Interview, April 14, 1999.

[25] "Two stove pipes" was a term often used to convey notions of dominant features on the landscape, of separate productive activities, and of unwanted side-effects.

[26] With thanks to Lynn Etheredge.

[27] Kathy Buto. Interview, April 15, 1999. Dan Waldo, Strategic Planning Office, HCFA. Interview, April 14, 1999.

[28] Following Aristotle's definition of "slaves by nature." Cf. Long (1954).

[29] Steve Pelovitz. Interview, April 27, 1999.

[30] Dan Waldo. Interview, April 14, 1999.

[31] Kathy Buto. Interview, April 15, 1999. In her view, planning needed to begin at a more aggregate level, which seem to make good sense since knowing what to "operationalize" may depend on further determination of the underlying problems, for instance, with a prospective payment system.

[32] Dan Waldo. Interview, April 24, 1999.

[33] The Waldo adaptation helped, for instance, to make manifest the seriousness of the Y2K problem.

[34] Donald Kosin, Office of General Counsel, DHHS. Interview, January 8, 1999.

[35] Ibid. The *Federal Register* requires preambles as a condition for publication, so that DHHS rules would normally have preambles. But HCFA put forth special efforts to make their preambles instructive and consistent with the regulatory texts.

[36] Ibid.

[37] Kathy Buto. Interview, April 15, 1999.

[38] Jean LeMasurier, deputy director, Plan and Purchasing Policy, HCFA. Interview, April 14, 1999.

[39] Ibid.

[40] Kathy Buto. Interview, April 15, 1999.

[41] Jean LeMasurier. Interview, April 14, 1999.

[42] Ibid.

[43] Kathy Buto. Interview, April 15, 1999.

[44] Cindy Mason, senior research analyst, Division of Demonstration Programs, HCFA. Interview, July 27, 1999.

[45] Ibid.

[46] Ibid.

[47] Ibid.

[48] Ibid.

[49] *Federal Register,* June 26, 1998, pp. 35032 ff.

[50] Cindy Mason, interview, July 27, 1999.

[51] P.L. 97-248.

[52] Patricia McTaggart, director, Quality and Performance Management, Center for Medicaid and State Operations, HCFA. Interview, May 4, 1999.

[53] Jeffrey Kang, director, Clinical Standards and Quality Office, HCFA. Interview, July 28, 1999.

[54] Congressional interest in the particulars was so low that much of the statutory text was "administratively written"—i.e., taken from HCFA drafts. Ibid.

[55] Peter Bouxsein. Interview, February 16, 2000. Bob Berenson, formerly director, Center for Health Plans and Programs, also made the same observation. Interview, June 28, 1999.

[56] In February, 1998, President Clinton ordered Medicare and Medicaid, among a number of other government-supported health programs, to comply with the patients' rights provisions of the "Consumer Bill of Rights and Responsibilities" contained in the interim report of the Quality Commission. *Health Care Policy Report,* March 2, 1998, p. 359.

[57] Jeffrey Kang. Interview, July 28, 1999.

[58] Jean LeMasurier. Interview, April 14, 1999. Donald Kosin. Interview, January 8, 1999.

[59] This early "roll-out" was not required by the "interim final rule" procedure, but it was customary and seen as fair to providers.

[60] Ibid.

[61] Ibid.

[62] Jean LeMasurier, interview, April 14, 1999.

[63] George Greenberg, senior Medicare program analyst, ASPE, DHHS. Interview, August 24, 2000.

[64] Nancy-Ann deParle. Interview, March 8, 1999.

[65] Both Kathy Means and Ed Grossman are credited with this suggestion, though both say that the idea was "around," and decline any particular credit.

[66] Philip Doerr, director, Premium and Financial Evaluation, HCFA. Interview, June 10, 1999.

[67] Kathy Buto. Interview, April 15, 1999.

[68] Philip Doerr. Interview, June 10, 1999.

[69] Ibid.

[70] Ibid.

[71] Ibid.72. Kathy Buto. Interview, April 15, 1999.

[73] Philip Doerr. Interview, June 10, 1999.

[74] Similar techniques were often used by ProPAC and PPRC, commissions that relied heavily upon building consensus.

[75] Philip Doerr. Interview, April 20, 2001.

[76] Kathy Buto. Interview, April 15, 1999.

[77] Philip Doerr. Interview, June 10, 1999.

[78] Barbara Wynn. Interview, May 13, 1999. Michael McMullin, deputy director, Center for Beneficiary Services, HCFA. Interview, April 28, 1999.

[79] According to one account, almost every major IOM donor called about the report, the principal supporter of the original report was especially uneasy, and Bruce Vladeck (as of March 1999) was not on speaking terms with Stan Jones, one of the authors.

[80] The term "navigator" was popular in much of the discussion at that time.

[81] L. Sue Anderson, Health Insurance Counseling Project, George Washington University. Interview, April 8, 1999.

[82] For instance, HCFA sought to review HMO beneficiary newsletters that were allegedly being used to mobilize the enrollees in HMO lobbying efforts. The health plans pleaded the First Amendment. See Pear (2000a).

[83] According to Carol Cronin, director of the Center for Beneficiary Services, their time schedule was demanding and Congress was highly prescriptive, but CBS "wanted the mandate." Interview, April 21, 1999.

[84] Michael McMullin. Interview, April 28, 1999.

[85] Ibid.

[86] National Medicare Education Program, meeting of the Coordinating Committee, Washington, D.C., March 10, 1999.

[87] Michael McMullin. Interview, April 28, 1999.

[88] Ibid.

[89] Carol Cronin. Interview, April 21, 1999.

[90] Meeting of the Coordinating Committee, March 10, 1999.

[91] Mike Hash, deputy administrator, HCFA. Interview, March 18, 1999.

[92] As HCFA develops new requirements for the health plans, these are often made known to the plans in the course of their annual ACR filings to establish the new premiums.

[93] Michael McMullin. Interview, April 28, 1999. *Health Care Policy Report,* March 2, 1998, p. 370.

[94] Ibid. L. Sue Anderson. Interview, April 8, 1999.

[95] Meeting of the Coordinating Committee, March 10, 1999.

[96] Geraldine Dallek, Institute for Health Care Research and Policy, Georgetown University. Interview, March 11, 1999.

[97] Bruce Vladeck, Mount Sinai Medical Center. Formerly, HCFA administrator. Interview, February 8, 1999.

[98] Hospitals that were not included in the hospital PPS and remained under the earlier system of payment established by the Tax Equity and Fiscal Responsibility Act of 1982 (P.L. 97-248)

[99] September 1 in order to allow a month before October 1, the beginning of the new fiscal year and of the new hospital payments.

[100] Barbara Wynn. Interview, September 6, 2000.

[101] Also, comments needed to be assembled for many elements already proposed. Ibid.

[102] Ibid.

[103] Ibid.

[104] Ibid., September 11, 2000.

[105] Ibid., May 13, 1999.

[106] Ibid. Kathy Buto. Interview, April 15, 1999.

[107] Rather than prescribing a PPS for mental health hospitals, the payments were "rebased," which means changing the historic base formula that runs from year to year, and is changed by annual percentage updates and specific modifiers that take account of such variables as regional labor costs, changes in the MEI, demographic factors, and so forth.

[108] Nancy-Ann deParle warned Congress and the administration that HCFA would not be able to do all the prospective payment systems on time. Staff persons in Congress were aware of this problem. Nancy-Ann deParle. Interview, May 8, 1999. Howard Cohen, Greenberg, Traurig. Formerly, majority professional staff, House Commerce Committee. Interview, June 6, 2000.

[109] Barbara Cooper, Alphonse Esposito. Interview, April 20, 1999.

[110] Janice Flaherty, deputy director, Chronic Care Policy Group. Interview, April 27, 1999.

[111] Alphonse Esposito. Interview, April 20, 1999.

[112] William Scanlon, managing director, Health Care Team, General Accounting Office. Scanlon believes that HCFA was oversold on these systems; that methodologies existed but had never been worked out; and that fully prospective payments systems might not be practicable in some instances, such as skilled-nursing facilities or home health care. Interview, September 23, 1998.

[113] Alphonse Esposito. Interview, April 20, 1999.

[114] MedPAC was also of this opinion. Cf. Medicare Payment Advisory Commission 2001:16).

[115] *Health Care Policy Report,* July 6, 1998, p. 1100.

[116] Ibid.

[117] Ibid. Stark's proposal would have gotten HCFA more direct authority over the intermediaries and leverage to make them move more quickly in getting their systems Y2K compliant.

[118] P.L. 106-113.

[119] Laura Dummitt, associate director, Health Care Financing and Systems, General Accounting Office. Interview, April 25, 1998.

[120] Alphonse Esposito. Interview, April 20, 1999.

[121] Imagine, for instance, asking VNA nurses working in an urban ghetto to collect the copays, and then hiring body guards to protect the nurses. Erik Sokol, assistant director for governmental affairs, National Association for Home Care. Interview, September 29, 1998.

[122] It was later reinstated, but has continued to be controversial.

[123] Tom Ault, Health Policy Alternatives. Formerly, director, Bureau of Program Development, HCFA. Interview, September 30, 1998.

[124] Ibid. Also, William Scanlon. Interview, September 23, 1998.

[125] ProPAC had also recommended an interim payment system (Prospective Payment Assessment Commission 1997:54).

[126] Payments were capped at 98 percent of year 1994. "Where the hell did that come

from?" queried one observer. The answer is that the formula got exactly the savings needed.

[127] The 15 percent was a default reduction if the PPS was not implemented by October 1999. The additional expenditures were to be offset by a small decrease in the update beginning in 2000 and by revenues from a "sin tax" on gambling. *Health Care Policy Report,* October 26, 1997, p. 1669.

[128] William Scanlon. Interview, November 23, 1998.

[129] Mandated, that is, as a condition of participation in the Medicare program. *Health Care Policy Report,* February 1, 1999, pp. 201–02.

[130] Erik Sokol. Interview, September 29, 1998.

[131] *Health Care Policy Report,* April 5, 1998, p. 574.

[132] Ibid., June 21, 1998, p. 1005.

[133] Ibid., March 11, 1999.

[134] Bryant Hall, legislative director, staff of Sen. Bob Graham. Interview, September 2, 1998.

[135] "Report and Recommendations to Congress," March 3, 1997, Ibid., p. 40.

[136] Ibid.

[137] Barbara Wynn. Interview, September 11, 2000.

[138] According to Bruce Vladeck, a version had been completed and was "sitting on the shelf," awaiting the resolution of some differences with OMB over copays. Interview, February 8, 1999.

[139] Margaret Sulvetta, Urban Institute. Interview, August 26, 1998.

[140] Some modest reductions were made.

[141] *Health Care Policy Report,* August 24, 1998, p. 1367.

[142] Thomas Hoyer. Interview, April 20, 1999.

[143] Ibid.

[144] *Health Care Policy Report,* January 25, 1999, p. 364.

[145] Steven Scheingold, Division of Program Analysis and Performance Measurement, HCFA. Interview, September 26, 2000.

[146] *Health Care Policy Report,* April 10, 2000, p. 566.

[147] Ibid., July 24, 2000, p. 1256.

[148] *American Society of Cataract and Refractive Surgery v. Shalala,* filed November 4, 1998. Health Care Policy Report, January 25, 1999, p. 364.

[149] Of which only $996 billion was "on budget." The remaining $1.9 trillion was excess Social Security and Medicare payroll taxes.

[150] *Health Care Policy Report,* July 12, 1999, p. 1141.

[151] Ibid., July 12, 1999, p. 1120.

[152] Ibid., September 13, 1999, p. 1427.

[153] In March, the Bipartisan Commission failed by one vote to gain majority support for its report. *Health Care Policy Report,* March 22, 1999, p. 491.

[154] Ibid., September 20, 1999, p. 1469.

[155] Ibid., May 13, 1999, p. 435.

[156] Ibid., June 14, 1999, p. 963.

[157] Ibid., p. 962.

[158] Mainly by underestimating the effect of FFS Medicare reductions, which reduced the AAPCC more than expected.

[159] Ibid., October 18, 1999, pp. 1624–25.

[160] Ibid., November 8, 1999. p. 1748.

[161] Originally, the bill had passed the House as part of a tax measure, but the Senate refused to consider it in this form.

[162] *Health Care Policy Report,* December 25, 1999, pp. 2016–17.

[163] *Juilliard v. Greenman,* 110 U.S. 421, at 458. (1884).

[164] *Health Care Policy Report,* May 21, 2001, p. 813.

[165] Ibid., April 16, 2001, p. 594.

[166] Ibid., August 31, 1999, p. 1392,

[167] Ibid., July 12, 1999, p. 1141.

[168] Bruce Fried, Shaw, Pitman. Formerly director of Office of Managed Care, HCFA. Interview, February 10, 2000. Carlos Zarabozo, Office of Strategic Planning, HCFA. Interview, July 14, 1999.

[169] *Health Care Policy Report,* July 12, 1999, p. 1142.

[170] Bruce Fried. Interview, February 10, 2000.

[171] Developing a risk adjuster required some way of measuring the intensity of resource use (or devising a plausible proxy) in order to estimate variations between patients. But HMOs, operating on a risk basis, spread risk across an average of patients and had less need for patient-specific data. Some plans, like Kaiser Permanente, maintained no encounter data. Others would have to develop it, often at great cost to themselves. HCFA would have the problem of trying to enforce such a mandate and get quality data in a timely fashion from health plans, some of them resentful and recalcitrant.

[172] Carlos Zaraboza. Interview, July 14, 1999.

[173] Ibid.

[174] Bruce Vladeck had long maintained that the FFS program subsidized MCOs both directly and indirectly, making the cost-saving advantage of MCOs largely illusory. There is no conclusive proof of favorable selection. Some studies show favorable selection; others that the advantage is temporary and disappears as plans "mature."

[175] *Health Care Policy Report,* August 17, 1998, p. 1348.

[176] Ibid., March 16, 1998, p. 451.

[177] Ibid., February 15, 1998, p. 279.

[178] Ibid., April 6, 1998, p. 598.

[179] Bob Berenson, formerly director, Center for Health Plans and Providers, HCFA. Interview, June 23, 1999. Berenson believed from the beginning that seven was too many, but said that HCFA officials were being pushed by ASPE to set a high level.

[180] The regulation was actually published on June 26, which made the situation even worse.

[181] In this instance, HCFA moved first and got some credit for a change Congress would have certainly made had HCFA not done so. *Health Care Policy Report,* April 19, 1999, p. 651.

[182] Bruce Fried. Interview, February 10, 2000. Mohit Ghose, Media Relations, American Association of Health Plans. Interview, October 4, 2000.

[183] *New York Times,* July 4, 1998, p. A1.

[184] *Health Care Policy Report,* September 14, 1998, p. 1452.

[185] Ibid., September 21, 1998, p. 1480.

[186] Ibid., November 2, 1998, p. 1713.

[187] Ibid., July 26, 1999, p. 1200.

[188] Ibid., July 3, 2000, p. 1300.

[189] Along with the Coalition for Medicare Choices.

[190] Mohit Ghose. Interview, October 4, 2000.

[191] *Health Care Policy Report,* August 17, 1998, p. 1348; April 26, 1999, p. 704; May 24, 1999, p. 844. It should be added that HIAA responded with sophisticated research and policy papers of its own.

[192] Ibid., February 15, 1999, p. 279.

[193] The Medicare/Medicaid and SCHIP Benefits Improvement and Protection Act of 2000 (BIPA). The legislation also permitted HMOs to reconsider decisions to withdraw after rates were announced. *Health Care Policy Report,* December 17, 2000, pp. 2016–17.

[194] As the program was being developed, it was referred to as CHIP. The legislation added the S, so that SCHIP has become the official title, though the program is often still referred to as "CHIP."

[195] Judy Moore, National Health Policy Forum. Formerly, director of the Medicaid program. Interview, October 12, 2000. Debbie Chang, deputy secretary, Maryland Department of Health and Mental Hygiene. Formerly, director of the Medicaid program. Interview, October 13, 2000.

[196] Judy Moore. Interview, October 12, 2000.

[197] Judy Moore. Interview, October 15, 1998.

[198] Debbie Chang. Interview, October 13, 2000.

[199] Ibid.

[200] They were also integrated into Waldo's monitoring system.

[201] Judy Moore. Interview, October 12, 2000. Debbie Chang. Interview, October 13, 2000.

[202] Judy Moore. Interview, October 12, 2000.

[203] This was a technique that had been used effectively by the Food and Drug Administration.

[204] More like one hundred different topics that were explored in considerable depth.

[205] Judy Moore. Interview, October 12, 2000.

[206] Debbie Chang. Interview, October 12, 2000.

[207] According to Chang, they all did, having no ready alternative. Ibid.

[208] "Crowd out" was the displacing of existing insurance by new coverage that was free or less expensive—for instance, employers withdrawing coverage or employees opting for a government program instead of a work-based policy. The limit on non-health-related expenditures was especially sensitive. Too tight and it would hamper state flexibility and experimentation. Too permissive and it opened the way for football stadiums and highways.

[209] Debbie Chang. Interview, October 12, 2000.

[210] HCFA's Medicaid operations staff could be used for much of this activity.

[211] For SCHIP, but not for Medicaid.

[212] Jennifer Ryan, technical director, SCHIP, HCFA. Interview, October 30, 2000.

[213] The President's Advisory Commission on Consumer Protection and Quality in the Health Care Industry—the "Quality Commission"—had issued a Consumer Bill of Rights and Responsibilities, with its interim report of November 20, 1997. On February 20, 1998, the Clinton administration directed federal health agencies, such as Medicare and Medicaid, to begin implementing the CBRR provisions for their beneficiaries.

[214] David Cade, deputy general counsel, Office of the General Counsel, DHHS. Interview, October 24, 2000.

[215] For instance, where provisions in Medicaid contracts had been customarily excluded and were understood to be so.

[216] Judy Moore. Interview, October 12, 2000.

[217] 63 FR 52040, September 29, 1998.

[218] Access and access standards were put in the statute under Section 4705, "Quality Assurance Standards."

[219] Judy Moore. Interview, November 2, 2000.

[220] Section 338.56(b)(3)(v); see also Rosenbaum and Darnall (1998:28).

[221] Section 438.104(b)).

[222] Judy Moore. Interview, November 2, 2000.

[223] *Medicaid Managed Care: Four States Experiment with Mental Health Carve-Out Programs,* GAO/HEHS-99-1218, September, 1999, p. 7. I am indebted to Dick Hegner for calling my attention to this publication as well as for perspectives on the problems of enforcing Medicaid requirements.

[224] Section 4707(e). The intermediate sanctions included civil monetary penalties (CMPs), suspension of operations or termination of contract, appointment of temporary managers, suspension of enrollment or payment, and allowing individuals to disenroll themselves. These intermediate sanctions, established earlier for the federal government, would in theory give the states more flexible and effective enforcement power than the drastic and clumsy weapons of contract termination and/or criminal prosecution.

[225] Section 4707(b)(4).

[226] 63 FR 52055.

[227] Ibid.

[228] Social Security Act of 1935, P.L. 74-620; Section 402(a)(4); Social Security Act of 1965, P.L. 89-97, Section 1902(a)(3); *Goldberg v. Kelly,* 397 U.S. 254 (1970); *Mathews v. Eldridge,* 414 U.S. 319, 1976. See Chasan-Sloan (2001).

[229] Note that the statute requires an internal "grievance procedure" only for MCOs. The regulation does not include MCEs or PCPs.

[230] Section 1852(g). Though the external review was only for coverage decisions.

[231] An interesting detail is that the regulation specified that a beneficiary could pursue the appeals process or seek a state hearing, or both, except that states could require aggrieved parties to exhaust their appeal remedies. This provision recognized the legal priority of the fair hearing, as well as supporting (by association) the appeals process.

[232] 63 FR 52154.

[233] Judy Moore. Interview, October 12, 2000.

[234] Ibid. Interview, August 9, 2001.

[235] Published in the *Federal Register* on January 19, 2001.

[236] SCHIP was also delayed, but it suffered, ultimately, a gentler fate than the managed care regulation.

[237] *Health Care Policy Report,* March 5, 2001, p. 330.

[238] Ibid., May 7, 2001, p. 733.

[239] These were especially administration priorities, not in the legislation, and were supported with reservations by some of the HCFA staff.

[240] A good argument can be made, of course, that Medicaid enrollees—because of their disadvantaged circumstances—need a more facilitative grievance system. But

states complained especially about the grievance system, and some of its provisions had little legal foundation or support among Republican legislators or within the new administration. Following the Medicare model in this instance seems reasonable.

[241] Amending a text is easy; improving it may not be.

[242] NGA Policy Position HR-32, "Health Care Reform Policy," adopted February, 2001.

[243] *Health Care Policy Report,* March 5, 2001, p. 230. See also Holahan (2001:17).

[244] Including, for instance, *Olmstead v. L.C. ex. rel. Zimring* 144 L.Ed(2d) 546 (1999), which held that states could be required to provide community-based rather than institutional care when appropriate for persons with disabilities.

[245] Andy Schneider. Interview, August 27, 2001.

[246] NGA Policy Position HR-32, op. cit., pp. 2-3.

[247] A general requirement of waivers is that they be "budget neutral," meaning, in this context, that the waivered program not cost more federal dollars than traditional Medicaid would have.

[248] One aspect of the Section 1115 waiver was that it was flexible and left enormous discretion in the hands of the secretary. See Lambrew (2001).

[249] Note that the "flexibility" savings would seem to be relatively small and especially if there were no relaxation of the budget neutrality requirement and continued maintenance-of-effort requirements with respect to mandatory Medicaid populations.

[250] Matt Salo, legislative director, Health, National Governors' Association. Interview, September 17, 2001.

[251] President Kennedy said that a major lesson he learned from the Bay of Pigs episode was never to trust the military's views of its own capabilities.

[252] Timothy Westmoreland, who came from the White House to be the Clinton administration's last director of the Center for Medicaid and State Operations, described his aim as including in the managed care regulation as much as possible of the CBRR, the patient protections in Medicare, and the secretary's special needs report to Congress. This was a different emphasis from that which guided the earlier proposed regulation (Council on Economic Impact of Health System Change 2001).

8

Old Business and New

Three issues largely dominated the health care debate from the fall of 1997 through the election and the year 2001. One was managed care reform, especially patients' bills of rights. Another was increased access to health care, including coverage for the uninsured and a pharmaceutical benefit for Medicare beneficiaries. The third was restructuring Medicare for the long term. Each of these topics included old business that had been considered prior to BBA 97 but had not been addressed or not fully resolved by this legislation. They were "new" business because they were considered in a changed context, they shifted attention to the private sector, or they contemplated increasing an entitlement. They are of interest because each is likely to remain part of the national agenda for some time and because they illustrate health care politics under conditions of weak mandates, thin majorities in Congress, and continuing struggle for electoral advantage. Examining these issues and the politics attending them helps bring the health care debate up to date and provides some guidance in anticipating how events may develop in the future.

Managed care reform or patients' bills of rights were the most persistently and sharply contested of all these issues. The proposed legislation was primarily intended for private sector HMOs and, for that reason, was not centrally relevant for Medicare or Medicaid. At the same time, this initiative was preceded by quality improvement mandates for both programs and represented, to some extent, the extension of this kind of protection to the broader public, especially as the administration mandated versions of patients' bills of rights for Medicare, Medicaid, the FEHBP, and other government programs. The controversy over managed care reform took time, used up energy and goodwill, and diverted attention from other agendas. It illustrates how Congress can be distracted by a policy enthusiasm of dubious merit, and it serves as a warning of the bitter fights that might ensue if Medicare itself were converted into a managed care program, especially one that became politically unpopular.

During this period, access to care—mainly for uninsured children and low-income workers—continued to be an issue, along with additional benefits for those already insured, especially the elderly. This topic grew in salience with the election campaigns of 1998 and 2000. Expansions of coverage also brought into renewed prominence issues of entitlement and of public vs. private control: of whether to use Medicare, Medicaid, or SCHIP as vehicles or to go the route of tax credits, MSAs, and small market insurance reforms. These debates opened new prospects, revived ideological cleavages, and revealed some of the limits of incrementalism, implying the need for more comprehensive and systematic solutions. Few were ready to say, even whisper, "national health insurance," except as an epithet, but the outlines of yet another distinctively American approach toward NHI were beginning to emerge, especially by the end of 2001.

A third cluster of issues, left as unfinished business by BBA 97, related to the long-term future of the Medicare program. The approach taken by BBA was to create a National Bipartisan Commission on the Future of Medicare, charged to report to Congress by March 1, 1999, roughly eighteen months after the passage of the statute. Although the commission failed to agree on a scheme, it did leave behind an endorsement of a premium support system modeled on the Federal Employee Health Benefits Program. That elicited a counterproposal from the administration also featuring premium support as a fiscal principle. Both recommendations included a pharmaceutical benefit. These initiatives articulated two distinctive approaches and helped clarify partisan differences in philosophy, though as the election campaign of 2000 revealed, without doing much to settle these differences—so that this particular controversy goes on much as it did prior to BBA 97.

This chapter explores some of the political *sequellae* of BBA 97 and their significance for the future of Medicare and Medicaid as well as several initiatives that developed as next steps beyond BBA 97. Over four years, none of these issues was even partially resolved. They became prominent campaign issues in the election of 2000 and agenda items for the Bush administration and the 107th Congress. Various factors help account for a lack of more positive outcomes: divided government and the lack of a working majority or a mandate; partisanship and the campaign mode of policymaking; the power of the Washington lobby; and the role of individual personalities, especially President Clinton and President Bush. However, one stark fact is that, despite four national elections and over six years of legislative struggle over Medicare, Medicaid, and related health care issues, Democrats and Republicans are little closer to an agreement or compromise over the fundamental, and largely ideological, issues they have fought over since 1995. The parties are as divided as ever over questions of entitlement, regulation vs. the market or private sector, and federal vs. state control. An optimistic view of the future would be that the electorate will grow increasingly disgruntled about the lack of progress and that a critical mass of politicians and activists will realize that only sound policy compromises are likely to work and last. A more pessimistic view is that the campaign mode of policymaking will continue, along with the virulent partisanship, the disreputable tactics, the deception, and the pseudo-solutions that pass for serious proposals. In that event, gridlock may again prevail, until the emergence of another health care "crisis,"[1] impels a new wave of reform.

I. MANAGED CARE REFORM AND PATIENTS' BILLS OF RIGHTS

The title for this section reflects a historic reality that the issue itself took various forms depending upon which faction was advocating the changes. Most of the headlines were about patient protection or a patients' bill of rights. Provider rights got less public billing but were a principal concern, especially in the House. Consumer information and choice were supported as a form of beneficiary protection and a stimulus for health competition. Both the administration and House and Senate leadership sought to combine patient protection with more general managed care reforms. Most of this was about regulating HMOs, not patient or provider protection in general. The ambiguity of the title acknowledges, in some measure, the various strands of opinion and interest that were involved.

Most of this controversy over patients' rights and managed care had little direct impact upon either Medicare or Medicaid, except that it occupied the attention of Congress and diverted effort from other substantive issues, including the plight of the uninsured, Medicare reform, and a pharmaceutical benefit. At the same time, the long-term consequences of this episode may be important for the future of managed care and, therefore, for both Medicare and Medicaid. It also is useful to illustrate the kind of health care politics that may increasingly characterize the future, with interest group mobilization, partisanship, and a campaign style of legislation, but a lack of effective leadership—so that gridlock is a likely and, sometimes, even desirable outcome.

The Quality Commission

One important impetus for a patients' bill of rights came from the administration, in the form of recommendations from the President's Advisory Commission on Consumer Protection and Quality in the Health Care Industry, generally known by its short title, the Quality Commission. How and why a commission on quality became important for a patients' bill of rights needs some explanation.

As is usually the case with large initiatives, timing and opportunity, calculations of political advantage, and the interests of various groups worked together. After the political struggles over BBA 95 had died down early in

1996, policy people and political appointees within the White House and executive agencies—in keeping with the president's own philosophy—began thinking about ways to move from a defensive posture to a more aggressive and positive agenda.[2] Agenda items for the coming election cycle were also needed, and since there was hope that President Clinton might win a second term, thought was being given not only to the usual campaign demagoguery but to policy proposals that would play well in a second term.[3]

Various interests and program developments made quality and consumer protection an attractive prospect. At the time, there was a robust and growing quality movement, supported both in the private sector and within government, especially by the DHHS and such agencies as AHCPR.[4] Presumably, managed care would continue to increase its share both in the private sector and for government programs such as Medicare and Medicaid, the FEHBP, and the Department of Defense. It was generally recognized—for instance, even in the House version of the Medicare Preservation Act of 1995—that managed care would require special measures to protect the plan enrollees. This would be especially true for poor, elderly, and frail Medicare and Medicaid beneficiaries. But it would also be important for the 70 percent. of the manufacturing workforce in managed care plans, many of them enrolled in substandard plans or with only one plan to choose, or under ERISA protected self-insured plans[5] that gave employees little effective recourse. Moreover, labor had an additional incentive to join in this effort since many trade union members were not only consumers of health care but providers who worked in hospitals and for state and municipal governments as nurses, aides, and administrative support and who wanted their jobs protected against arbitrary plan dismissals or staff reductions.

In the initial White House planning, there was no particular emphasis upon a patients' bill of rights. The September 5 executive order[6] establishing the commission specified quality and consumer protection. It provided that the secretaries of Health and Human Services and the Department of Labor should serve as cochairs, but no special mention was made of patients' rights as such, even less of a bill of rights. At the time, the patients' rights movement was still taking shape. Moreover, patients' rights as such raised a number of issues that were both complex and controversial, such as who would be covered, what specific rights would be created, what their contours should be, the enforcement mechanisms and sanctions to establish, and the amending of ERISA, which since its passage in 1974 had become a domain unto itself. Policy people who were knowledgeable about the issues and the work of advisory commissions thought at the time that such an assignment might be timely but could overtax the commission. There was also some question of constitutional propriety since a patients' bill of rights, depending upon how it would be structured, could be a big and untidy expansion of federal power into affairs previously regarded as a matter for the states or for private dispositions.

A delay in starting the commission's work was an important factor. The quality and consumer protection issues were popular with some, alarming to others, and many wanted a say in this matter. One result was that the White House was deluged with over six hundred applications for board appointments, all of which had to be read and evaluated. In addition, labor lobbied for larger representation, leading to other balancing appointments and the eventual expansion of the commission from twenty to thirty-two directors.[7] Not until March 26, almost seven months after the first executive order, was the advisory panel finally appointed.

Meanwhile, President Clinton had developed a lively interest in managed care reform and patients' rights. While in California, working the crowds, he had asked people "How many of you think your health plan is okay?" When he saw the number who "sat on their hands" rather than raising them, he realized the political potential of this issue.[8] He also believed, on the merits, that HMO quality and patients' rights had been too long neglected and that HMOs would need to change in order to survive.[9] Upon returning from his western trip, he began supporting patients' rights, for instance, by directing DHHS to step up its campaign against "gag orders" in Medicare and Medicaid health plans and by endorsing or calling for legislation on patients' rights. A short time afterward, at a White House ceremony announcing the executive order that increased the membership of the commission, he directed the members to give top priority to a patients' bill of rights.

The executive order called for an interim report. On November 20, 1997, this report was delivered to the president in the form of a Consumer Bill of Rights and Responsibilities. As the title suggests, this submission was not so much a general interim report as it was a patients' bill of rights, addressing most of the issues that were then receiving attention in Congress and among advocacy groups. The commission version also had a distinctive approach. It sought to correct acknowledged abuses in ways that still allowed HMOs to manage. Much reliance was put upon alternative ways of protecting consumers, such as providing more options and improving quality and consumer information. While speaking of "rights," a divisive issue of enforcement was largely sidestepped by specifying only minimal requirements for internal appeals and an impartial external review. There was a studied (and prudent) lack of specificity about many of its provisions—leaving the details to private orderings, the states, the Congress, and the administration.

The commission completed the rest of its report within the year allotted. Despite the scope of the assignment and the large and pluralistic board, it was a consensus document, with no minority report.[10] Essentially, the commission stuck to a central theme of assessing and improving quality in health care, including the Consumer Bill of Rights and Responsibilities in a separate addendum. Experts in the field, regardless of partisan affiliation, acknowledge the work as exceptional in quality and scope, an achievement attributable largely to years of antecedent governmental and private efforts in quality improvement, to the *esprit* of the commission, and to the high level of competence and professionalism of the staff and staff leadership. In an era of partisan wrangling, it was a notable exception. Unfortunately, it received little attention in the subsequent disputes over patients' rights.

Both the president and the Congress were eager to fill in the details and responded quickly to the commission's interim recommendations. On January 14, 1998, House and Senate Democrats met with President Clinton for another White House ceremony, which called for enforceable legislation to codify the Consumer Bill of Rights and Responsibilities.[11] They said that they would seek bipartisan collaboration with Rep. Charlie Norwood (R., Ga.), who had introduced a bill with similar provisions,[12] which had gotten 218 sponsors in the House, 120 of whom were Democrats. In his State of the Union address, late in January, President Clinton gave the Consumer Bill of Rights a prominent place, urging quick action by Congress. In February, some weeks before the commission's final report, he ordered Medicare and Medicaid to comply with the CBRR provisions and directed all 350 health plans participating in the FEHBP to implement a number of its guarantees.[13] Over the next two years, he urged Republicans to pass a "genuine" bill of rights and threatened a veto for any bill that fell short in its guarantees.

As early as January 1998, patients rights was predictably developing into one of those minor catastrophes that had everything: complexity along with passion and ideology; a failure of both party leadership and bipartisanship; House and Senate deadlocked; and distrust between the president and Congress. Even though the outcome may have been foreseeable, like a neurotic quarrel, there seemed little possibility of getting beyond the wrangling, the ploys, and the counterploys, to avert the ultimate debacle.

Patients' Rights in Congress

Prior to 1997, there was little stir in Congress over a patients' bill of rights, though as managed care gained increased political salience the amount of latent interest in patients' rights quickened. Advocacy groups lobbied for legislation and a number of states passed laws that dealt with particular HMO abuses. Within Congress, bills sprouted in clumps dealing with such topics as "gag" rules, standards for emergency care, privacy, and coverage. Senator Edward Kennedy and Rep. John Dingell cosponsored a comprehensive bill; and Rep. Pete Stark introduced a version of his own. In 1997, though, health policy was mostly taken up with the Balanced Budget Act, and for much of the year patients' rights as such were less visible than other managed care issues, such as quality of care or payment formulas.

The most important patients' rights initiative developed in the House, supported by a bipartisan coalition led by three second-term Republicans who were themselves health care professionals turned legislators: Tom Coburn (Okla.), Gregg Ganske (Ia.), and, especially, Charlie Norwood (Ga.). When BBA 97 was under consideration in the Commerce Committee, this same trio—a physician, a surgeon, and a dentist—joined by Democrats, got a number of far-reaching patient protective measures written into the Medicare + Choice program. Norwood, who was profoundly committed to this project, was strategically placed with memberships on the Commerce Committee, with jurisdiction over health, and the Education and Workforce Committee, critical because of ERISA. His bill, introduced in April with more Democratic than Republican cosponsors, quickly became the lead proposal for those seeking comprehensive reform. By September, with bills in House and Senate and the administration's Consumer Bill of Rights and Responsibilities nearing completion, patients' rights were a highly visible political issue and perceived as a major threat, both to the managed care industry and to the Republican leadership agenda.

Norwood's bill, the Patient Access to Responsible Care Act, or PARCA, was the most comprehensive and the most drastic version of patients' rights under consideration. It would cover 162 million employees in managed care plans, not just the 48 million in the industry self-insured ERISA plans. To health plans and many employers, PARCA seemed intended to destroy the concept of managed care as such by its guarantees of access, limits imposed on selective contracting and control of providers, and opportunities to sue for damages in state courts. Where the administration's Consumer Bill of Rights and Responsibilities was meant to balance rights and responsibilities, PARCA came down almost entirely on the side of the patient. It was protective of professional autonomy and the doctor-patient relationship and, in that respect, tilted heavily toward traditional gildlike privileges of providers. According to one count, the bill had over three hundred new mandates, imposing costs and administrative burdens upon health plans, and creating new grounds for lawsuits.[14] An actuarial report by Milliman and Robertson estimated that PARCA would increase managed care premiums nationally by 23 percent;[15] other estimates predicted that five to nine million Americans would lose their health care insurance.[16] Clark Havighurst, a widely respected antitrust authority, observed that PARCA, with its regulations and concessions to professional control, was profoundly anticompetitive and likely to produce its own perversities in addition to increasing costs.[17] Nevertheless, a Kaiser Foundation poll showed that 86 percent of Americans supported the bill, although that support dropped to 68 percent when the poll assumed a $5 to $10 monthly increase in premiums.[18]

By February 1998 there were—depending on how one counted—seven or eight patients' bills of rights ranging across a wide spectrum of political philosophy. In addition to members' offerings, the Republican leadership in the House and Senate appointed task forces to develop their own versions. Like a tropical storm or a prairie fire, patients' rights gathered force in 1998, a sharply contested midterm election year. Driving this issue was a strong populist appeal and the uniting of anti-HMO and patients' right sentiment from both parties. At the same time, it conflicted with the broader, more moderate agenda of the Republican leadership.

Within Congress, the Republican leadership was concerned about their overall political strategy in an election year. They recognized the need to respond to the patients' rights issue. They were also increasingly worried about a scheme they imputed to President Clinton and the Democrats of moving incrementally toward universal coverage or national health insurance: objectionable in itself and competing with their own desire to claim some of the access issue for Republicans. They preferred to combine some recognition of patients' rights with attempts to broaden coverage and access through private sector programs such as MSAs and small business purchasing pools. More drastic patients' rights initiatives—Norwood's PARCA, the administration's Consumer Bill of Rights—or the Kennedy-Dingle version—would undermine such an effort, possibly ceding both issues to the Democrats.[19]

The Republican leadership also understood the importance of getting as many inside the tent as they could and invited Norwood to join the task force. Norwood and supporters of PARCA realized, for their part, that they might improve their chances with leadership support. Working together they assembled a compromise bill,[20] much like the multicommittee, aggregative health insurance bill developed by a similar task force in 1996.[21] A major concession by Norwood was giving up the right to sue managed care plans in state courts. The Republican leadership agreed, for their part, to broaden coverage and to require a stronger system of internal and external appeals. They added a scheme to encourage risk-pooling for individuals and small employers and a hastily contrived innovation, "Health Marts," that would have allowed an array of choices—including PPOs, PoS options, and MSAs—under a multiplan arrangement similar to the FEHBP. Included in the task force version were several familiar add-ons: raising the limits on MSAs, and lowering ceilings on malpractice awards. Each of these could be a "sweetener" or a "poison pill," depending upon circumstances or one's point of view.

Although the leadership Patient Protection Act was the bill most likely to pass Congress, it ran into trouble from almost every quarter. Nine House Republicans had already crossed the aisle to support a Democratic version. Health plans and employers charged that the leadership version went too far and had too many mandates, and patients' advocates that it offered too little protection. Because of the tenuous compromises on which it rested, it was brought to the floor without committee action.[22] It passed on July 24 with a six-vote margin, after a Democratic version lost by only five votes. Even before it passed, the White House announced on July 23 that President Clinton would veto the bill in its existing form, because it failed to cover enough people, did not provide adequate patient protection, and contained "unnecessary and irrelevant provisions that undermine the chances for a bipartisan agreement."[23]

As it turned out, the White House statement was moot, since even the Patient Protection Act would have been unacceptable to the Senate. In the Senate, there was a companion bill to PARCA and a Chafee-Lieberman proposal similar to the House Democratic bill. But the version developed by a leadership task force in the Senate was radically different from PARCA or even the House Republicans' Patient Protection Act. The task force version rested squarely on the premise that regulation was not a good way to remedy HMO abuses and, as Senator Nickles put it, that health resources "should be used for patient care, not to pay trial lawyers."[24] Their version applied primarily to the forty-eight million in ERISA self-insured plans, contained fewer specific protections, and ruled out any increase in plan liability, especially suits in state courts.

To understand future developments, it is important to be aware that the Senate leadership version incorporated strong convictions, widely shared among Republicans. One was the view, pithily enunciated by Senator Nickles, that lawsuits are costly, disruptive, and may not be the best way to improve patient care. A second was that patients' rights ought to be approached in a way that upset existing arrangements the least, especially the ERISA exemption and the long-established primacy of the states in regulation of the insurance industry. In keeping with this philosophy, the leadership bill, acknowledging the problems created by federal preemption, applied a number of core protections to the ERISA plans, but otherwise left specific patients' rights up to the states. It extended a system of internal and external appeals of coverage decisions to the seventy-five million Americans in "fully insured plans," in this respect, reaching beyond the forty-eight million in self-insured ERISA plans. No rights to sue were included. For Senate Republicans, most of whom supported this version, this bill provided a workable and available remedy, protected the big, flagship ERISA plans, and kept the federal government from encroaching on local tort law and the insurance business. At the least, it would seem a prudent way to proceed in this murky area.

The situation within the Senate was complex. Republicans almost certainly had the votes to pass the leadership version, but they believed that the issue would benefit the Democrats in the election. They also feared, realistically, that their own bill would be used by Democrats to score points and would be chewed to bits with unlimited amendments during the floor debate. Therefore, the task force took its time. Democrats, with no leadership version to debate, sought to get their own bill to the floor by attaching it to other legislation. At one point, the Republicans agreed to a debate, but only if floor amendments were limited to three for each side, a proposal that Democrats rejected. Similar maneuvers continued through August into September. By the end of September, with the campaign trail beckoning and the Senate agenda crowded with must-pass legislation, patients' rights proponents were turning their attention to next year and to pinning the blame on their adversaries. The 105th Congress ended without a patients' rights bill reaching the Senate floor.

The election of 1998 left the partisan divide of Republicans and Democrats in the Senate at 55–45, the same as before; but it reduced the Republicans to a slim edge of five in the House, leaving them, practically speaking, without a governing majority. Even though patients' rights had figured prominently in the campaign, the election provided no mandate for either party on the issue.[25] The 106th Congress opened with renewed declarations from Republicans and Democrats about their intentions to fashion a bipartisan patients' rights bill. However, the bipartisan sentiments soon dissipated, followed by two years of wrangling and a stalled conference committee that lasted an entire session of Congress and finally died in December 2000 without reporting a bill.

This time around, the Senate moved before the House, introducing in January a slightly modified version of their leadership bill of the previous year. Efforts to produce a compromise version failed, largely over whether an MSA add-on would be included,[26] so that, again, the alternatives were the Nickles leadership bill and the Democratic proposal, similar to the earlier Norwood bill.

Within the House, efforts by the Commerce Committee and by the Republican leadership to work out a moderate compromise were defeated by a bipartisan coalition of patients' rights enthusiasts. Norwood and Dingle, sponsors of the two chief alternatives to the leaderships' Patient Protection Act, then put together a compromise proposal of their own bill. This bill became the lead proposal, strongly supported by Democrats and insurgent Republicans, but the version most objectionable to the Republican leadership.

When brought to the floor, Norwood-Dingle roundly defeated a leadership alternative in a bipartisan vote of 275–151 margin of 124 votes made possible by the defection of 68 Republicans. Though proclaimed a victory for bipartisanship, it was of a disturbing sort, moved largely by patients' rights issues with the most populistic appeal and unrestrained by the usual institutional checks or considerations of programmatic consequences. Moreover, Republican supporters of Norwood-Dingle mortgaged the future of their own bill in two ways. One was by defying their own party leadership; and the other was by passing a bill radically at variance with the Senate version. These acts went against strong party and institutional norms.

Since the two bills were far apart, especially on key issues, Republicans and Democrats in both chambers had strong incentives to put party loyalists and strong negotiators on the conference committee. The Senate appointed its conferees first, with Don Nickles as chair, and six more Republicans. Roth and

Moynihan, the chairman and ranking member of the Finance Committee, who would normally have been a part of the conference because of the tax provisions, were excluded because they had collaborated on a bipartisan compromise proposal.[26] The only representatives from the Finance Committee were Nickles, the chairman, and Phil Gramm (R., Tex.), whose own patients' rights bill was a minimalist version. The House Republicans took a similar approach, excluding from their conference both Norwood and Ganske, the main proponents of the House bill. Only one Republican conference member, Michael Bilirakis, had voted for Norwood-Dingell. This created an anomalous situation in which the House bill would be represented by Republican conferees who voted against it. At one point, the Democrats offered Norwood a position on their delegation, but he declined. Democrats, for their part, appointed more typical slates, but mostly partisan stalwarts.

The House did not appoint its conferees until November 3, so that a first meeting was not held until February 10, 2000. It may have set another record as the longest conference in American legislative history. The conference opened informally with declarations about everything being "on the table" but with a preemptive statement from Don Nickles that the right to sue was not open for negotiation and a resolution from the House that urged the conference to get on with it and adopt the Norwood-Dingell version—portents of what was to follow.

Following a common conference practice, the conferees adjourned while staff sought agreements on consensus proposals that could be adopted at a next meeting. When the conference reassembled on March 2, almost a month later, the staff aides reported that the only issue on which they had been able to reach consensus was access to pediatric care, having narrowly failed to agree on emergency care and direct access to obstetrician-gynecologists.[27] The conference adjourned again, while the staff continued to work on "consensus" items, and to move at a glacial pace on the major issues of the right to sue, the definition of medical necessity, and the scope of coverage.

As the deadline retreated from March 31 to late April and then May, various attempts were made to move the process ahead. An inner group of conferees began meeting intensively with the staff and were able to reach an agreement, in principle, on the outlines of an external appeals provision. Charlie Norwood proposed an amendment to his own plan limiting it to the fifty-six million in self-insured plans, and President Clinton met with the conferees and offered his services and those of his staff in a bid to speed the negotiations.

By the time of the mid-May White House meeting, the conference was foundering. Of the twenty-two major issues that required merging in the two bills, only two had been completely resolved: access to pediatricians and nondiscrimination against health providers.[28] By then each side was accusing the other of stalling.[29] Conferees would appear at closed sessions and announce their positions but refuse to negotiate. Democrats began boycotting the closed sessions and sought to restart the conference by passing their own bill in the Senate, failing by only one vote to attach their version to a defense authorization bill. With Democratic conferees effectively outside the process, the Republicans continued on their own, inviting Charlie Norwood to join the conference to broaden their support and to help broker a compromise. After Norwood, they tried again with John Shadegg (R., Ariz.), coauthor of a more centrist Republican version.

Though any positive outcomes were obscured by the partisan rhetoric and procedural maneuvering, the conference made some progress, reaching a compromise on the most critical issue, the right to sue. At this point, though, they no longer had a bill that would pass. President Clinton had promised to veto similar legislation. Neither House nor Senate Democrats would support the access provisions of the bill; and House Republicans would balk without them. And the right to sue went too far for the AMA, the health plans, and a number of Senate Republicans.

After the August recess the conference ceased to function. There was talk of another Norwood compromise effort and of an attempt in the Senate to attach a bill—which Senator Nickles vowed to stall using dilatory parliamentary procedures. Nobody declared the conference over. It expired silently with the 106th Congress.

Patients' Rights—Year Six.   As the new Congress assembled, a number of legislators had hopes that a patients' bill of rights might be more successful in this session. A bipartisan majority in both houses supported the concept and were generally agreed about who should be protected and the substantive rights to be included. The remaining item—the biggest of all—was the right to sue, but even on this controversial issue, the final offer from the previous year seemed to have the essential elements for a workable compromise.[30] Also the closeness of the election and precarious status of any governing majority might dispose Congress to conduct its affairs with less partisanship and demagoguery. Much would depend, of course, upon the newly elected president, his agenda, and political style.

President Bush's priorities and political style were, of course, critical in determining the evolution of events. He had said, during his campaign and after the inauguration, that he wanted a "patients' bill of rights he could sign." George Bush, as Texas governor, though, had worked for "tort reform," which generally means reducing causes of action and curbing lawsuits, not increased tort liability. He had vetoed one patients' bill of rights and allowed another to become law without his signature. He regarded lawsuits as a poor way to reform HMOs or to protect patients. When he said a bill he "could sign," he meant one with a limited (or no) right to sue HMOs, providers, or employers. He was also well aware of the popular support for such legislation, and the political damage he might suffer from vetoing such a bill. Therefore, he wanted an alternative to the leading proposals-which were Dingell-Norwood in the House and Kennedy-Edwards in the Senate, bills that were similar in their provisions and that had robust "right to sue" provisions. Both had strong support. Dingell-Norwood had passed the House the year before with a lop-sided bipartisan majority, and the Kennedy-Edwards bill soon gained the support of John McCain (R. Ariz.), giving it increased support and symbolic importance.

White House staff recognized the importance of a proactive response to this situation. Early in the new administration, Bush aides reached out to Charlie Norwood and sought to persuade him to wait until he had seen what kind of alternative Bush was prepared to support. White House staff worked with Sen. Bill Frist (R., Tenn.) to develop a Senate alternative to the McCain-Kennedy-Edwards bill, and urged President Bush to sharpen his veto threats and make it clear that he supported neither the conservative Nickles version nor the bipartisan McCain-Kennedy-Edwards bill.[31] These efforts were modestly successful. Representative Norwood did refrain from cosponsoring his own bill, but Senator Frist gained little support for his alternative, in part because of the relatively detached attitude of President Bush.

By March, the initial momentum for a patients' bill of right had slowed, with another lengthy stalemate seeming the most likely prospect. In the House, Gregg Ganske replaced Norwood as a sponsor, but without Norwood's active support and the president's opposition, the bill lost much of its appeal. Within the Senate, McCain-Kennedy had strong bipartisan support and might well win a majority of the Senate in a debate; but the Republican leadership refused to allow the bill to be brought to the floor. In May, Senator McCain threatened to attach his bill to Bush's education bill as a way to revive some interest in patients' rights. He never carried out his threat, but his actions prompted Senator Frist to release his own version, which was quickly endorsed by President Bush.[32] The alternatives now seemed to narrow: either gridlock or give the president a patients' rights bill he could sign.

This situation changed radically after May 24, when Senator Jeffords (R., Vt.) declared himself an independent, adding that he would vote with Democrats for organizational purposes. Even with a majority of only one member, the Democrats could organize the Senate and control the agenda—which, practically speaking, translated into great power to shape what substantive legislation, if any, would pass. After the Memorial Day recess, the Democrats moved quickly and efficiently to pass McCain-Kennedy on June 29 by a lop-sided vote of 59–36—a majority that showed depth of bipartisan support but also the new majority leader's effectiveness and the Democrats' tactical skill and partisan unity.

The Republicans found themselves embarrassed for lack of an alternative. Even before the Senate floor debate began on June 21, President Bush had vowed to veto McCain-Kennedy or any bill closely similar to it. Meanwhile,

Rep. Charlie Norwood had failed to win significant concessions from the Bush administration in his search for a moderate compromise and said that he would now endorse the Ganske-Dingell bill, the successor to his earlier version and substantively almost identical with the Senate's McCain-Kennedy. Confronting these equally objectionable alternatives, the Republican House leadership hoped to pass a compromise bill to take to the conference. The president had need of this bill to avoid the political damage of vetoing popular legislation or the loss of prestige from backing down on a pledge to veto.

It came down primarily to George W. Bush and Charlie Norwood. President Bush would veto any bill with rights to sue as expansive as Ganske-Dingell, or so it seemed to Norwood and many of his supporters. House Republicans welcomed the president's veto strategy, but feared the electoral consequences of defeating a popular bill. Without Norwood's support, though, the House Republicans lacked the votes to pass the leadership's preferred alternative, which was the Fletcher-Peterson bill.[33] Still twenty votes short, House Republicans planned to delay floor action and a final vote until after Labor Day, beyond the month-long August recess. Meanwhile, President Bush—returning from a trip to Europe—intensified administration lobbying of Congress and especially negotiations with Representative Norwood (Pear 2000b). The first of these efforts bore little fruit, but the one-on-one negotiations with Norwood did produce a bill[34] that the president "could sign," which passed the House by a partisan vote of 226–202, and that Norwood defended as the best possible legislative outcome, given the circumstances.

The best possible turned out to be not good enough. President Bush, in a Rose Garden speech after the House vote, declared that Republicans had broken "six years of gridlock in the task of protecting patients' rights from arbitrary medical decisions by bureaucrats."[35] A Republican congressman observed that passage of the Fletcher bill was 90 percent of the way and that just the act of going to conference would be "95 percent of the way there."[36] Representative Norwood worked to mend fences with his former colleagues[37] and urged the conference to reach a quick agreement upon a final version.

Senate Democrats did not take the same view of this process. Sen. John Edwards (D., N.C.), a sponsor of the Senate bill, observed, "Having a law that will be signed by the president isn't the goal."[38] When Congress returned from its August recess, Senate Democrats made no move to name conferees. After the September 11 terrorist attacks, attention shifted from health issues. Senator Daschle cancelled a preconference meeting with Richard Gephardt, the House minority leader, and later said that a conference would go forward only if it would be free of "contentious debate" and likely to yield "amicable compromise."[39] No further action was taken on these bills in the 2001 session.

In the course of six years, the two opposing camps managed to narrow their differences over the patients' rights to be protected, who would be covered under the act,[40] and the right to sue in both federal and state courts. They continued to disagree over the division of jurisdiction between federal and state courts, caps on damages, and the appeals process. But the lengthy saga had important side benefits. Republicans were able to check a policy that seemed wrongheaded to them and avoid some of the blame for defeating a popular initiative, and Democrats could exploit a popular agenda item over six years, divide Republicans, and divert them from mischief—such as restructuring Medicare. It may even be that the American people will benefit from this outcome rather than, for instance, seeing either the House or the Senate bill passed and then having to live with it.

II. BEYOND THE BALANCED BUDGET ACT: RHETORIC AND THE FUTURE

Health care politics generally revolves around the three major issues of cost, quality, and access. In national politics, the common pattern has been to alternate between a primary concern with cost containment and one of expanding access, especially for the uninsured. BBA 97 appeared to settle, for a time, what the federal government proposed to do about Medicare and Medicaid cost containment, and it made a substantial down payment on increased access for mothers and children, though it provided almost nothing for the remaining forty-three million uninsured. Quality of care, not generally a hot political topic, got plenty of response when presented as patients' rights and attacks on HMOs. Also during this period attention shifted to increased access because—for Democrats especially—it seemed the appropriate next step on the health care agenda, it suited campaign politics, and a budget surplus was projected.

The previous discussion of patients' bills of rights or managed care reform provides an illustration of how ideological issues, partisanship, and narrow parliamentary majorities can lead to gridlock. Most of the issues dealt with in this section involve proposals that were typically not marked up, debated, or voted upon. In other words, they were promoted largely as rhetoric and political tactics: to gain a point or counter the opposition, to stake out a position, or to bolster a long-term strategy. Advocates of these measures would, of course, have welcomed a legislative opening and an opportunity to turn their proposals into law. But there were no such opportunities—largely because of disagreements about how to extend access or to "reform" Medicare. As a consequence, there were few incentives to craft pragmatic compromises that could gain majority support. Over time, the partisan positions became more clearly and fully articulated—but they also tended increasingly to diverge.

Developments of this sort usually do not have sharply defined beginnings. Still, the cessation of immediate hostilities over the Balanced Budget Act of 1995 and the subsequent passage of HIPAA (Kassebaum-Kennedy) at the beginning of August 1996 serve as approximate markers. By then the Democrats, in the Congress and the administration, were seeing opportunities to go on the offense and were thinking about the election of 1996. It was in this context that President Clinton announced his quality initiative. He also said, during a Rose Garden occasion on August 2, that he still believed in the goal of universal coverage, but that it would have to be reached incrementally, "in a sort of a step-by-step basis."[41]

President Clinton's avowal, repeated on subsequent occasions, both made some history and grew in importance because of subsequent events. It was an election year. About the same time as Clinton's statement, both the White House and Democrats in Congress came forward with incremental proposals to expand access, especially for children and unemployed workers. A month later, Clinton announced his plans for a quality commission. This initiative was quickly denounced by Representative Thomas as "a political ploy in an election year,"[42] and by other Republicans as a wedge issue intended to divide Republicans while the president pursued his own agenda—which was to increase access to health care. In this context, Dick Armey, the House majority leader, expressed his view that Clinton had never given up on his goal of "a government run single payer system."[43]

The November election was seen by Democrats as a partial endorsement of this strategy and by at least some Republicans as a wake-up call. In his first major speech after the election, Clinton called for bipartisan collaboration to balance the budget and for a Medicare buy-in for early retirees. Other proposals would follow.[44] Conservative think-tanks and Republican leadership groups began saying they needed to respond to these Democratic initiatives with an agenda of their own that dealt with access issues. In the Senate, Trent Lott, for instance, declared that Republicans should have "alternatives and positive proposals" to counter the Democrats and prevent them from accomplishing, "a slice at a time," what they "were trying to do with the big health care package" of 1994.[45]

Early in 1997, both Republicans and Democrats began with modest incremental packages. These initiatives were soon shoved aside by the Balanced Budget Act, the big event for the year. Scarcely had that legislation been signed, though, when Clinton picked up on the incremental strategy, asking for Medicare buy-ins to cover temporarily unemployed workers and early retirees. In the same speech, to the Service Employees International Union, he called for legislation to protect health care consumers and patient privacy, and to prevent health insurance discrimination based upon genetic testing.[46] Access measures like these plus the Patients' Bill of Rights comprised much of the Democratic health care agenda in the new Congress.

Although 1998 was an election year and the congressional Republicans were aware of the need for an attractive health care agenda, they got off to a slow start in the new session. The House especially was distracted by the Monica Lewinsky scandal and the looming prospect of an impeachment battle. Some wanted to see what recommendations would be produced by the Bipartisan Commission on the Future of Medicare. Within the House, there were increasing divisions between hard-line conservatives and moderates, and there were important differences, in both the House and the Senate, over how to approach the issues of access and of patients' rights.

The Republican leadership, generally, would have preferred that the issue of patients' rights simply go away and that increased access be achieved through a combination of tax credits and/or insurance reform—but not through incremental additions to Medicare and Medicaid, the two big entitlement programs. The Republican approach, which had more merit than suggested by a casual appraisal, would provide a procompetition and less regulative alternative, reduce dependence on employer-sponsored insurance, and get the government, Republicans especially, out of the politically distasteful business of micromanaging medical care.

In 1998, as noted above (see p. 336), the House Republican leadership appointed one of its multijurisdictional task forces to develop an alternative to Norwood's PARCA. One part of their strategy to make their own Patient Protection Act more acceptable to their own membership and business constituency was to include some access features, such as risk pools for the small businesses and the self-employed,[47] and HealthMarts, which adapted an FEHBP approach for a larger market. This leadership initiative did not get under way until March 1998, by which time PARCA and the administration's own Patients' Bill of Rights had gained political momentum and were dominating the health care agenda. The Patient Protection Act, which was the only significant Republican access initiative for the year,[48] passed the House with a six-vote margin and then expired at the end of the session when the Senate failed to pass a counterpart of its own.

A charge made by Republicans was that Clinton and the Democrats hoped to gain by an incremental strategy what they had failed to get in their ambitious health care reform attempt of 1993–94. Some, including Trent Lott, also saw their sponsorship of patients' rights as a divide-and-conquer strategy— dividing Republicans and diverting their legislative energies from a sensible and moderate attempt to provide coverage for the uninsured to a futile and misguided patients' rights boondoggle. True or not, these beliefs may have shaped behavior in some important ways.

In general, Democrats never denied that they believed in universal access to health care and in moving incrementally toward that goal. What they did deny was that they were trying to resurrect the Health Security Act, either in part or in its entirety.[49] Similarly, the Democratic quality and patients' rights initiatives were in part campaign ploys, but they were also needed managed care reforms.[50] To be sure, Democrats mourned little over the Republican mismanagement of these issues, but they were as surprised as the Republicans by the astonishing persistence and legislative successes of Norwood and his allies. It would be closer to the truth to say that the Republicans brought these calamities on themselves than that they were ambushed by the Democrats.

It is of interest to examine the situation and consider how it might have seemed to Republicans at the time. They had lost, by and large, on structural reform of Medicare, which remained an entrenched, single-payer entitlement system with administered pricing, and mere gestures in the direction of pro-competition or private market features. The quality provisions made it, if any-thing, more impervious to reform of the kind Republicans had in mind. Also, Medicare and Medicaid, as legislative vehicles, provided many opportunities for extending benefits and coverage: adding drugs and long-term care, and covering youth and early retirees, the unemployed, and the working disabled. Even if the ultimate goal might be unclear or not even under consideration, the Democrats were, in fact, increasing entitlements and expanding a single-payer system far beyond its original conception.

The Democratic strategy, pushed especially by President Clinton, empha-sized incremental extensions of the Medicare and Medicaid entitlements, with some use of tax credits. In his 1999 budget, released on February 1, the pres-ident reiterated a 1998 proposal for Medicare buy-ins for those aged sixty-two to sixty-five—many of them early retirees—who lacked group insurance, He offered the same option to displaced workers between fifty-five and sixty-five years of age. Then in midyear came the administration proposal for a pre-scription drug benefit for Medicare enrollees. Medicaid initiatives included a program to extend coverage to the working disabled. In addition, states would be allowed to cover home and community-based long-term care up to 300 percent of the FPL. Most important was proposed coverage for low-income children to age twenty-one. This initiative was extended in the following year with FamilyCare, a program to provide coverage for parents of children enrolled in either Medicaid or SCHIP. This single program was expected to cover over four million people in the next ten years.[51]

The administration initiatives made some use of tax credits. Workers tak-ing advantage of the buy-in proposals would receive tax credits equal to 25 percent of the premium; small firms that participated in purchasing coalitions or insurance pools would get a 20 percent tax credit; and tax credits would be used to help families pay for long-term care. The central thrust of the admin-istration proposals, though, was to increase the Medicare and Medicaid enti-tlements or add to coverage and/or benefits under the existing entitlements. In so doing, they were extending programs originally intended for the elderly, disabled, and poor to cover the uninsured—broadening the entitlements into new and unexplored territory.

From the Republican point of view, there was an abundance of reasons for not liking this thrust of the Democratic proposals. In the most immediate sense, it extended entitlements. It would either increase taxes or put new burdens upon existing revenue streams in a year in which Republicans were advocating a 10 percent across-the-board tax cut. It would further extend the single-payer administrative or "bureaucratic" model rather than making steps toward a procompetition, market-oriented, and "modernized" version of Medicare, and it was a categorical, incremental approach, that left out most of the uninsured, despite the universalistic concerns expressed for their plight.

Timing was important in this situation. After the passage of the Balanced Budget Act of 1997, both parties were seeking to stake out their health policy agendas for the future. For the Republican leadership—thwarted by the patients' bill of rights controversy—this need grew in urgency with the passing months. Partisan politics and gridlock meant that little of substance was likely to be accomplished in 1999 or 2000, so that strategic positioning for the campaign became still more important. By 1999, Congress was getting used to a budget surplus. In that environment, tax cuts had a new appeal. It also made sense, both from a policy and a political perspective, to think again about tax cuts and about the forty-three million[52] or so without health insurance—not just those with a favored categorical status.

Countering a Democratic emphasis on entitlements, the Republican agenda was tax credits and deductions and private sector, market-oriented support for private insurance. Some of their schemes, such as MSAs and risk pools for small business and the self-employed, go back even before the Balanced Budget Act of 1995. Most of these earlier initiatives were repeated with modifications, but the 1999 session loosed a cascade of tax-related proposals—Republican, bipartisan, and Democratic. Several related approaches were made part of an overall tax-reduction strategy by Republicans and tied in with other private sector, market-oriented insurance reforms.

The Armey plan, "Fair Care for the Uninsured," was the most visible of these proposals, both for its basic policy provisions and because of its sponsorship by the House majority leader. It also had some bipartisan support. Pete Stark, the ranking Democrat on the Health subcommittee, joined with Dick Armey in a *New York Times* statement supporting the initiative, though later he refused to cosponsor it because of disagreements over details. This bill, which followed closely a model advocated by the first President Bush and by the National Association of Health Underwriters, would have created a refundable tax credit[53] of $800 per adult and $400 per child up to an annual family maximum of $2,400 for persons, not otherwise insured, to purchase health insurance from a qualified plan. The maximum, later raised to $3,000, was an amount calculated by the NAHU to avoid "crowding out" employment-based insurance (Guenther 2001; see also Gruber and Poterba 1995). One interesting feature was a provision that unused tax credits would be pooled to create a "safety net" block grant that states could use to create an insurance fund for high-risk individuals or to develop other ways to cover the uninsured.

Aside from its bipartisan appeal and indications of White House support, this proposal had a number of attractive features. One was its relatively low cost. There was an element of fairness, since it provided a tax benefit to those without the automatic tax exemption that came with employer-based coverage. It could be easily combined with MSAs, insurance pools, or a Health-Marts option. It could be income related and targeted toward the poor, or used to spread risk. It could even serve, in a version proposed by Rep. Bill Thomas, to sever completely the ties between the employer and health insurance and create the foundation for universal individual coverage.

The larger vision behind this proposal was appealing, and profoundly so to many Republicans. It offered a way to extend health insurance to the uninsured, including some of their own strongest and most deserving supporters: the hard-working self-employed and small-business people. It empowered individuals and small groups, creating incentives for them to manage their own affairs and to become informed consumers of health care, who would make their own choices between quality, access, and ultimate cost. Finally, it was a nonregulative, nonbureaucratic, decentralizing, and individualistic way of extending health insurance.

There may be an important and unpleasant truth underlying this particular vision. Americans have never been well schooled in the responsibilities that go along with social or health insurance. They like the benefits of health insurance but not the sacrifices that make it work. They want the lowest premiums but the latest technology and "miracle" drugs. For a time, managed care and HMOs seemed like a relatively painless way to control costs. Now, neither managed care nor administered prices seem adequate. It may be that more effective cost constraint is impossible without some way of motivating individuals to take greater responsibility for their own health and for the costs of the medical care they receive. Tax credits are an imperfect instrument, but if used both to empower and to create incentives they could make a vital contribution.

Coming up with an attractive concept is still a long way from developing an acceptable way of implementing it. Tax credits would, by themselves, purchase little for an isolated individual, and restricting their use to an acceptable health plan would still leave a tax credit scheme vulnerable—like MSAs and like most risk pools—to high administrative costs and favorable risk selection. Many would be unable to buy adequate health insurance with subsidies of the size being discussed. With a low subsidy, the take-up rate—the number using the tax credit—might be so low that few would benefit while the per capita expenditure by the government would be unacceptably high.[54] If the subsidy were raised, the scheme would run into serious crowding-out problems, which would displace employer insurance and could seriously threaten the stability of the employer-based system. A study by the Lewin Group, for instance, estimated that a tax credit that paid half of the premium—about the amount in several proposals—would be used by only seven million of the uninsured. According to their estimates, it would take a tax credit of 80 percent to reach as many as 14.6 million of the uninsured.[55] At that level, the crowding-out problem would become intolerable. In this context, some experts began talking again about individual or employer mandates as a way to get the uninsured enrolled. That would probably take comprehensive insurance reform to develop acceptable offerings to be purchased.

An incremental Democratic strategy of building upon Medicare and Medicaid had its problems too. Adverse selection and dividing the risk pool, though much less of a threat, could still occur—for instance, with individual buy-ins or with risk selection under state programs. Crowding out as well as low participation rates would be an issue, both for Medicare and Medicaid or SCHIP. Furthermore, these programs built upon historically established categories and brought with them the traditional problems of gaps in coverage, need for outreach, and complicated eligibility requirements.[56] In the aggregate a relatively small minority of those eligible were likely to be enrolled. There were also political difficulties. Extending coverage to those over eighteen years of age, for example, was not nearly as appealing, politically, as covering pregnant women and children. States might also be reluctant: a proposal to cover the families of Medicaid and SCHIP children, for instance, had not been popular with the states—i.e., when made available as an option under Section 1931.[57] Aside from the fact that the Democratic proposal did little to cover the rest of the uninsured population, the Republican majority in both House and Senate were adamantly opposed to major entitlement extensions— even more so because some Republicans saw them as pieces of a larger, covert strategy to move toward a single-payer system of national health insurance.

The incremental strategies of both Democrats and Republicans failed with few minor exceptions. Since both were intended largely for campaign positioning and debate, the fact that they failed as legislative initiatives is not surprising nor was their failure especially important. However, the interpretation of these events may be of larger significance, especially in revealing some limitations of incremental approaches and the way in which structural issues intrude forcefully as these limits begin to be reached.

An important tie-in with structural issues, for both Republicans and Democrats, was that the incrementalism was often and by calculation strategic in nature, contributing to more comprehensive objectives, such as a preserving a particular vision of Medicare or advancing a broad procompetition, private sector philosophy. With the semipermanent political campaigning on both sides, even minor and relatively innocent incremental proposals often acquired a high political valence or seemed inspired by a partisan plot to gain advantage. When incrementalism was itself part of a campaign, it did not have to go far or gain much momentum before it gave rise to alarm and met with resistance.

Increasing access by increments was also the kind of endeavor that rather quickly began to raise larger issues of structural and comprehensive reform. From the nature of the enterprise, increasing access can result in crowding out and uneven participation or risk selection. Such problems then generate a need—or a demand—for mandates or for inducements to get insurers to continue their coverage, and for ways to increase the risk pool, curb risk selection, or otherwise provide for the high-risk groups. So, inevitably, incremental approaches to access tend to reach limits—economic, structural, and political. In this context, both Democrats and Republicans began talking once again about such topics as tax credits, employer and individual mandates, and strategies for universal coverage—but mostly as campaign rhetoric rather than as legislative proposals they would develop in detail and make a serious effort to pass.

The Bipartisan Commission

The National Bipartisan Commission on the Future of Medicare was included in BBA 1997 primarily as a concession to members in both houses who were concerned that not enough had been done to assure the long-term solvency of the Medicare program, especially with the enormous drain that would be created by the retirement of the baby boom generation, rising medical expenses, and a declining ratio of contributors to beneficiaries. In one brief sentence, the commission was also directed to "make recommendations regarding a comprehensive approach to preserve the program," but the primary thrust of Section 4021 was preservation of fiscal soundness, not a restructuring of Medicare.

Under the circumstances, not much was expected of the commission. With a report due in March 1999, about a year of working time remained—a short period in which to hire staff, establish an agenda, develop task force reports, and reach final recommendations. Moreover, BBA 97 had just dealt comprehensively with cost containment and the trust fund seemed safe until at least 2008. Therefore, the two major concerns that had generally driven Medicare reform—the budget deficit and threats to the trust fund—were much diminished. As the appointments were being discussed, pundits observed that there was neither time nor a political climate that would support major structural changes. Under the circumstances, even prominent policy brokers who strongly favored such reforms said that the commission could might best use its time in seeking to improve the finances of the traditional FFS program and perhaps investigate a "defined contribution" alternative, but otherwise try to educate the general public about some of the long-term problems.[58]

Several members, like Senator John Breaux, the chairman, and Representative Bill Thomas, urgently wished to move on structural reform. Of the initial seventeen appointees, eight were already strongly committed to a defined contribution approach or premium support. Two others were sympathetic or open to considering such an option. Those opposed to this agenda protested that there was no pressing need for structural reform and that other options should be considered, but there was neither time nor staff resources to explore alternatives in any depth, and the minority had no systematically developed alternative of its own. For that matter, the advocates of structural reform—most of whom already shared a commitment to a defined contribution—did not explore alternatives either: they simply took the Federal Employees Health Benefits Program (FEHBP) as a template, modifying it in some particulars.

The most important recommendation of the commission was for a comprehensive restructuring of Medicare, with "premium support" as the method of financing. Administration of the system would be modeled on the FEHB program, with the traditional fee-for-service program included as one of the competing plans. Private plans would be required to offer a "high option" that would include a benefits package equal at least to that under the FFS program, but otherwise could vary benefits, copays, and deductibles, subject to approval by a governing Medicare board. The government contribution would be limited to the computed national average premium for a standard benefits package, adjusted for risk and geographic variations, and updated annually. Costs would be held down by consumer incentives and by a competitive bidding process, supervised by the Medicare board. The board would also monitor plan offerings and activities with respect to such matters as actuarial and fiscal soundness, quality and performance, and adverse selection.[59]

The commission proposal was quickly denounced, especially by Democrats who were veterans of the 1995 BBA struggle, as a "defined contribution" under a different name. One critic pointed out, as a dubious merit, that it would at least be more direct in its action, since the commission proposal would quickly force beneficiaries into managed care plans, while the Medicare Preservation Act, with its complex look-back scheme, would drive out FFS providers first, with beneficiaries to follow.[60] By way of further comparison, the Medicare Preservation Act of 1995, especially in the House version, was deliberately gentle with beneficiaries, while the commission proposal would increase the eligibility age from sixty-five to sixty-seven, and endorsed copays as a desirable way of constraining costs.

An important procedural requirement for the commission, imposed by Congress in the original legislation, was a " supermajority" of 11 votes of 17 to approve the final report. This provision had come from the White House, at the insistence of Gene Sperling, who feared the partisan tendency of such a commission and wished to build in some extra protection.[61] As a result, with eight Republicans and two Democrats—John Breaux and Bob Kerrey—favoring a defined contribution or premium support, only one person was needed for a majority. Among the other members of the commission, Stuart Altman—a former chairman of ProPAC and earlier a sponsor of a Medicare HMO alternative—and Laura Tyson—an economist and former chairwoman of Clinton's Council of Economic Advisers—were both favorably inclined toward managed care options. Since either of them could complete a majority, they were in a strong bargaining position.

One way that their leverage was exerted was in support of a pharmaceutical benefit. Although there was already a Democratic bill in Congress and a number of states were legislating in this field, the original version of the commission proposal had no pharmaceutical benefit, except for a requirement that Medigap plans cover drugs. As the commission sought agreement on its draft version late in January 1999, several members, including Stuart Altman, said that they could not agree to the premium support concept unless a prescription drug benefit were also included.[62]

Discussion of the pharmaceutical benefit went on for some time, with the commission eventually announcing an agreement of this issue on March 8, 1999, roughly one week before their final meeting. Though this inclusion was an important addition to entitlements, the plan itself was tough on beneficiaries and gentle toward the drug companies. Basically, it would require both FFS and managed care plans to offer beneficiaries a "high option" choice with prescription benefits, but without controls on prices and no limits on cost sharing, except for a required stop-loss or catastrophic limit. Drug coverage options would have to pay for themselves, without any across-the-board subsidy, which both Altman and Tyson had urged.[63] Pharmaceuticals for low-income beneficiaries would be included in comprehensive coverage for all *eligible* individuals below 135 percent of the FPL, a provision that still left this group subject to the exceptions and local variations of Medicare and Medicaid coverage for the poor. The plan was grudging, exposed Medicare beneficiaries to heavy deductibles and copays, with new savings coming from the beneficiary, not the provider side.

During this same period, the commission was wrestling with the issues of long-term solvency and how to finance the plan. An interesting perspective was contributed, along the way, by a Congressional Budget Office report in February that said the commission proposal was "clearly promising," but lacked enough detail to estimate its ultimate potential for cost saving. CBO commented that much of the success of the plan would depend on how well the private sector performed in holding down its costs and whether the Medicare oversight board would have sufficient leverage to restrain the "benefit creep" in these private plans, which were being driven by such factors as explosive medical technology and rising consumer expectations. CBO further observed that adapting the FEBHP model to Medicare beneficiaries would be a "formidable challenge," taxing the administrative capabilities of such a board.[64]

A final meeting, scheduled for March 3, was postponed for a week while the commission members sought agreement on financing issues. The major sticking point was President Clinton's recommendation that 15 percent of the projected budget surplus be set aside in order to extend Medicare solvency from 2008 to 2020. Republican members of the commission objected, saying that the Clinton proposal was an "accounting gimmick" that would pour more money into a failed program. Democrats, on the other side, said that the money would sustain Medicare while Congress considered the reform recommendations.[65] On this issue, neither Stuart Altman or Laura Tyson would budge. So, the commission proposal went down by a vote of 10–7, one vote short of the required supermajority. Even that was not the end. At the request of the chairmen, the commission agreed to postpone a last, final decision until March 16, when they would meet briefly in the afternoon and vote again. The result was the same: ten in favor, seven against.

The budget surplus issue was a surprise to outsiders,[66] even seen as a politically motivated pretext for defeating the plan despite its substantive merits. Yet, the underlying issue was the same that proved critical with the Medicare Preservation Act of 1995: whether the new scheme would preserve the traditional FFS program as a viable option or whether it would gradually undermine it. Committing some of the budget surplus to Medicare would provide some insurance—extending solvency, affirming a commitment to the program, and buying time for thoughtful deliberation and for other options to be developed.

Assessing the Bipartisan Commission is difficult. It provided Republicans and some procompetition Democrats with a plausible proposal for restructuring Medicare that was, on the whole, easier to defend publicly than the earlier Medicare Preservation Act of 1995. It has served to advance public debate by giving visibility to some of the issues and problems and articulating proposed solutions within a single scheme. It also stimulated the administration to put forward a comprehensive proposal of its own.

As an exercise in bipartisan collaboration, the commission was a dismal failure that, at best, provides cautionary lessons for the future. Essentially, it was an episode in the continuing political struggle over the future of Medicare, not a serious effort to come together in a genuine bipartisan way. Most of the appointees were major players in that conflict, with strong political and program commitments of their own. Unlike the earlier Quality Commission, little attention was paid to the kind of agenda, staffing, and procedures that would promote problem-solving and work toward an ultimate consensus. Instead, it became a vehicle for advancing, on another level, the policies held by individual stakeholders, who ended far apart and as separated along partisan lines as when they began.[67] Ironically, the main task with which the commission was charged—to deal with the "long-term financial condition" of the Medicare program—was the major issue on which they were unable to reach a consensus and upon which the commission foundered.

The CBO report suggests some dubious assumptions or possible weaknesses in the commission proposal. One is a supposition that the extent and nature of competition among health plans will act as a major cost restraint. CBO was skeptical, especially given industry trends toward consolidation and the inflationary pressures upon managed care plans. Despite the lack of systematic evidence or even persuasive argument, confidence in the efficacy of market competition to constrain the costs of managed care plans seems to be an unexamined belief based upon occasional behavior, a few regional examples, or faith. The commission plan also spoke of "risk adjustment" by the Medicare board as though monitoring or correcting for either risk aversion strategies or adverse selection would be a technically simple and administratively easy task. The contemporary experience of HCFA (CMA) with implementing a managed care risk adjuster indicates that it is likely to be neither; and CBO's caveat about the board's lack of "leverage" (read, administrative muscle and political clout) to deal with the problem seems much in point. Along with CBO, other observers were concerned about the role of the marketing board, especially with respect to such critical activities as implementation of the new system, negotiating with private plans, and monitoring and enforcement activities.[68]

Ultimately, the Bipartisan Commission on the Future of Medicare seemed to be less about Medicare as most people knew it, than about the inclusion of Medicare in a competitive scheme without making clear how that scheme itself would work, or how Medicare—for the more than 85 percent remaining in the FFS program—would be continued or improved in future years.

Despite the defeat of the commission proposal, it was soon resurrected, first as a Breaux-Thomas initiative, and later as the Breaux-Frist Medicare Preservation and Improvement Act,[69] which was first unveiled on November 9, 1999. The basic FEHBP template remained, but Breaux-Frist was kinder to beneficiaries. It provided a more generous pharmaceutical benefit, available to all Medicare beneficiaries. It dropped the increase in the age of eligibility from sixty-five to sixty-seven. Cost-sharing was reduced. The bill was never debated on the floor of either house, but it became unofficially the Republican policy and was adopted, in general terms, by George W. Bush in his campaign for the presidency.

The election of 2000 produced a 50–50 tie in the Senate and an initial wariness about proceeding with controversial and divisive initiatives such as Breaux-Frist. A weighty reason for going ahead, according to Senator Frist, was the election of a Republican president committed to the commission proposal for reform of Medicare. In other words, the Republicans would be redeeming a campaign pledge, now, with the power and prestige of the president on their side. Steep increases in the cost of prescription drugs were a second major factor, making a pharmaceutical benefit even more critical for seniors. The high cost of this benefit would strengthen the argument for restructuring Medicare (Toner 2001a). In this way, the drug benefit—a popular Democratic issue—could be embraced by Republicans and turned to their advantage. Senator Frist did not make the additional point, though it was obvious, that this approach would articulate well with the larger Republican strategy of reducing taxes and disbursing the surplus.

When the Breaux-Frist initiative was revived, early in 2001, it came in two forms. One was the original Medicare Preservation and Improvement Act (S 357), proposing a complete restructuring based on the FEHBP model. The second, the Medicare Prescription Drug and Modernization Act of 2001 (S. 358)—often referred to as Breaux-Frist II—took an incremental approach. The traditional FFS program would remain, much as it was—a defined benefit, under HCFA and the secretary of DHHS. Managed care plans, though, would be administered by a newly created Medicare Competition Agency, established as an independent agency with a commissioner and a board.[70] Managed care contracts would be awarded through a competitive bidding process that increased incentives and risk but remained tied to a "county specific per capita cost." Minimal administrative reforms were proposed for the FFS program, though the salary of the HCFA administrator would be raised. A comprehensive drug benefit was added that was not especially generous to FFS beneficiaries,[71] but would provide a good basis for bipartisan negotiation.

Taken together, the two versions of Breaux-Frist contained proposals similar to those made earlier by President Clinton and by Sen. Bob Graham and were seriously considered by the Democratic members of the Finance Committee. Democrats were concerned, however, about the implications of considering managed care provisions before the pharmaceutical benefit, about the size of the drug benefit, burdens on beneficiaries, and the incentives for risk selection in the latter program.[72] They also thought that too much attention was being given to managed competition and not enough to reforming Medicare for the more than 85 percent of the beneficiaries still enrolled in and preferring to remain in the traditional FFS program.[73] Still, they continued to work with Republicans on the Breaux-Frist proposals even after the May 24 turnover. Forecasts about the economy and the need to use Medicare and Social Security surpluses to augment revenues, however, made an expensive pharmacy benefit increasingly hard to entertain. And without a pharmacy benefit, Breaux-Frist in either version, lost most of its bipartisan appeal. After September 11, major restructuring of Medicare was abandoned for that session of Congress.

The President's Plan to Modernize and Strengthen Medicare

On March 16, 1999, a few hours before the Bipartisan Commission took its final vote, President Clinton announced that he would offer an alternative. In part, this move was preemptive,[74] especially in its timing, since the Congress had made clear that it would move quickly on the commission's proposals. The administration was also looking forward to the year 2000. Major elements of the plan that was subsequently developed had been included two months earlier in the State of the Union Address: especially the reform of Medicare, a pharmaceutical benefit, and committing some part of the budget surplus to assure long-term solvency of the Medicare program.

The president said at the time that "our commitment is clear," which was a signal to the administration to get busy.[75] With a tight schedule, there was no time for information and proposals to bubble up from HCFA, to do the more than seventy iterations for the drug program, or to get the usual administrative clearances. The plan was developed at the top level, primarily by White House staff,[76] though with a working group drawn from HCFA's Office of Legislation. It was the kind of product for which presidential priorities, timing and strategic political calculations, and getting a few big numbers right were most essential. Relying largely on political appointees within the White House also protected the career civil servants from being embroiled in political controversy.[77]

A key feature of the Clinton plan, announced on June 29, was the "competitive defined benefit," an *entitlement* that guaranteed to every Medicare recipient a standard benefit package, including prescription drugs. Plans within the system would compete, but on a somewhat different footing. Following the defined-benefit concept, beneficiaries would receive actuarial equivalent benefits under either FFS or managed care. Initially, managed care plans would be paid 4 percent less, an amount estimated from rates for 2003.[78] A payment adjustment would be made for geographic cost differences. Plans would then compete on price and quality, but not by varying basic benefits—a practice that, in the administration's view, tended to encourage benefit creep and risk selection. To assure that competition would be based on price and not on risk selection, the risk adjustment system mandated under BBA 97 would be fully implemented by 2004.[79] If a plan could deliver the defined benefits for less, beneficiaries who chose that plan would receive 75 percent of the savings, with 25 percent returned to the federal government. Plans could offer more benefits, but only as an addition to the basic package. Beneficiaries who chose the more expensive options would have to pay for them, either out-of-pocket or through improved Medigap policies.

A second major element of the Clinton plan was to "modernize" and strengthen the traditional FFS program. It would be strengthened with new administrative authority, adopting the "prudent purchaser" concept urged by HCFA (see pp. 193–94) and several administrative reforms supported by the General Accounting Office, some already in use by large indemnity insurers and other government programs, such as the Veterans Administration and CHAMPUS. Among these were, for example, FFS primary care and disease case management, selective contracting with preferred providers and "centers of excellence," and competitive pricing of Part B supplies and services. These administrative changes would give HCFA freedom to manage more efficiently. They did raise some questions about HCFA's role as a major or sole purchaser of medical supplies and services, and about the kind of political stir this would occasion. However that may be the proposed measures stopped short of using commanding market power to leverage lower premiums from health plans.[80]

The "modernization" part applied mostly to benefits, including some familiar administration perennials as well as a new prescription drug proposal. The plan would allow beneficiaries between the ages of sixty-two and sixty-five to buy into the program for about $300 per month. It would eliminate copays and deductibles for all preventive services covered by Medicare. The major addition was, of course, the prescription drug benefit, to begin in 2002, and estimated to cost $118 billion over ten years. Also included was $7.5 billion for hospitals, to be gotten by carving out DSH payments to managed care plans and delaying for two years the implementation of payment adjustments for transfer patients.[81] These expenditures would be partly offset by a 20 percent copay for clinical laboratory services,[82] by indexing the Part B deductible for inflation, and from savings realized when patients chose lower priced plans.

The Medicare prescription drug benefit—to be added as a new Part D—would pay half of drug costs, without any deductible, up to a limit of $5,000 a year. Premium costs would begin at $24 a month and rise to $44 a month when fully phased in by 2008. After the $5,000 cap was reached, beneficiaries could claim a 10 percent discount on prescriptions, an amount typically received by large purchasers. The premium would be eliminated for beneficiaries with incomes below 135 percent of the federal poverty line; and premiums would be subsidized for those between 135 and 150 percent of the poverty level. Incentives would be created for employers who maintained a prescription benefit equivalent to the one offered by Medicare. Guidelines for the program would be established by HCFA, but actual administration would be through private sector pharmacy benefits managers, entities that could be roughly described as managed care plans for drugs.

A comment on the president's drug benefit is that it seems unexciting and less than generous to beneficiaries. Coverage began at $2,000 a year and only gradually rose to $5,000 a year,[83] after which beneficiaries would be eligible for a less than overwhelming 10 percent discount—which many pharmacies would have given them anyway. Moreover, there was no catastrophic limit—especially important to elderly patients with chronic and often severe conditions.

The proposal was written with an awareness that it would face stiff opposition, both within Congress and from the drug companies. Also, like other entitlements, it could be improved upon incrementally. For instance, the draft version had a provision, later dropped, that would have issued Medicare beneficiaries a card allowing them to get the price discounts available to Medicaid plans.[84] This discount card, with its tie to Medicaid prices, could have been an important provision in the proposed legislation.[85] The proposal was stiffly opposed by the pharmaceutical companies because of its direct monetary implications, and because it would have exposed their pricing practices to public view. It was dropped in the final version and the insipid 10 percent discount substituted; but the earlier version suggests what the future might hold. Moreover, as various plans were debated over the next year, Democrats in Congress came up with their own proposals to fatten the benefit. For instance, under a version unveiled by Senator Graham in June 2000, beneficiaries would pay an initial $250 deductible, but thereafter no limits would be imposed. Above the deductible, Medicare would pay 50 percent up to $3,500, then increase payments to 75 percent, and after the out-of-pocket reached $4,000 would pay any additional drug expenses.[87] Although the benefit would be administered by pharmaceutical benefit management plans, the government would be exercising oversight over coverage and costs, much as it has done with Parts A through C of the Medicare benefit.

The other major proposal in the president's plan was to commit $794 billion—about 15 percent of the anticipated budget surplus over the next fifteen years—to extend solvency of the trust fund from 2015 to 2027. About $45.5 billion of this amount would help pay for the pharmaceutical benefit, the rest of which would be financed by savings from plan competition and administrative efficiencies.[94] For a president with a strong awareness of the relation between budget surpluses and deficits and the ups and downs of the business cycle, this gesture would seem to be symbolic rather than based on sound expectations. But it was important as a marker, affirming an intention to use a substantial part of the budget surplus to shore up entitlements and to make "investments" in human capital and other priority programs rather than disbursing the surplus with tax cuts. The initiative illustrated again a Democratic tendency to "institutionalize" the future, or lock in the options for Medicare.

A Republican criticism of the president's "Plan to Modernize and Strengthen Medicare" was that it committed still more dollars—in this instance $750 billion—to prop up a "failed" program. Wrapped in the partisan rhetoric of the moment, that appreciation is likely to be dismissed, but it deserves closer attention.

The administration and the congressional Democrats have, especially since 1995, given more attention to increasing entitlements and defending the Medicare (and Medicaid) programs from attack than to effective cost containment. Such an approach reflected their own priorities as well as recognizing the political reality that Medicare was being attacked—both the entitlement as such and the fee-for-service program specifically. In general, their defense of the program has been politically successful—so far, at least. The president's plan, though, with $795 billion to assure solvency—even acknowledging the baby boomer issue—suggests that, fiscally, there continues to be a problem.

One of the most important differences between the president's plan and the proposal of the Bipartisan Commission is the competitive treatment of Medicare. Under the commission proposal, Medicare competes with the whole array of managed care plans. With the president's plan, it is given a separate status and assured support by a defined benefit. So that Medicare can compete on equal—even advantageous—terms, a pharmaceutical benefit is added and the whole scheme conditioned upon the successful development of a managed care risk adjuster. If such a risk adjuster were developed and successfully implemented, it would help assure more adequate compensation for those providers and institutions that care for the high-cost chronically and severely ill patients. In these respects, the president's plan "equalizes" competition between the FFS program and managed care, and it would address adverse selection and the burden of costly patients—by paying for the disproportionate expense,

Cost containment suffers. Even taking the administration's own estimates at face value, the projected savings under the president's plan are modest. Savings of $39 billion, the largest single amount, would come not from the president's plan itself, but by extending the life of cost-saving provisions already legislated by the BBA 97. Even these savings were partially offset by a $7.5 billion give-back to providers, mostly hospitals. The whole array of private sector "prudent purchaser" techniques, including a preferred provider option, were estimated at $25 billion over ten years. Ten-year savings for the "competitive defined benefit" were only $8 billion. The grand total was $72 billion over ten years. Against this was a $7.5 billion give-back, $118 billion for the pharmaceutical benefit, and $795 billion for the trust fund.

One question that the president's Plan brings to mind is whether administered pricing may not be approaching its political limits as a cost saver, It was notable, for instance, that neither with respect to the managed care premium nor for the pharmaceutical benefit did the administration propose to use its single-payer advantage to negotiate lower prices. Managed care plans were left free to set their own premiums. And the administration, through Gene Sperling, specifically denied that any "accumulated bargaining power" would be used to seek cost savings from the pharmaceutical benefit.[88] This behavior suggests an awareness by the administration that the advantage a "prudent purchaser" might theoretically have as a single payer would soon be curtailed by political opposition if used to negotiate steep price cuts.

The cost containment measures legislated by BBA 97 have proven politically difficult to implement and have led to an alarming number of plan withdrawals[89] from Medicare participation and to a series of give-backs over two years totaling $41 billion, with threats of more to come. Meanwhile, the difficulty of securing encounter data to develop a managed care risk adjuster has slowed progress along that path to a crawl.[90] Whatever technical promise administered pricing may have, its political capacity to exact savings seems increasingly limited, especially given the effectiveness with which providers, consumers, and politicians can join in lobbying the government for relief.

Yet Democrats remain committed to this approach—and build upon it and entrench it with layers of regulation—because they do not see a politically viable alternative that will also protect the poor, the disabled, and the frail elderly with affordable care of acceptable quality. In so doing, they gain a comparative advantage in regulatory techniques and in defending the status quo, but often overlook its limitations and hidden costs: regulatory burden, fraud and abuse, programmatic conservatism, and difficulty of reform.

Republicans and economists of the procompetition, market-oriented variety, for their part act as though competition in the healthcare market place were a natural state or mode of behavior, prevented mainly by the intrusion of regulation. In so doing, they fail to acknowledge how unusual and contrived such behavior is and the amount of regulation and persistent surveillance that is needed to make an approximation to such a market work, even as partially and intermittently as it does. They also make light of or ignore the special difficulty risk selection poses for programs like Medicare, in which—to remind the reader again—70 percent of the patient care costs are occasioned by 10 percent of the beneficiaries.[91] So far, managed care enthusiasts have yet to make the case that a restructuring of Medicare based on a defined contribution or premium support will assure adequate care for these most vulnerable beneficiaries.

Despite these differences, there has been significant progress: in clarifying underlying issues, narrowing differences in policy, and working together across party lines. President Clinton's "Plan to Modernize and Strengthen Medicare" gave increased visibility and programmatic importance to Medicare's special responsibility for the most vulnerable and costly beneficiaries. Two years later, Senator Graham's "Medicare Reform Act of 2001" set forth in detailed, legislative language what quality care for the severely and chronically ill might entail,[92] including the administrative reforms needed to address this challenge. Both plans emphasized negotiation as an important cost containment device but also acknowledged the importance of competition, proposing new ways to increase its role.[93] One important initiative— scarcely noticed amidst the rhetoric—was the proposal in Clinton's plan for a "competitive defined benefit," a step that acknowledged the need for cost-containment measures that put a greater burden on beneficiary demand. Taken together, these steps helped to bring differences between Democrats and Republicans within the range of negotiation.

From the other side, Breaux-Frist II made some important concessions, as well as laying down a Republican marker or two. It put on the table a serious proposal for a pharmaceutical benefit. It also acknowledged the entitlement status of Medicare, retaining a defined benefit and tying managed care premiums to a modified version of the ACR. Managed care would be organized separately, but as a single-head agency, not a board. In effect, there would be a structure similar to FEHBP for MCOs, but FFS Medicare would not be included and would continue to be supported separately as an entitlement. These concessions impressed Finance Committee Democrats sufficiently that they continued working with the Republicans until September 11 imposed new priorities and time constraints, postponing Medicare reform for another year.[94]

Gridlock?

According to William Safire, "gridlock" was first used to describe the traffic congestion that resulted from a 1980 transit strike in New York City. The term was immediately extended to politics—first, to the perennial legislative logjam, but later, and increasingly, to the inability of congressional partisans to agree (Safire 1993:305). It is used in this latter sense in the present context.

Surveying Medicare and Medicaid legislative attempts following BBA 97, it is tempting to label all of them casualties of gridlock. Nothing of consequence passed, except for give-backs, regulatory relief, and postponements of statutory deadlines. Six years of bickering over patients' rights ended with a stalemate in 2001 when the Senate refused to appoint conferees. Attempts to increase access by extending Medicare or using Medicaid or SCHIP funds to cover the unemployed or uninsured failed with minor exceptions, largely because of ideological differences over entitlements, calculations of strategic advantage, and distrust of others' motives. What appeared to be a moderate, well-intentioned, and bipartisan effort to restructure Medicare stalled, in part, because of ideological differences and maneuvering for political advantage[95] Even the retrograde effort to upset the political settlement reached by BBA 97 for Medicaid was thwarted largely because of a failure of Congress to take action and a procedural technicality.

Before judging this period to be an unrelieved wasteland, though, one should remember that deserts are, for that matter, not one barren stretch but contain areas that sustain life or can be cultivated. Much the same can be said about Medicare-related policy in the period since 1997. It was not a coherent episode, but independent initiatives and adaptations, some of which were important steps forward.

The most egregious example of gridlock was the patients' bill of rights: six years and two bills passed but with Republicans and Democrats so opposed that the Senate boycotted the conference. This would seem to be an instance in which a combined pathology of divided government, partisanship, and the campaign mode of legislation blocked any constructive outcomes. It is plausible, though, that a federal patients' bill of rights was not a good idea to begin with[96] and that both parties got what they wanted most: the Republicans no legislation but political cover; and the Democrats, a popular policy initiative and a good wedge issue with which to divide Republicans and deflect attacks on Medicare or Medicaid. In fact, considerable progress was made in deciding the substantive rights that needed to be protected. Even with respect to the divisive right to sue, differences were narrowed to a short list of "must haves" and "can't stands," which could, in the future, shorten the time elapsed in getting from rhetoric to serious negotiation. Though virulent, the six-year period of gridlock was useful. Moreover, it was not "pernicious" in the sense employed by Kevin Phillips and Thomas Friedman.[97] Except for the time consumed and the diversion of effort, it did not spill over into other areas of Medicare or Medicaid policy or reduce the disposition or capacity to negotiate differences.

Putting an issue on the table even though no bill is passed or even marked up can be another form of progress. For instance, President Clinton put on the table a "competitive defined benefit" along with the drug benefit. The competitive defined benefit was an important concession, indicating that structural reform of Medicare was open for discussion. Increasing the drug offering and accepting the entitlement status of Medicare was a similar gesture made in Breaux-Frist II. Such concessions can widen and deepen bipartisan discussion and lead to serious negotiation, even though no bill is passed. On this point, it seems a pity that Senator Graham's Medicare Reform Act of 2001 was not marked up and debated along with Breaux-Frist I and II. It could have been the best opportunity yet for the wider American public to gain some understanding of the underlying issues.

Developing proposals for markup and legislation can be an educative and winnowing process, especially when it leads to detailed formulation and reformulation of policies. The Medicare Reform Act of 2001 is a case in point. A concern of Senator Graham's had been that not enough was being said, in the discussion of Medicare reform, about administrative reform of the FFS program, which was still the option chosen by more than 85 percent of the beneficiaries.[98] In developing a bill for mark-up, the Senator and his staff set forth, comprehensively and in legislative language, a Democratic version of administrative reform that raised significantly the question of what reform should include, articulated this aspect of Medicare policy for Democrats, and put on the table a serious proposal for Republicans to consider. From one perspective, the outcome was another instance of gridlock. From another perspective, this initiative could significantly raise the level of future debate.

The malignant effects of gridlock are often exaggerated, in part, because the mortality reports are overstated.[99] Initiatives that are rejected often do not die and may be more successful later or in another setting. For instance, some of the 1999 access proposals that seemed, at best, in a state of suspended animation were revived by the recession and the debates over various stimulus packages. Except for the Consumer Bill of Rights and Responsibilities, the recommendations of the Quality Commission were largely ignored. Two years later, this initiative was renewed by the Institute of Medicine and much of its work incorporated in Senator Graham's bill for Medicare reform (Institute of Medicine 2001). Subsequent iterations may improve these policy initiatives or gain more support for them. In any event, they provide additional opportunities to evaluate them, which in this turbulent and raucous political environment can be valuable.

To be sure, gridlock exists and is harmful. Four years with no significant Medicare or Medicaid legislation is not a trivial matter, but it is important to be aware that gridlock is an overused and abused term and that the extent and consequences of gridlock are overstated. Like the desert, there are life and opportunity not apparent to the untrained eye. One reason for studying the policy process during these relatively barren patches is to gain a sense for what is alive, what adaptations are possible, and how progress can be made.

NOTES

[1] Both Thomas Friedman (2000) and Kevin Phillips (1994:Ch. 5) distinguish between ordinary gridlock, in which partisans are unable to reach working agreements because of the fundamental nature of their differences, and a pernicious, wasting gridlock, in which a diminishing system capacity makes agreements increasingly difficult, despite desire on both sides to reach them.

[2] Chris Jennings, deputy assistant to the president for health policy. Interview, June 9, 1999. Jack Ebeler, Robert Wood Johnson Foundation; formerly, deputy assistant for health policy, DHHS. Interview, September 11, 1998.

[3] Jack Ebeler. Interview, September 11, 1998.

[4] Agency for Health Care Policy and Research. Since renamed as the Agency for Healthcare Research and Quality.

[5] Employers that self-insured, e.g., large "Fortune 500" plans, could generally be sued only in federal courts, pretty much for contract violations only, not for medical malpractice.

[6] EO 13017.

[7] Jack Ebeler. Interview, May 21, 1999.

[8] Chris Jennings. Interview, May 30, 2000.

[9] Ibid.

[10] Like the HCFA "neg-reg" task force, the Quality Commission made use of consensus building techniques similar to those employed by ProPAC and PPRC.

[11] *Health Care Policy Report,* January 19, 1998, p. 127.

[12] HR 1415; S 644.

[13] *Health Care Policy Report,* March 2, 1998, p. 359.

[14] Ibid., January 5, 1998, p. 29.

[15] *Hearing on H.R. 1415, The Patient Access to Responsible Care Act (PARCA),* hearing before the Subcommittee on Employer-Employee Relations of the Committee on Education and the Workforce, House of Representatives, 105th Congress, First Session, October 23, 1997, p. 275.

[16] *Health Care Policy Report,* January 16, 1998, p. 174.

[17] Ibid., p. 240.

[18] Ibid., May 22, 1998, p. 780.

[19] Republicans in both House and Senate expressed the fear that politics was driving this issue and that President Clinton, especially, saw it as a wedge issue to divide Republicans while he pursued his own agenda. Ibid., March 2, 1998, p. 365.

[20] HR 4250, Patient Protection Act.

[21] HR 3301, Health Care Availability and Affordability Act of 1996.

[22] *Health Care Policy Report,* July 27, 1998, p. 1205.

[23] Ibid., p. 1205.

[24] Ibid., July 13, 1998, p. 1125.

[25] Along with the election results of 1998, the distribution of popular preferences was an important factor. According to a voter survey released by the Kaiser Family Foundation and Harvard University, 73 percent of the voters in the November election said that saving Medicare was a top priority, 61 percent that coverage for the uninsured was, while only 54 percent supported managed care reform or patients' bills of rights. When shifting from the general proposition to specific proposals, though, voters divided sharply along partisan lines over how to reform Medicare or to extend insurance; but large majorities of both Democrats and Republicans favored specific patients' rights, such as the right to sue HMOs. In other words, patients' rights still included "hot buttons" that could be pushed by politicians from either political party, even though voters lacked a consensus about what to do and, as events proved, Congress was unable to agree either. *Health Care Policy Report,* January 25, 1999, p. 174.

[26] The tax provisions (including an expansion of MSA demonstrations) did not go through the Finance Committee, which lacked the votes to pass them. They were added on the floor by the leadership. Ibid., October 25, 1999, p. 1659.

[27] Ibid., March 6, 2000, p. 385.

[28] Ibid., May 15, 2000, p. 764.

[29] Tom Daschle, the Senate minority leader, said that the Republican leadership was protecting members with tough elections from politically dangerous votes. Trent Lott suspected the White House of encouraging Democrats not to reach an agreement and to keep the debate alive as an election issue. In this respect, the patients' rights issue provides a good illustration of the campaign mode of legislation and how it can foster gridlock.

[30] Norwood's September compromise proposal seemed reasonable and as close as Congress ever came to an agreement. In addition to lack of majority support in either house, there were other difficulties, such as lack of time and of an amendable vehicle to which the legislation could be attached. *Health Care Policy Report,* October 16, 2000, pp. 1696–97.

[31] *Washington Post,* July 23, 2001, p. A-1.

[32] *Congressional Quarterly,* May 19, 2001, p. 1159.

[33] HR 2315, Patients' Bill of Rights of 2001, HR 2315.

[34] The amendments agreed upon by Bush and Norwood would be turned into legislative language and offered as amendments to the House bill (Pear 2001b).

[35] *Congressional Quarterly,* August 4, 2001, p. 1901.

[36] Ibid., July 14, 2001, p. 1692.

[37] Some of whom, and especially Democrats, felt betrayed by his unilateral negotiations with President Bush and failure to consult with or even inform them.

[38] As quoted in *Congressional Weekly,* August 4, 2001, p. 1900.

[39] *Health Care Policy Report,* September 24, 2001, p. 1425.

[40] Both bills covered all Americans in private or employer-sponsored insurance plans. The Senate bill also covered enrollees in Medicare, Medicaid, and other federal health plans.

[41] *Health Care Policy Report,* August 12, 1996, p. 1309.

[42] Ibid., p. 1403.

[43] Ibid., p. 1403.

[44] Ibid., January 12, 1997, p. 85.

[45] Ibid., December 16, 1996, p. 1909.

[46] Ibid., September 22, 1997, p. 1441.

[47] Initially, Multi-employer Welfare Arrangements (MEWAs) in a bill sponsored by Rep. Harris Fawell (R., Ill.), the ERISA Targeted Health Insurance Reform Act of 1996 (HR 995); these MEWAs were modified and renamed Association Health Plans (AHPs) in the Expanded Portability and Health Insurance Coverage Act (EPHIC) of 1997.

[48] Representative Thomas was considering some tax credit provisions, but biding his time until the Bipartisan Commission filed its report.

[49] Chris Jennings. Interview, June 9, 1999.

[50] Jack Ebeler. Interview, May 21, 1999.

[51] *Health Care Policy Report,* January 24, 2000, p. 119.

[52] Forty-three million was the estimate at the time. According to Census Bureau figures, the number of uninsured dropped to 38.7 million in 2000, though it may be again on the rise.

[53] The "refundable" feature was later changed to make funds available quickly.

[54] *Health Care Policy Report,* April 12, 1999, p. 608.

[55] Ibid., November 15, 1999, p. 1816.

[56] Many of these categorical problems would disappear if eligibility were based solely on income. Cf. Feder, Levitt, O'Brien, and Rowland (2001:30).

[57] *Health Care Policy Report,* January 31, 2000, p. 175.

[58] Ibid., November 3, 1997, p. 1654.

[59] *Building a Better Medicare for Today and Tomorrow,* National Bipartisan Commission on the Future of Medicare, http://thomas.loc.gov/medicare/bbmtt31599.

[60] Bill Vaughan, administrative assistant to Rep. Pete Stark. Interview, March 1, 2001.

[61] Chris Jennings. Interview, May 30, 2000.

[62] *Health Care Policy Report,* February 1, 1999, p. 195.

[63] *Congressional Quarterly,* March 20, 1999.

[64] *Health Care Policy Report,* March 1, 1999. Also Gail Wilensky, "HCFA Governance and Medicare Reform," testimony presented to the Committee on Finance, U.S. Senate, May 4, 2000, p. 5.

[65] *Health Care Policy Report,* March 15, 1999, p. 454.

[66] *Congressional Quarterly,* March 13, 1999, p. 610.

[67] Comments from two commission members are illuminating. According to Debo-

rah Steelman, a Republican member, "We never got past the religious, ideological components, the belief systems. It's like the Middle East, abortion, civil war." Rep. Jim McDermott (D., Wash.) said, "It was wired from the start to move every senior into managed care, and they didn't want to look at anything beside that." As quoted from Toner (2001a).

[68] Testimony by Gail Wilensky and Representative Stark before the Senate Finance Committee, May 4, 2000.

[69] The title may sound familiar. In 1995, it was the "Medicare Preservation Act."

[70] The CMA was similar to the Social Security administration in several respects: the commissioner would be appointed for six years and removable by the president for cause. The board was bipartisan and had staggered terms.

[71] For FFS beneficiaries there was a $250 annual deductible, copays up to 50 percent, and they would pay 75 percent of premium costs. Initially, annual coverage was capped at $2,100, though there was an annual limit of $6,000 out-of-pocket expense. FFS plans would be administered by PBMs, without enough supervision—according to Democrats—to insure against risk selection.

[72] Lisa Layman, senior policy advisor to Sen. Bob Graham; formerly staff of Sen. John Chafee. Interview, December 6, 2001. The pharmaceutical benefit would be largely administered by pharmacy benefits managers—risk-bearing entities that would have strong incentives to avoid or shift risk.

[73] Lisa Layman. Interview, Dec. 6, 2001.

[74] Jeanne Lambrew, Office of Management and Budget, formerly, senior health policy analyst, National Economic Council. Interview, August 25, 1999.

[75] Ibid.

[76] The chair was Gene Sperling, director of the National Economic Council. Jeanne Lambrew. Interview, August 25, 1999.

[77] Ibid.

[78] Depending on budget constraints, this differential might be phased out.

[79] President's Competitive Defined Benefit Proposal, White House release, June 29, 1999, p. 3.

[80] The proposals were later developed, more fully and systematically, in Title I of Senator Graham's Medicare Reform Act of 2001 (S 1135).

[81] *Health Care Policy Report,* July 9, 1999, p. 1069.

[82] In addition to deterring use, a copay would help to keep track of payments and to control fraud and abuse.

[83] One important reason for these limits was concern with "crowd out."

[84] Jeanne Lambrew. Interview, August 25, 1999.

[85] Lambrew said it might have been the most important part of the benefit.

[86] Medicare Outpatient Drug Act of 2000 (S 2758). An attempt to bring this proposal to the floor by attaching it to the Labor-HHS Appropriations Act was defeated, 44–53. *Health Care Policy Report,* June 26, 2000, p. 1058.

[87] Ibid., July 5, 1999, p. 1070.

[88] Ibid., p. 1069.

[89] In addition to 1.6 million that had already been dropped by health plans, another 536,000 were dropped as of January 1, 2002 (Pear 2001a).

[90] The Medicare/Medicaid and SCHIP Benefits Improvement and Protection Act of 2000 (BIPA), the second major give-back legislation, extended the phase-in of the

risk adjuster from 2004 to 2007. *Health Care Policy Report,* December 25, 2000, p. 2019.

[91] For Medicaid, the problem is similar, with seven million "dual eligibles" accounting for 35 percent of the program costs.

[92] S 1135 moved considerably beyond the president's proposal in systematically addressing this issue. It stressed especially the importance of quality and coordination in caring for the gravely and chronically ill, working with AHRQ and IOM, and incorporating many recommendations from the Institute of Medicine (2001).

[93] Senator Graham had been a long-time supporter of more competition, especially in the traditional, FFS part of the program. In fact, his proposals for competitive adaptations would probably have given pause to a good many providers and even Republican supporters of competition. Lisa Layman. Interview, December 6, 2001.

[94] Ibid.

[95] For example, marking up a pharmaceutical benefit before restructuring Medicare seemed to be bad policy to Republicans. To Democrats, reversing the order would be using a drug benefit to promote Medicare amendments that did not stand on their own merits. Merging the Part A–Part B accounts might have had fiscal and programmatic advantages. To Democrats, though, it would burden beneficiaries and radically change the solvency status of the trust funds. Democrats also thought Republicans were uncritically supportive of private sector PBMs These issues mixed ideology, policy, and tactical considerations, adding to the controversy.

[96] Greater emphasis on quality and less on patients' rights and lawsuits to back them up might have been a more constructive way to go.

[97] See note 1.

[98] Lisa Layman. Interview, December 6, 2001.

[99] Consider in this respect the incremental and aggregative tactics discussed in Chapter 5. Some bills are loaded with "poison pills," "sweeteners," or items included for purposes of bargaining. Trashing these parts may not be gridlock, but progress toward a resolution.

9

Postscript

The terrorist attacks on the United States in the fall of 2001 have already had profound effects upon domestic policy: diverting attention to foreign affairs, changing the political valence of many activities, and obligating money and resources to urgent new needs. As with the attack upon Pearl Harbor or the assassination of President Kennedy, these events sharply separate life before them from life after them. A discontinuity of this magnitude, with many policy initiatives altered or put on hold, shows how unforeseen events can change expected outcomes. It has created a hiatus in Medicare and Medicaid policy-making, with uncertainty about when or on what terms discussion of these matters will be resumed. One fairly safe prediction, though, is that the underlying problems with these programs will not vanish because of a temporary lack of attention. Some may continue to grow worse during this interval, such as the rising cost of pharmaceuticals or access to managed care in rural areas. For Medicare and Medicaid, this interim is probably just that, a temporary delay in the pursuit of various policy objectives. It is also an opportunity and a challenge that may or may not be used for our common benefit: to take stock, get reoriented, and think about how to confront the future.

A central topic in this book has been the partisan dispute over the Medicare and Medicaid entitlements and, underlying that, the Republican commitment to reduce the size of the federal government and a Democratic determination to defend entitlements pretty much as they are. One possibility for the future that merits some consideration—though not betting much—is that Republican conservatives might moderate their commitment to reducing the size of government and changing the status of entitlements and that Democrats would seriously consider how to reform Medicare and Medicaid for the long term. We are in the midst of a protracted international crisis. Such times often foster bipartisanship and that mood could persist afterward. Shared sacrifice and successes in meeting public objectives may tend to increase the legitimacy of government. Immediately after the September 11 suicide bombing, there was a surge of bipartisanship and suggestions that differences over the reform of Medicare might be quickly resolved, aided by a new spirit of burying divisive issues and getting on with combating terrorism. Desirable or not, this access of comity quickly disappeared as partisan differences broke out over tax cuts to stimulate business recovery and bailouts for multinational corporations vs. health insurance for unemployed workers. For the present, neither the Republican nor Democratic leadership shows signs of moderating their entrenched positions on Medicare or Medicaid.

One possibility, worth considering in some depth, is that partisan strife over Medicare and Medicaid will revive, much in its earlier form, and that the Republicans will succeed in their long-term effort to transform these entitlements: Medicare into a defined contribution similar to the FEHBP and Medicaid into a modified block grant. At present, initiatives in this direction seem checked, except for efforts by the DHHS and CMS to proceed along administrative lines with waivers and demonstrations. Yet, the near success, under the new administration, of the Governors' Plan for Medicaid and the bipartisan Breaux-Frist Medicare reform proposal shows that these remain strong initiatives that could yet succeeded.

This prospect has been discounted on the ground that neither the driving force nor the urgency for restructuring Medicare or Medicaid continues to exist. Since 1995, much of the impetus for change has come from rising program costs, threats to trust fund solvency, and the budget deficit. As the economy continued to grow, especially from 1997 through 1999, budget surpluses and declining baselines diminished these pressures and, with those developments, the alleged need to restructure Medicare or Medicaid. For a time, there was almost an embarrassment of riches, with President Clinton proposing a pharmaceutical benefit and setting aside 15 percent of the surplus to extend the solvency of the Medicare trust fund and Congress bestowing "give-backs" upon providers and finding ways to compensate for Medicaid DSH funds. The major concern was what to enhance, not what to cut.

While Democrats were looking for program enhancements, Republicans were concluding it was time to cut taxes and made this a central campaign issue. In office, they immediately pushed for a huge tax reduction schedule, ranging from $1.3 trillion to $2.1 trillion,[1] back-loaded and extending over ten years. This proposal was defended with the argument that Democrats, if they had the money, would simply spend it and that the people, not government bureaucrats, were the best judge of how to use their own money. Soon, with the support of Federal Reserve Chairman Alan Greenspan, Republicans added a second argument—as the economy began to soften—that a stimulus package was needed. This was a theme that won over a number of Democrats, although they pushed for shorter-term tax relief and subsidies targeted toward middle and lower income levels.

Leaving aside the rhetoric and fiscal prudence of this tax legislation, it is likely to have great long-term significance for Medicare and, possibly, Medicaid as well. Among the purposes of the legislation—other than tax relief—was to keep the federal government out of mischief by reducing the size of the surplus and to impose greater fiscal and budgetary discipline. A 4.2 percent cap was set for the overall increase in discretionary spending, the most stringent limitation in recent years. Entitlements were not included. Both Republicans and Democrats pledged to respect the trust funds, except that actuarial surpluses could be used to further pay down the debt. As the economy slipped toward recession, though, Congress began debating the use of Social Security trust funds for a stimulus package. After the terrorist attacks—which imposed direct costs and further weakened the economy—both the Social Security and Medicare trust funds were generally regarded as available to help meet the emergency. Meanwhile, Democrats and Republicans argued over what had caused the surplus to decline, but even optimistic accounts conceded that it would probably be gone by 2002.

The return of budget deficits would strengthen the central role of the budget reconciliation process. The success of President Bush and the Republicans in passing a major tax reduction package demonstrated that a deficit is not necessary to make the reconciliation process a powerful fiscal instrument. However, deficits create a need, add impetus and legitimacy to the reconciliation procedures, and are especially suitable for this bloody work since they facilitate the coordination of taxes, appropriations, and programmatic changes. Moreover, these procedures are not subject to a filibuster in the Senate.

Medicare and Medicaid were not featured in this round, which was about tax cuts and discretionary spending, but these entitlements could become prime targets for future deficit reduction efforts, much as they were in 1995 and 1997. Health care costs generally are projected to go up by 12–14 percent in the coming year, a rate of increase that will reverberate through the health care system, including Medicare and Medicaid. Additional costs associated with the terrorist attacks and the recession may add several percentage points to that amount. States will be hard-pressed by economic recession, swelling unemployment, and increased health and security demands. Cost increases of this magnitude, especially if they continue, make Medicare and Medicaid of central importance for budget and deficit reduction strategies. They also upset existing calculations; create hardships for providers, beneficiaries, and taxpayers; mobilize political protest; and require accommodations and adjustments along with cost containment and budget cutting. For deficit reduction, in other words, there are a number of reasons to target Medicare and Medicaid and to use a budget reconciliation procedure.

Another consideration that would make the reconciliation strategy attractive is that both the Medicare and Medicaid programs may require structural reforms that go beyond incremental tinkering. The continuing plan withdrawals from Medicare+Choice reflect deep lying sources of disaffection and raise fundamental questions about the role of managed care in the Medicare program. The aborted Governors' Plan for Medicaid will probably acquire new relevance because of the recession and the added strains upon local governments imposed by international terrorism. Reconciliation procedures provide a way of amending programs and their financing that is comprehensive and makes it relatively easy to repair the machinery while it is operating.

The budget reconciliation process is also a good vehicle for dealing with controversial and technical issues, under divided government, and with slender or bipartisan majorities, conditions that have obtained with respect to Medicare and Medicaid over much of their history and especially during the last seven years. In the summer of 2001, before the terrorist attacks, a modified version of Breaux-Frist was gaining bipartisan support within the Senate Finance Committee. Part of the governors' plan was already being administratively implemented and, with modifications, more of it might gain legislative support. Each of these initiatives would be a good candidate for an omnibus reconciliation bill that could shape them to increase support and add leverage for change. The first of these would transform Medicare into a defined contribution system similar to the FEHBP. The second would turn Medicaid into a modified block grant. To be sure, the new version of a defined contribution or "premium support" would be quite different from the Medicare Preservation Act of 1995. And the governors' plan would be only a partial change in the entitlement status of Medicaid, but the principle sought with respect to entitlements in 1995 would be established in large measure.

Both of these initiatives had stalled by the August recess and were put on indefinite hold after the September terrorist attacks. Congress is not likely to do much substantively about these deeply divisive issues in an off-year election. The election of 2002 could change little, leaving Democrats with a bare majority in the Senate and Republicans marginally in control of the House. Assuming that present economic trends continue, initiatives along the line of Breaux-Frist II and the governors' plan might be appealing to Republicans and moderate Democrats, and they could well succeed, especially if senators Baucus, Graham, and Rockefeller weaken in their opposition to Breaux-Frist and a deal could be negotiated on the Medicaid match. Though speculative, these contingencies illustrate two of the ways the reconciliation process can be instrumental: offsetting expenditures and putting pressure on holdouts and peeling away their supporters.

For a time, the surge of patriotism and unity after the September attacks led not only to predictions of a bipartisan "national" government but to apprehensions on the part of Democrats that President Bush would be a shoo-in for a second term and that Democrats would probably lose the Senate in 2002. Several Democratic senatorial hopefuls withdrew because of this belief and the difficulty it posed for campaign fund-raising. These attitudes and behavior prompted the distinguished historian, Arthur Schlesinger, Jr., to write a piece for the New York Times entitled "Democracy in Wartime,"[2] in which he declared himself "astonished" by the view that the terrorist attacks were bound to favor the incumbents. He pointed out, for example, that eleven months after Pearl Harbor under the leadership of Franklin Roosevelt, the Democrats lost fifty seats in the House and eight in the Senate in the mid-term elections of 1942. In 1950, five months after the beginning of the Korean War, Republicans gained twenty-eight seats in the House and five in the Senate. Similar gains by the opposition party were scored during the Vietnam and Persian Gulf wars. The point being that not only are Democrats—and other Americans—ignorant of their own history but Democrats might gain in the House and Senate in 2002 with the prospect they could control both houses of Congress.

Democrats in control of the House and Senate—with a Republican in the White House—would have strong incentives to use the reconciliation process, much as they did under the Reagan administration, to amend and micromanage Medicare and Medicaid. They would also be confronting a president running for a second term. By then, increases in health care costs and the number of uninsured could be good campaign issues raising a prospect for another NHI proposal.[3] In that event, some of the proposals that were developed in 1999 and 2000 might provide a way, either independently or as additions to Medicare, Medicaid, and SCHIP, to extend coverage and access to care that would be less ambitious or risky than the more comprehensive 1994 model.

These various scenarios are sketchy and hypothetical, but the analogy of a scenario is helpful, since in Medicare and Medicaid politics much is known about roles, procedures, policy options, and political context. Within these constraints, there are usually several plausible scenarios, not a dozen. Thinking them through serves to exclude the unreasonable, interpret events as they unfold, and reach agreement about the investment of time and resources. The same exercise can also help distinguish rhetoric from viable policy and identify weak or missing elements of a policy initiative.

Major legislative action with respect to Medicare and Medicaid will probably be postponed until after the election of 2002. Whether Democrats or Republicans win the election, the instruments of policy with respect to these entitlements are likely to be much the same as they were in the past—employing the budget reconciliation process, but with complementary incremental and aggregative strategies. By then, however, five years will have elapsed since BBA 97 was enacted, with little change in policy or party rhetoric. Meanwhile, the health care industry will continue evolving and there will be several years of additional experience with implementing the act. There are dangers in thinking that we can pick up where we left off. One pitfall is to be mistaken about where we did, in fact, leave off—about what was or was not accomplished. Another is not to take account of intervening change. Some attention to each of these may be useful in guarding against lapses of this sort.

A major legacy of the 1990s was to stir up controversy about the role of government, federalism, entitlements, and markets, and leave most of the policy issues unresolved. This statement is especially true with respect to

Medicare—where we are little closer to a solution or some kind of viable peace treaty than in 1995 when this saga began. In some respects, the underlying problems have gotten worse and our capacity to resolve them has diminished.

Some notable progress has been made since 1995. Federal and state fraud and abuse legislation and enforcement are much more effective and have become powerful instruments for cost containment and to fight the growth of corruption. Quality improvement and prospective payment systems have become generally accepted norms. The Medicaid and SCHIP amendments would seem to represent for this entitlement something of a political and federal settlement—that could be a workable and even durable compromise reconciling fundamental differences. It should be noted, in passing, that these accomplishments represented, in different ways, instances of bipartisan collaboration.

I. MEDICARE

Medicare as a single-payer, federally administered entitlement is in a category by itself, because of the degree of federal involvement and Medicare's symbolic and strategic importance. As we have seen, BBA 97 purported to be a grand compromise but was not—in the sense of a compromise with respect to fundamental policy differences. As one result, many who thought in 1995 that Medicare needed basic restructuring believe that job remains to be done. In addition, some key provisions of BBA 97 seem not be work as well as hoped, leading to an unstable situation likely to require extensive intervention.

Trends in managed care are one such destabilizing factor. Most earlier policy proposals for major structural changes in the Medicare program have assumed that HMOs (or MCOs) would, in principle, save money for Medicare, earn a surplus, and aggressively recruit Medicare enrollees. None of these assumptions now seems reliable. Because of the AAPCC-based payment formula, the proposition that HMOs would save money for Medicare was one of those notions never really tested. Now, with the contemporary regulatory burden, the threat of lawsuits, and the cost of new drugs and technology, many HMOs doubt that they want Medicare's business, especially when they can do better for themselves and with less fuss, insuring a non-Medicare clientele. We have already noted how extensive plan withdrawals combined with an aggressive lobbying and public relations campaign by HMOs created a minor panic in the Congress and the enactment of two give-back bills to remedy the "excessive" corrections in BBA 97. Amid projections of plan withdrawals affecting several hundred thousand more enrollees in 2002, the House Ways and Means Committee put together a third rescue package but this initiative died in the Senate.[4] At the very least, these events are a warning that the expected role of HMOs in Medicare and their willingness to play it can no longer be taken for granted.

A similar kind of situation may obtain with respect to the prospective payment systems put in place by BBA 97 to contain costs on the FFS side of Medicare. These systems were legislated hastily, while they were still in process of development, and calibrated to meet specific deficit reduction targets. Unlike the hospital PPS or the physician fee schedule, they did not have behind them years of congressional involvement and "buy-in" to the process. Generally, they were based on payment mechanisms that were less refined predictors of resource use or costs and therefore shifted more risk to the providers. These factors both prompted and strengthened appeals to Congress to postpone implementation and to ease the pinch of payment reductions. We have noted the results in 1999, in the election year of 2000, and beyond.

A disturbing development has been the tendency of Congress, in its various rescue missions, to disregard the advice of its own staff agencies and to increase payments or bestow give-backs upon hospitals, HMOs, and other providers despite contrary views expressed by MedPAC, CBO, and the GAO. Unfortunately, the conclusion drawn by some providers may be that it is more profitable to lobby the Congress than to make their case on technical grounds or seek to operate with greater efficiency. In earlier days, the providers' lobby and their champions in Congress had on occasion almost overwhelmed the technically based prospective payment methodology for Medicare hospitals and physicians. Following such orgies, Congress would repent and sometimes take measures to improve and protect the process. There seem to be few second thoughts in the contemporary Congress.

These developments raise serious doubts about cost containment strategies for Medicare, since neither managed care nor administered pricing is likely to achieve what its supporters hoped. Meanwhile, health care costs rise, with CMS announcing a 10 percent increase in FY 2001 for Medicare.[5] To these considerations, add that most Republicans and some Democrats regard a fundamental restructuring of Medicare as unfinished business, left over from 1997, and it seems likely that this initiative will be a prominent agenda item when Congress and the Bush administration turn their attention again to domestic affairs, such as health care and the environment.

As late as September 2001, it looked as though a modified version of Breaux-Frist might clear the Senate Finance Committee and gain enough bipartisan support to break the deadlock over restructuring Medicare. Ostensibly, the sticking point was that not enough was allocated for the pharmaceutical benefit. Mention of this specific item, though, should serve as a reminder of other issues still dividing the two parties, such as a defined contribution (premium support) vs. a defined benefit; risk selection and structuring competition between FFS and managed care plans; effectiveness and fairness in cost containment; and assuring long-term solvency.

The litany of differences is similar though not identical to that confronting Congress and the administration in 1995, creating an eerie sense of having been here before and of reliving an unpleasant part of the past. Yet, we are not likely to repeat the past, in part because the policy environment has changed, even though partisan commitments and a number of the fundamental issues remain the same.

Unlike 1995 and 1997, there is no looming "bankruptcy" of the Medicare Trust Fund, nor is there yet a budget deficit. Medicare is currently running a surplus and the trust fund is solvent until 2015 or 2030. Predictions are that the projected budget surplus will be exhausted sometime early in 2002 and we will again be in a deficit position. If the international crisis and the recession continue, though, the deficit is likely to be seen as a justifiable borrowing against the future, not as a moral defect in our political and fiscal behavior. Both the Social Security and the Medicare trust funds might be tapped to help pay for the war and stimulate the economy but, following the same kind of argument, depletion of these trust funds should be seen as borrowing, not as evidence of the actuarial weakness of Medicare. Simply put, the fiscal argument for restructuring Medicare is likely to lose much of its political appeal and driving force, especially in the near future.

In other ways, revamping Medicare may be a more challenging task than it was in 1995. Aside from the lack of a political mandate and fiscal pressure to drive change, payment mechanisms that seemed to be reliable cost savers have proven to be politically more difficult to implement and less effective than expected. This development is likely to sharpen the issue of how to contain costs including the redistribution of burdens as between providers and beneficiaries. Medicare politics from 1995 to the present demonstrates that such an effort provokes an enormous amount of organized resistance and legislative conflict. Absent governing majorities in one or both houses of Congress or more bipartisan consensus about common goals, this kind of conflict may be impossible to resolve.

Early in the new administration, there was talk about bipartisan collaboration in restructuring Medicare, but partisan mobilization and campaign-style legislation soon returned as the dominant mode for domestic politics, with emphasis upon strategic and tactical advantage, message and spin. One probable consequence for Medicare policy is that—like adverse parties in a marital or labor dispute—neither side will be able to admit a weakness in its own position or concede strength in its opponent's, although one or both might be essential for moving toward serious discussion. In fact, there are several admissions or perceptions of this sort that could have a decisive effect on the future of Medicare policy.

One such is a recognition that administered pricing is not, by itself, an adequate method of cost containment. Administered pricing in the Medicare program works well as a device to cut provider payments but not—given political realities—to curb beneficiary demand for expensive medical care and high-tech pharmaceuticals, services, and procedures. In general, the prospective payment systems were designed that way—to ratchet down on inputs, but to allow beneficiaries to choose, in large quantities, the best and often most expensive course of treatment or providers. The consequence has been inflationary pressure on the demand side, with constraints on the supply side largely borne by providers who take their case to the politicians and, over time, seem to win more and more.

An important contribution of BBA 95, BBA 97, and the Bipartisan Commission was to direct attention to the long-term cost push of such factors as consumer demand, the baby boom generation as well as the general aging of the population, and the impact of new technology and pharmaceuticals. They also mentioned the unmentionable, which was more sharing of the cost containment burden by Medicare beneficiaries. Defenders of administered pricing, mostly Democrats, tacitly acknowledged the existence of a serious problem by their repeated attempts to earmark part of the budget surplus for extending Medicare trust fund solvency, but they disagreed with the prescription, and especially that turning the Medicare entitlement into a defined contribution was either necessary or the best way to save the program.

Advocates of managed care are right in seeing that capitation is an important part of a solution. If well structured, managed care could provide a uniquely American way to ration care by imposing a tolerable amount of restraint on both providers and beneficiaries. Other benefits would be sharing risk and reducing in some measure the unseemly political economy of micromanagement. Assuming that these statements are true, then critics of HMO are doing a disservice if they drive MCOs out of the program or make it impossible for them to perform their useful functions of rationing care and sharing risk.

Supporters of procompetition schemes could help by acknowledging, for their part, that market competition, as applied to Medicare MCOs, is likely—in the short run and perhaps indefinitely—to be imperfect, spotty, and inadequate by itself to constrain costs, assure a broad array of choices, or provide affordable, quality care to those who need it most. Like a Sorelian myth,[6] the "hidden hand" of market competition is a useful idea to unite partisans and inspire action, but even assuming that such a "market" could be made to work, getting there would probably take a decade or more.[7] This would be an "administered" market, with marketing and quality standards, a risk adjuster, competitive bidding,[8] and negotiations over participation and access. Moreover, many decisions would be painfully redistributive leading to appeals to Congress and formula fights, fixes, and bailouts.[9] This is not to say that moving somewhat in the competitive direction would not be a good thing, assuming that it is feasible, only that "administered competition" is not a complete solution and may not be that different or that much better than administered pricing.

If the two opposing sides ever made a serious effort to find common ground, it might even be possible to reach an agreement on the Medicare entitlement itself that would protect those with greatest need but have beneficiaries share more of the burden. Much of the reason that defined contribution schemes are resisted is not that they impose a greater burden upon beneficiaries in general, but that they might put intolerable burdens upon some, seem likely to encourage risk selection, gradually destroy the FFS program, and abandon the chronically and severely ill. An undertaking on both sides to assure appropriate care for this latter group but to charge other beneficiaries more for unneeded care going beyond the level appropriate for their condition would be one way of working around this impasse. In practical terms, risk selection could be reduced by frequent calibration of the managed care risk adjuster and negotiating with MCOs willing and able to assume larger numbers of high-risk patients. The federal government could provide an alternative and a public yardstick through programs such as Centers of Excellence, PACE, and additional FFS managed care initiatives.

There would be some nonobvious benefits to such a scheme. Associating a number of the flagship managed care plans would help keep quality high and encourage private sector innovation. It would also spread risk and foster the ethos of social insurance. The direct involvement of the federal government in this venture would serve as an earnest of the commitment to provide continuing care for all Medicare beneficiaries through the last stages of life.

Achieving Medicare reform that would be workable, durable, and broadly acceptable is likely to be a lengthy and technical process. Even if Congress and the president were able to reach a quick agreement on some compromise version, for example, of Breaux-Frist II and a Democratic retread of Clinton's "competitive defined benefit," it would take years to work out the details of the legislation and the payment formulas, develop the regulations, revive and restructure Medicare+Choice, implement competitive bidding, collect data and get a risk adjuster working, modify and calibrate the prospective payment systems, develop new information materials and services, establish working relationships with the providers, devise protocols for monitoring the system, and so forth. The point is that all of this will require years of technical and largely cooperative endeavor. An important corollary of this proposition is that this decade-long enterprise will require staff with experience, competence, and a will to make the program work, including staff on the Hill, in HCFA (CMS), and in GAO, CBO, and OMB. One telling indicator of the seriousness of efforts to reform Medicare, as opposed to dismantling it, is the quality and numbers of staff deployed in pursuit of the objective. In this respect, recent trends are discouraging: modest bipartisan efforts to increase funding and powers of HCFA (CMS)[10] offset by decline in congressional staffs.

The history of Medicare, the political clout of the stakeholders, the rooted and conflicting principles involved, and the American form of government pretty much assure that a reformed Medicare will be a compromise: long on negotiated trade-offs and short on logic or coherence. Cooperation across party lines and good staff work can help make the final product fair and workable.

How durable such an effort will be depends on factors such as demography, medical technology, felt needs, trends in the economy, and how successfully a revised Medicaid statute can bound conflict as it accommodates change.

Of great importance for health policy in America are the attitudes about what constitutes fair treatment. In relation to Medicare, "social insurance" is sometimes invoked as a supporting ideology that could defend the entitlement as well as encourage positive attitudes toward sharing and responsibility, but this notion has surprisingly little resonance with the American people as compared, for instance, with the Germans, the British, or the Canadians. Americans respond strongly to issues of fairness: what is fair (or unfair) to beneficiaries or providers. As we have seen, a populist fervor can be aroused over "slashing" Medicare to provide tax cuts for the rich (Kaiser Commission on Medicaid and the Uninsured 2001:1). Less dramatically, though, casting so much of the public debate in terms of "fairness" makes redistributive decisions difficult and tends to invest "entitlements" with even greater sanctity—without a like emphasis upon personal or corporate responsibility. There is good reason to insist that Medicare and Medicaid are entitlements: they need to be defended. But the American people should also be educated about the correlate responsibilities that go with the entitlement.

II. MEDICAID

The situation with respect to Medicaid is simpler to characterize but more uncertain. For a time after the passage of BBA 97, Medicaid seemed to be one of those rare instances in which the federal government reached an elegant, sane, and durable solution for a difficult set of problems. The balance between flexibility and beneficiary protections embodied in the Medicare legislation of 1997 did not depend upon an explicit agreement, but it did express an underlying philosophy that informed the efforts of key participants; and it seemed, if not a contract, at least a good foundation for future progress. This "settlement," if one may call it that, is at serious risk in part because of the election of 2000 and the NGA's *Health Care Reform Proposal,* but probably even more because of the downturn of the economy and the after-shocks of September 11, 2001.

The governors' plan would have used Section 1115 waivers to extend coverage to the unemployed by reducing optional Medicaid benefits and collecting an enhanced match from the federal government. The fiscal effect would be to shift resources from Medicaid programs to benefit the unemployed and to channel quite a large amount of money from the federal government to the states. In two ways, this initiative went contrary to the settlement achieved in the Medicaid amendments of 1997. One was that it represented another try on the part of the NGA to restructure Medicaid—not bad in principle, but distressing in its opportunistic disregard for a hard-won bipartisan compromise. As events transpired, Congress showed no interest in supplying the funds and OMB held to the requirement of budget neutrality. So far, the administration's HIFA demonstration waivers have met with little response. But economic trends, especially since September 2001, will almost certainly prompt further efforts of a similar character.

Two reminders help provide perspective on the importance of the economy for Medicaid policy. One is that BBA 97 was passed when times were good: the economy was booming, the deficit and Medicaid baselines were declining, and unemployment was low. A second is that Medicaid programs face cost inflation pressures similar to those confronting Medicare as well as aggravating factors that depend upon the fiscal situation of the states within the federal system. Put these two together, and it is easy to see why governors think they have grounds for some relief.

Demography and technology afflict Medicaid much as they do Medicare. Demography is a problem for states, in the form of increasing numbers of elderly, disabled, and aliens, many of them requiring special care. States are hit by expensive technology and drugs and increasing intensity of care. The beneficiary lists also continue to grow, especially when there is an economic downturn. Recession is especially hard on the states. Tax revenues drop just at a time when benefits such as welfare, Medicaid, and employment services are most needed. Debt often cannot be incurred because of constitutional limitations, and taxes are hard to raise because of concerns about their impact upon the poor or how they will affect recovery. States have declining resources to meet increasing needs and little capacity to change the situation. Not without reason, they turn to the federal government for money and for easing of constraints.

In August 2001—even before the terrorist attacks of September 11—the National Association of State Budget Officers noted that half the states reported they were in or near recession. The association projected a meager 2.7 percent increase in state overall expenditures, though Medicaid was expected to rise by 8.9 percent.[11] September 11 added to the states' plight with further downturns in the economy and tax revenues, more unemployment, and increased resources devoted to domestic security, public health, and future contingencies.

As governors and legislatures sought ways to respond to the fiscal crisis, Medicaid expenditures were a natural target. Short-term responses were, generally, of the familiar sort and moderate, involving some cost cutting and minor program changes: freezes on staff and travel expenses; tightening enrollment procedures and discouraging expansion; lower increases in provider payments; copays and some benefit reductions. Looking ahead, governors foresaw extended and deepening budget troubles, and they renewed demands familiar from the past: for greater flexibility, an enhanced match, help with the dual eligibles, even a "swap," that would allow states to care for only the acute populations and transfer responsibility for dual-eligibles and long-term care to the federal government.[12]

One effect of the terrorist attacks and the recession could be that the governors' plan of 2001 would develop new impetus as a way to address the health care needs of the unemployed and to ease the states' fiscal crunch.[13] If the Republicans were to regain full control of Congress after the election of 2002, this plan might find favor in Congress with a less enhanced matching formula. This partial restructuring, abetted by the lax waiver policy of the current administration could turn Medicaid into an entitlement in name only, and the entitlement that began in 1965 as an afterthought would pretty much disappear with little thought or controversy at all.[14]

Another possibility is that the Democrats, in an off-year election, might retake the House of Representatives. Even if they lost the Senate, they could easily block further structural changes in Medicaid and, through the budget reconciliation process, incrementally amend and enhance the entitlement. The latent power of that engine of change was demonstrated during the Reagan administration when a Democratic House used a series of budget reconciliations to restructure Medicaid between 1984 and 1990 and to develop the Medicare Fee Schedule over nine years, despite the opposition of the administration and Republican control of the Senate from 1980 to 1986.

Several final comments. The entitlement status, as such, remains enormously important not just as a promise, but in practical consequence as well. Somewhat like the American Constitution, keeping Medicare and Medicaid as entitlements helps to bound controversy, restrain intemperate majorities, and protect those with little political power. This security provides opportunity to experiment safely, to undo mistakes, and to invest the entitlement with new vigor—as the history of Medicare and Medicaid reform illustrates in rich detail. Over time, we have devised ways to work with these entitlements, creating institutions of government that can be used to mobilize collective power, restructure whole programs, or modify them in detail. These institutions can be readily employed either for partisan warfare or for collaboration in difficult, protracted technical ventures. We have tried the first alternative. Let us hope we have the good sense and will to try the second.

NOTES

[1] The higher figure includes debt interest that would not be retired and other costs.

[2] *New York Times,* October 3, 2001, p. A-23.

[3] Health insurance for the unemployed and uninsured was a make-or-break issue in the second stimulus package debated at the very end of the 2001 session of Congress.

[4] In large part because of a belief that HMOs were already adequately paid. HMOs protested that the Senate was relying on figures that were ten years out of date. About the only successful initiative was a demonstration program involving five small HMOs in risk-sharing between these plans and CMS.

[5] A growth rate of 10 percent seemed alarming, especially when considered against the background of a 1 percent decline in Medicare expenditures in 1999. By way of comparison, in 2001 FEHBP announced increases of more than 13 percent. Private plans posted increases of 20 percent and more. Marilyn Moon [1995] has argued that Medicare generally outperformed the private sector over a ten-year cycle. Bruce Vladeck (1999) adds that Medicare supported the private sector with a number of subsidies and still performed better on cost containment. Nevertheless, 10 percent was a shock in comparison with −1 percent; and some observers said it was time for another round similar to BBA 97.

[6] Sorel (1912). Sorel (1847–1922) was a French revolutionary syndicalist who believed that the "myth of the general strike" would unite workers and move them to deeds of heroism. It never did.

[7] Kathleen E. Means, senior public policy adviser, Patton Boggs, LL. Formerly staff of Senate Finance, House Ways and Means. As quoted in *Health Care Policy Review*, February 26, 2001, p. 284.

[8] Assuming that managed care plans will accept "competitive bidding" with any bite to it—which is a sizeable assumption. It is wise to remember in this context that managed care plans have shown they can live without Medicare.

[9] Bruce Vladeck (1999:35) argues that regional and local interests can be adjusted with a defined contribution or voucher program almost as easily as under the present system. He mentions the internal revenue code as an instructive example of how legislators can address particularistic interests despite the legislative constraint of generality.

[10] Most of the recent "administrative reform" efforts sought to raise comfort levels for providers rather than increase the powers or funding of CMS. Even these failed to survive the end-of-session crunch.

[11] The progress of this debate is instructive. In 1995, when Democrats attacked the Medicare reductions as "tax cuts for the rich," Republicans then said that they were saving Medicare by restructuring it and extending solvency. This response did not entirely counter the fairness issue, but it helped. After BBA 97, the argument was that an FEHBP model would give Medicare beneficiaries the same kind of plan that members of Congress had—and what could be unfair about that? Democrats then began talking more about risk selection—a topic they had avoided in 1995 because they thought it too abstract and technical for public debate. As one benefit, more Democrats now believe risk selection is an issue that can be sufficiently appreciated by a wider public.

[12] Dick Hegner, senior research associate, National Health Policy Forum. Interview, November 8, 2001.

[13] Though some in Washington say that the states have "been partying too long" and need to share the burden with the rest of us. Ibid.

[14] Ironically, this outcome would return Medicaid to the second-class status with which it began. It would be a comment on who and what gets sacrificed in a time of hardship. The distinguished Canadian economist Robert Evans, commenting on American health policy, said that he found Americans "amazing." They would, he said, spend millions to save a few polar bears in the Arctic regions, but when it came to needy health care recipients, they did not care how many go overboard, as long as they "don't have to hear the splash."

Appendix A

TITLE IV—MEDICARE, MEDICAID, AND CHILDREN'S HEALTH PROVISIONS

SEC. 4000. AMENDMENTS TO SOCIAL SECURITY ACT AND REFERENCES TO OBRA; TABLE OF CONTENTS OF TITLE.

(a) AMENDMENTS TO SOCIAL SECURITY ACT—Except as otherwise specifically provided, whenever in this title an amendment is expressed in terms of an amendment to or repeal of a section or other provision, the reference shall be considered to be made to that section or other provision of the Social Security Act.

(b) REFERENCES TO OBRA—In this title, the terms 'OBRA-1986', 'OBRA-1987', 'OBRA-1989', 'OBRA-1990', and 'OBRA-1993' refer to the Omnibus Budget Reconciliation Act of 1986 (Public Law 99-509), the Omnibus Budget Reconciliation Act of 1987 (Public Law 100-203), the Omnibus Budget Reconciliation Act of 1989 (Public Law 101-239), the Omnibus Budget Reconciliation Act of 1990 (Public Law 101-508), and the Omnibus Budget Reconciliation Act of 1993 (Public Law 103-66), respectively.

(c) TABLE OF CONTENTS OF TITLE—The table of contents of this title is as follows:

Sec. 4000. Amendments to Social Security Act and references to OBRA; table of contents of title.

Appendix B
HCFA/CMS

The Health Care Financing Administration was created in 1977, early in the Carter Administration, by the merger of the Medicare and Medicaid programs and their related medical care quality staffs. This step was part of a sweeping reorganization of the Department of Health, Education, and Welfare. It was also prompted by a desire to separate the medical programs from welfare and to prepare the way for national health insurance. At that time, most of the Medicare and Medicaid personnel were moved to one end of Social Security Boulevard, outside of Baltimore, though a number of the top officials had and have second offices in Washington, D.C., in the downtown complex of the Department of Health and Human Services. This is a relatively small agency of about 4,500 employees, but in the year 2000 oversaw annual expenditures of $370 billion. On July 1, 2001, the name of the agency was changed to Centers for Medicare and Medicaid Services in order to emphasize, according to an official release, priorities of responsiveness to beneficiaries and providers and quality improvement. Though small, HCFA/CMS has been assigned many new responsibilities over the years and especially by BBA 1997. It has not gotten commensurate administrative funding or staff authorizations—which has been a chronic problem. The agency's activities can be summarized under three main headings.

IMPLEMENTATION OF THE PROGRAMS

HCFA/CMS administers the Medicare program and shares with state agencies the administration of Medicaid and SCHIP. For Medicare, the agency contracts *directly* with the carriers and fiscal intermediaries that administer claims and the managed care organizations that participate in Medicare+Choice; for Medicaid, it works *indirectly* through state Medicaid agencies and SCHIP authorities. Several functions are similar for both programs and they share in some activities, but they have remained separate with little overlap in personnel. Some of the implementation activities are as follows:

- Develop the policies and write the rules that implement legislation and mandates from the Congress and the Administration; contract with and supervise the carriers and fiscal intermediaries; contract with the Medicare MCOs; review Medicaid and SCHIP State agency plans, plan amendments, waiver applications, and provider contracts; write manuals, develop forms, procedures, and software to guide providers or third parties; issue statements of operational policies and state Medicaid director letters; organize or sponsor conferences and training sessions with providers, State officials, professional bodies, or other stakeholders; consult with a variety of advisory committees.
- In consultation with professional groups and advisory committees, amend, update, and oversee administration of a number of fee schedules and prospective payment systems.
- Assure and improve quality of care; collaborate in development of standards of quality and performance; set agendas for the PROs; work with state quality improvement systems and with state and private accreditation agencies; monitor quality in a variety of subordinate programs such as skilled nursing facilities, home health care organizations, and clinical laboratories.
- Oversee claims processing and the monitoring of fiscal integrity by the carriers and fiscal intermediaries; supervise the settlement and adjudication of disputes; implement the comprehensive fraud and abuse legislation of 1996 and 1997; educate providers through the program integrity initiatives; work with other federal authorities and with state and local officials to curb fraud and abuse; make recommendations for sanctions to the inspector general.
- Inform beneficiaries and providers about benefits, program activities, and responsibilities; as mandated by BBA 97, organize and supervise each year an annual Medicare+Choice "election"; approve "campaign" materials and monitor election practices; develop user-friendly and culturally sensitive materials, including multilanguage publications, 1-800 "hot lines," and internet web-sites. Collaborate with the States in developing similar programs, especially for Medicaid managed care.

A vital but low-visibility part of implementation is "operations," to use the earlier terminology. Operational activities supply the forms, instructions, computer software, manuals and instruction letters needed for providers to file claims and get paid, for institutions to meet conditions of participation and comply with regulations, and for beneficiaries to know their rights and make intelligent choices. Operations runs the mainframe computers, keeps the vast data files in order, and helps others to use them for research, systems design, and to maintain program integrity or identify fraud, waste, and abuse.

PROVIDING DATA, INFORMATION, OR
POLICY RECOMMENDATIONS TO OTHERS

In addition to informing beneficiaries and providers—exhaustively and in detail—about benefits or program requirements, the agency is charged with various other information and reporting responsibilities:

- Provide data, information, and policy recommendations for other DHHS component agencies.
- Develop and share statistics, data, actuarial projections, and research findings with other agencies, states, and private parties.
- Respond to requests for testimony, reports, briefings or policy advice from Congress, congressional agencies, or the Administration.
- Complete the numerous studies and reports mandated by Congress.

PLANNING AND DEVELOPMENT

The agency also maintains a large research and development component. It is expected to

- track actuarial, demographic, and macroeconomic trends and assess their impact on beneficiaries, providers, and the health care industry;
- perform and sponsor research and development, especially into new service modalities, methods of payment, and improvements in health care delivery;
- develop and implement strategies for updating and expanding data and information systems.

As the list of activities suggests, HCFA/CMS engages in little direct administration. Mostly, it writes rules and operational policies and oversees their implementation. To estimate and respond to future needs, it has its own actuarial staff and research and demonstration capability. It maintains a huge database and automated information system, an invaluable resource in itself. But much of the program activity is carried out by contract or liaison with consultants and research enterprises, provider groups and health care plans, state agencies, medical schools, and universities. This mode of administration has some disadvantages: delay, dependence on what is available, and various transaction costs. At the same time, it gives the agency flexibility in development and access to a vast and varied outside expertise and capability. In recent years, three of the biggest challenges for the agency have been the outpatient prospective payment systems, the quality initiative, and the consumer information system, all of which required flexibility and skill in contracting and working with outside sources.

In addition to the Baltimore and Washington offices, HCFA/CMS has a regional office in each of the ten HHS regional cities. Since 1997 these have been grouped into four regional consortia. About one-third of the 4,500 agency employees are in the regional offices, with activities divided between supervising the carriers and fiscal intermediaries; helping monitor and implement managed care activities; maintaining program integrity and combatting fraud and abuse; working with state and private agencies on accreditation and on Medicaid state plans; and providing information to beneficiaries and providers. Unlike the Social Security Administration (SSA), the agency has few field representatives working outside the regional offices, although the SSA still provides some help with Medicare enrollment and information. The Baltimore office sets policy and keeps in touch with the regions through frequent communication, including telephone conference calls. Opinion differs about the quality of the regional offices, but there is a consensus that, overall, quality is lower than that in Baltimore and that performance varies from region to region.

On November 7, 1996, HCFA announced the reorganization that later figured prominently in the implementation of BBA 97. This reorganization developed integrally from the Strategic Plan of 1994 and emphasized a beneficiary orientation and more "partnering" with providers. Figure B-1 shows the organization as it existed prior to that time and Figure B-2 shows the details of this reorganization. The major changes were to combine managed care and FFS administration under one division of Health Plan and Provider Operations; strengthen relations with beneficiaries and combine this function with the existing Bureau of Program Operations; put Medicaid and regional activities under a new division of State Operations; and upgrade clinical and quality standards. The Office of Research and Demonstrations was abolished as a separate entity, though the activities continue. Underlying objectives of this reorganization, not apparent from the organization charts, were to bring policy development and operations closer together, to strengthen beneficiary relations, and to create three main divisions headed by political appointees, reporting directly to the Administrator. According to rumor, another purpose was to bring the managed care and FFS programs together so as to make any future "two HCFA's" proposal difficult to implement.

Within weeks after the appointment of the new administrator, Thomas Scully, another HCFA reorganization was announced in June 2001(Figure B-4). Although this reorganization is still in process, several important differences are apparent. The new title, "Centers for Medicare and Medicaid Services," emphasizes a commitment to a "culture of responsiveness." The restructured "centers" follow "major lines of business," so that the FFS Medicare program again stands by itself and beneficiary information and choices and plan management are put together within the Center for Beneficiary Choices. Goals to be sought include (1) enhancing the Medicare education program, (2) creating a culture of responsiveness, (3) Medicare contracting

ORGANIZATIONAL CHART

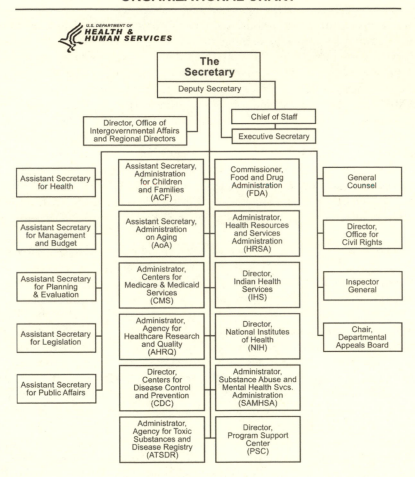

Figure B-1

reforms that emphasize flexibility, incentives and competition, and contractor evaluation. The new structure reflects, in some measure, the private sector and decentralizing preferences of the Bush Administration. It could be adapted to another "two HCFA's" proposal or to an FEHBP model for restructuring Medicare.

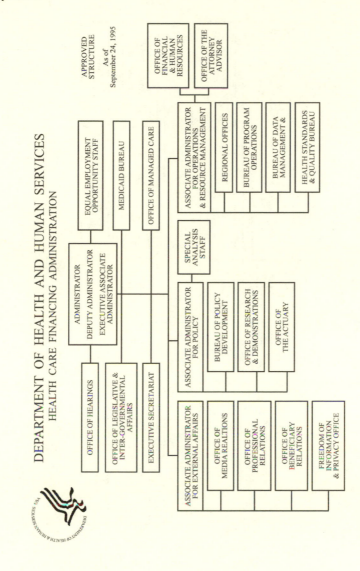

DEPARTMENT OF HEALTH AND HUMAN SERVICES
HEALTH CARE FINANCING ADMINISTRATION

APPROVED STRUCTURE
As of September 24, 1995

ADMINISTRATOR
DEPUTY ADMINISTRATOR
EXECUTIVE ASSOCIATE ADMINISTRATOR

OFFICE OF HEARINGS

OFFICE OF LEGISLATIVE & INTER-GOVERNMENTAL AFFAIRS

EXECUTIVE SECRETARIAT

EQUAL EMPLOYMENT OPPORTUNITY STAFF

MEDICAID BUREAU

OFFICE OF MANAGED CARE

OFFICE OF FINANCIAL & HUMAN RESOURCES

OFFICE OF THE ATTORNEY ADVISOR

ASSOCIATE ADMINISTRATOR FOR EXTERNAL AFFAIRS

OFFICE OF MEDIA REALTIONS

OFFICE OF PROFESSIONAL RELATIONS

OFFICE OF BENEFICIARY RELATIONS

FREEDOM OF INFORMATION & PRIVACY OFFICE

ASSOCIATE ADMINISTRATOR FOR POLICY

BUREAU OF POLICY DEVELOPMENT

OFFICE OF RESEARCH & DEMONSTRATIONS

OFFICE OF THE ACTUARY

SPECIAL ANALYSIS STAFF

ASSOCIATE ADMINISTRATOR FOR OPERATIONS & RESOURCE MANAGEMENT

REGIONAL OFFICES

BUREAU OF PROGRAM OPERATIONS

BUREAU OF DATA MANAGEMENT &

HEALTH STANDARDS & QUALITY BUREAU

Figure B-2

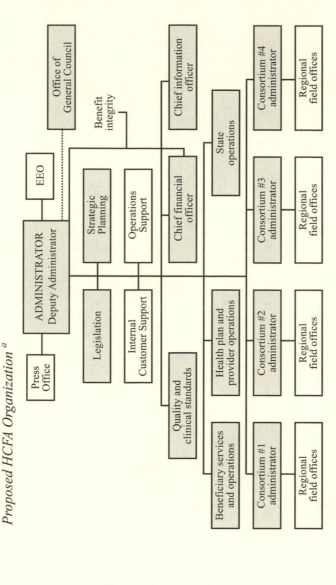

Proposed HCFA Organization [a]

a. Shaded boxes would be members of the Executive Council

Figure B-3

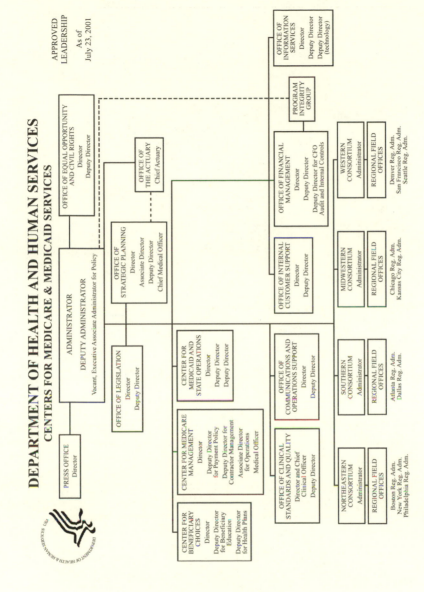

DEPARTMENT OF HEALTH AND HUMAN SERVICES
CENTERS FOR MEDICARE & MEDICAID SERVICES

APPROVED LEADERSHIP
As of July 23, 2001

ADMINISTRATOR
DEPUTY ADMINISTRATOR
Vacant, Executive Associate Administrator for Policy

PRESS OFFICE
Director

OFFICE OF EQUAL OPPORTUNITY AND CIVIL RIGHTS
Director
Deputy Director

OFFICE OF THE ACTUARY
Chief Actuary

OFFICE OF INFORMATION SERVICES
Director
Deputy Director
Deputy Director (technology)

OFFICE OF LEGISLATION
Director
Deputy Director

OFFICE OF STRATEGIC PLANNING
Director
Associate Director
Deputy Director
Chief Medical Officer

PROGRAM INTEGRITY GROUP

CENTER FOR BENEFICIARY CHOICES
Director
Deputy Director for Beneficiary Education
Deputy Director for Health Plans

CENTER FOR MEDICARE MANAGEMENT
Director
Deputy Director for Payment Policy
Deputy Director for Contractor Management
Associate Director for Operations
Medical Officer

CENTER FOR MEDICAID AND STATE OPERATIONS
Director
Deputy Director
Deputy Director

OFFICE OF FINANCIAL MANAGEMENT
Director
Deputy Director
Deputy Director for CFO Audit and Internal Controls

OFFICE OF CLINICAL STANDARDS AND QUALITY
Director and Chief Clinical Officer
Deputy Director

OFFICE OF COMMUNICATIONS AND OPERATIONS SUPPORT
Director
Deputy Director

OFFICE OF INTERNAL CUSTOMER SUPPORT
Director
Deputy Director

WESTERN CONSORTIUM
Administrator

REGIONAL FIELD OFFICES
Denver Reg. Adm.
San Francisco Reg. Adm.
Seattle Reg. Adm.

MIDWESTERN CONSORTIUM
Administrator

REGIONAL FIELD OFFICES
Chicago Reg. Adm.
Kansas City Reg. Adm.

SOUTHERN CONSORTIUM
Administrator

REGIONAL FIELD OFFICES
Atlanta Reg. Adm.
Dallas Reg. Adm.

NORTHEASTERN CONSORTIUM
Administrator

REGIONAL FIELD OFFICES
Boston Reg. Adm.
New York Reg. Adm.
Philadelphia Reg. Adm.

Figure B-4

Glossary

ACRONYMS

AAPCC	adjusted average per capita cost
ACR	adjusted community rate
AHRQ (AHCPR)	Agency for Healthcare Research and Quality
APC	ambulatory payment classification
ASPE	Assistant Secretary for Planning and Evaluation, DHHS
BBA	Balanced Budget Act (1995, 1997)
BBRA	Balanced Budget Refinement Act of 1999
BIPA	Medicare, Medicaid, and SCHIP Benefits and Improvement Act of 2000
CBO	Congressional Budget Office
CBRR	Consumer Bill of Rights and Responsibilities
CMS	Centers for Medicare and Medicaid Services
CPR	customary, prevailing and reasonable
CPT	Current Procedural Terminology
CR	continuing resolution
DCG	diagnostic cost group
DGME	direct graduate medical education
DRG	diagnosis related group
DSH	disproportionate share (adjustment)
EITC	Earned Income Tax Credit
EPSTD	Early and Periodic Screening, Diagnosis and Testing
ERISA	Employee Retirement Income Security Act (1974)
FAcct	Foundation for Accountability
FEHBP	Federal Employee Health Benefits Program
FIM-FRG	Functional Independence Measure-Function Related Group
FQHC	Federally Qualified Health Center
GAO	General Accounting Office
HHA	home health agency

HCFA	(CMS) Health Care Financing Administration (Centers for Medicare and Medicaid Services)
HCPCS	HCFA Common Procedure Coding System
HEDIS	Health Plan Employer Data and Information Set
HIFA	Health Insurance Flexibility and Accountability Demonstration Waiver
HIPAA	Health Insurance Portability and Accountability Act of 1996
HMO	health maintenance organization
HRSA	Health Resources and Services Administration
IMD	Institution for Mental Diseases
IME	indirect medical education (expense)
IPS	interim payment system
JCAHO	Joint Commission on Accreditation of Healthcare Organizations
MCO	managed care organization
MEI	Medicare Economic Index
MedPAC	Medicare Payment Advisory Commission
MSA	metropolitan statistical area; Medical Saving Account
NCQA	National Committee for Quality Assurance
NGA	National Governors' Association
OASIS	Outcome and Assessment Information Set
OBRA	Omnibus Budget Reconciliation Act
OMB	Office of Management and Budget
PACE	Program of All-Inclusive Care for the Elderly
PAYGO	Pay-as-you-go
POS	point-of-service plan
PPO	preferred provider organization
PPRC	Physician Payment Review Commission
PPS	Prospective Payment System
PRO	Peer Review Organization
ProPAC	Prospective Payment Assessment Commission
PSN	provider service network
PSO	Provider Sponsored Organization
QARI	Quality Assurance Reform Initiative
QISMC	Quality Improvement System for Managed Care
QMB	Qualified Medicare Beneficiary
RBRVS	resource based relative value scale
RUG-III	Resource Utilization Groups, version III
SCHIP	State Children's Health Insurance Program
SLMB	Specified Low-Income Medicare Beneficiary
SMI	Supplementary Medical Insurance Program (Medicare Pt. B)

SNF   Skilled Nursing Facility
SSI   Supplemental Security Income
TEFRA   Tax Equity and Fiscal Responsibility Act (1982)
Y2K   year 2000

TERMS

Adjusted Average per Capita Cost (AAPCC):   an actuarial estimate of the amount required to serve a Medicare population within a geographic area (county), adjusted for age, sex, institutional, and disability status

Adjusted Community Rate: rates for individual health plans contracting with Medicare based upon their estimates of the costs of providing services to Medicare enrollees and adjusted so that the plans do not receive a higher rate of return for these beneficiaries than they do for their commercial members

Adverse Selection: when an insurer is selected by a larger share of high-risk enrollees than statistically expected. Favorable selection is to get a smaller share

Ambulatory Patient Classifications: recent system that classifies outpatient procedures and services into payment groups

Assignment: agreement by a physician or provider to accept the Medicare allowed charge as payment in full, i.e., to forgo balance billing

Authorization: act of Congress, required by the Constitution, that provides the legal authority for appropriations to initiate or continue an agency or program activity

Balance Bill/Extra Bill: physician or provider charges that exceed those paid by Medicare or other third-party payer

Baseline: projection of future spending and revenues under assumed economic conditions and participation rates, with no change in current policy; usually projected annually and for five years by the CBO, with amendments during the year

Behavioral Offset: allowance made for expected response to limits on payment rates, for instance, change in a fee schedule

Block Grant: grant typically awarded to a state or local government, distributed according to formulas established by law, to support broadly categorical activities or programs with a minimum of restrictions, set-asides, or mandates; often contrasted with more narrowly defined or targeted "categorical" or "project" grants

Boren Amendment: after Sen. David Boren (D., Okla.); enacted in two stages, in 1980 and 1981, this Medicaid legislation had, as one aim, allowing states more flexibility to develop their own payment methods for nursing homes and hospitals; it required that hospital payments take into account a "disproportionate share of low income patients with special needs"; the amendment(s) also required that rates for hospitals and nursing facilities be "reasonable and adequate" to meet the costs of "effective and economic" operation; the legislation gave rise to a large number of lawsuits and was resented by many governors; repealed by BBA 1997

Budget Enforcement Act (BEA) of 1990: the most important act currently governing budget procedures

Budget Neutrality: requirement that changes in policies or payments be offset by reductions or increased revenues so that budget totals are not increased

Budget Resolution: annual resolution by Congress setting forth spending, revenue, and deficit targets for the next five fiscal years; the first year is binding and guides, in principle, the activities of all other congressional committees, but especially the authorizing, tax-writing, and appropriations committees; in principle, this resolution outlines the tasks and major priorities that guide the reconciliation process

Bundling: combining a number of services and/or procedures into a single package for coding, billing, or payment

Capitation: payment of a fixed amount per person for a period of time rather than compensating by salary or fees for specific services or procedures

Capped Entitlement: benefit available to all who are eligible, but in which a government limits the amount it will contribute; capped entitlements were proposed in the Reagan administration and again in 1995

Carrier: under Medicare, a private contractor (typically an insurance company) that processes claims for physician services paid under Part B

Case-Mix Index (CMI): index (number) that measures the severity of cases experienced by a provider

Centers of Excellence: HCFA demonstration that negotiated contracts with "centers of excellence," such as medical schools or clinical centers for high-quality programs of treatment for specially difficult and costly cases; this approach was adopted and broadened somewhat in its application by BBA 97

Competitive Bidding (Pricing): method used to set a price for a specified population and benefits soliciting competitive bids and then determining the price or contribution the payer will make; frequently used in the private sector; adapted for HCFA demonstrations

Conversion Factor: in a fee schedule, a multiplier that is used to convert the relative value scale into the dollar amounts paid to a provider

Coinsurance: cost sharing in which the insured party and the insurer share a specified ratio of the approved charges after a deductible has been met; under Medicare, for instance, the carrier pays 80 percent and the beneficiary pays 20 percent of Medicare approved charges

Copayment: amount paid by the covered party for a covered service

Cost Reimbursement: payment on the basis of audited costs (rather than "charges"), especially for Medicare hospital providers prior to the hospital inpatient PPS

Current Procedural Terminology (CPT): coding system developed by the American Medical Association and widely used as a basis for payment

Customary, Prevailing, and Reasonable (CPR): terminology for the charge limits under Medicare prior to implementation of the Medicare Fee Schedule in January 1992; adopting a method widely used in the private sector, Medicare would pay a physician based on the lesser amount of his or her actual or customary charge or the charge prevailing in the carrier locality

Debt Ceiling: legal limit on the amount of federal borrowing. Often increased temporarily or permanently especially in the course of budget negotiations

Deductible: amount of approved medical expenses an insured party must pay before receiving payments under an insurance scheme

Defined Benefit Plan: pension or health plan that promises the beneficiary benefits of a certain level—for example, the current Medicare FFS program

Defined Contribution Plan: plan to which an employer or public agency makes a monetary contribution and typically allows the benefits to vary—for example, the Federal Employee Health Benefit Plan

Diagnosis Cost Groups: clinical classification system based on diagnoses and demographic data that can be used to predict costs associated with a particular individual, and could provide the technical basis for a managed care risk adjuster; HCFA (CMS) has been attempting to implement one variant, the PIP-DCGs, or the Principal Inpatient Diagnosis Cost Group methodology

Diagnosis Related Groups (DRGs): methodology developed for classifying cases by diagnosis (or procedure); used as the basis for payment for inpatient hospital stays under the Medicare Prospective Payment System since its implementation in 1984

Discretionary Spending: spending that is controllable through the appropriations process—in contrast to mandatory spending, mostly for entitlements

Disproportionate Share Adjustment (DSH): payment adjustment for Medicare or Medicaid hospitals that serve a high volume of low-income patients

Dual Eligible: persons eligible for Medicaid coverage who, because of poverty, age, or disability have some supplemental coverage under Medicare

Early and Periodic Screening, Diagnosis and Treatment (EPSDT): Medicaid program established in 1967 that mandated certain services for "categorically needy" persons under 21 years of age, and included screening for mental or physical illnesses and conditions and treatment for those illnesses or conditions discovered; a federal mandate that was (and still is) considered onerous by states and has been difficult to enforce

Encounter Data: description of the diagnoses or services provided when a member visits a health plan provider; such information is especially important for the development of a managed care risk adjuster

Entitlement Program: program that requires the payment of benefits to all who meet the eligibility requirements, such as Medicare, Medicaid, Social Security, and veterans pensions

Employee Retirement Income Security Act (ERISA):   enacted in 1974, primarily to protect pension benefits, ERISA was extended to health plans; under the so-called ERISA preemption, regulation of large, self-insured or "ERISA" health plans are largely exempt from state regulation and from most lawsuits, especially for denial of benefits or malpractice

Exempt or Excluded Hospitals: hospitals or hospital units not included under the Prospective Payment System, often called "TEFRA" hospitals because they came under this earlier legislation; the most important categories are psychiatric, long-term care, children's and rehabilitation hospitals and separate rehabilitation or psychiatric units within hospitals—in all, more than 3,500 entities

Federal Medical Assistance Percentage (FMAP):   federal share (percentage) of a state's expenses that will be paid by the federal government; originally, the FMAP varied according to the per capita income within the state, with a minimum FMAP of 50 percent and a maximum of 83 percent

Federally Qualified Health Center (FQHC):   health center in a medically underserved area that is eligible for Medicare and Medicaid cost reimbursement

Fiscal Intermediary: under Medicare, a private contractor, that has contracts to make payments for Part A and some Part B services

Functional Independence Measure–Function Related Group: patient classification system used to classify patients and measure outcomes; considered as one basis for a prospective payment system for skilled nursing facilities

Graduate Medical Education (GME):   medical training following medical school, including internship, residency, and fellowships

Gramm-Rudman-Hollings: Balanced Budget and Emergency Deficit Control Act of 1985; especially important in providing mandatory procedures for budget deficit reduction, targeting Medicare and Medicaid among other programs

Health Care Financing Administration (HCFA):   unit within the U.S. Department of Health and Human Services with primary responsibility for the Medicare and Medicaid programs; established in 1977; renamed the Centers for Medicare and Medicaid Services in June 2001

Health Maintenance Organization (HMO):   organization that acts as an insurer, manages care, and provides comprehensive health services to members for a prepaid, capitated amount; "group" or "staff" models provide care exclusively through a "closed panel" of providers; independent practice association (IPA) models provide care through individual physicians or hospitals that typically contract with the HMO for only part of their services; "network" models make use of various arrangements with individuals and groups of providers; currently, there are many variants on these basic types, including PPOs, PSOs, and various POS arrangements

Indirect Medical Education Adjustment (IME): payment adjustment added to the DRG payments, based on the ratio of interns and residents to the number of inpatient beds

Intergovernmental Transfers (IGTs): one of several means employed by states to maximize their Medicaid matching funds; states would overpay Medicaid eligible facilities and, in turn, receive back transferred funds that they would use for a variety of purposes, including other health programs or additional matching funds; other schemes included provider donations or taxes and maximizing Medicaid DSH payments

Interim Payment System (IPA): payment system established for home health agencies by BBA 1997 that was to last from October 1, 1997, until October 1, 1999; it was regarded as onerous and unfair by the agencies

Look-back: type of sequester created by the Budget Enforcement Act of 1990; use of this mechanism figured prominently in BBA 95

Mandate (Federal): enforceable federal requirement imposed upon a state, local government or private party

Mark, Markup: legislative stage at which the text of a bill is discussed and amended; the committee or subcommittee chair normally decides which bill to consider, which then becomes the "chairman's mark"

Market Basket Index: index of the annual change in goods and services used by providers employed especially for setting prospective payments

Medicare+Choice: program created by the Balanced Budget Act of 1997 that provided an array of choices among coordinated care health plans; separate from the traditional FFS Medicare program

Medicare Cost Report: annual report required of institutions participating in the Medicare program, including total costs and charges, costs attributable to Medicare, and Medicare payments received; long regarded as onerous by providers, but considered an important source of data and a monitoring tool by HCFA (CMS)

Medicare Economic Index (MEI): index of physician inputs and expenses constructed by the federal government and used since 1975 to limit prevailing charges for Medicare services

Medicare Fee Schedule: fee schedule for Medicare physician payments, in effect since January 1992

Notice and Comment: stage in the informal rule-making process during which interested parties are notified that they may comment on the proposed rule; especially important, in law, are the quality and responsiveness of the explanations and justifications the agency then gives

Nursing Facility: provides institutional care—a "nursing home"—for elderly Medicaid beneficiaries who need it and who qualify with respect to assets and income; the Omnibus Budget Reconciliation Act of 1997 (OBRA 97), sometimes referred to as the "nursing home reform act," changed the official terminology from "nursing home" to "nursing facility"

Outlier Payments: payments for cases deviating from the norm, for instance, in expense or length of stay

Participating Physician, Supplier: physician or supplier who agrees in writing to take assignment of all Medicare claims for a year

Peer Review: review of the work of providers by other health care professionals, usually within the same specialty or subspecialty, especially with respect to its quality and necessity

Peer Review Organization (PRO):   organization under contract with the HCFA to review the medical care provided to Medicare beneficiaries

Per Capita Cap (PCC):   proposed cap on expenditures per Medicaid beneficiary, as opposed to an aggregate cap for a whole area; the PCC would limit the rate of increase using Medicaid beneficiary categories such as sex, age, disability, and poverty level; it retained the concept of entitlement and would help avoid interstate distribution issues, but would lock in historic inequities; proposed earlier in the Reagan administration and again in 1995 and 1996

Point-of-Service Plan (POS):   plan combining features of managed care and of FFS insurance; enrollees can opt for "plan" providers or for providers outside the plan at the time the service is needed; usually, for going outside the plan a substantial deductible and copays will be charged, though often with a "catastrophic" limit

Preferred Provider Organization (PPO):   plan that contracts with one or more panels of providers who provide services based on a negotiated fee schedule or a discount from usual charges; PPOs offer more freedom of choice than the typical managed care plan, often with incentives for patients to use PPO providers; they vary widely in selectivity of providers and the amount of control exercised over them

Program of All-Inclusive Care for the Elderly (PACE):   originally a HCFA demonstration that used managed care contracts to provide comprehensive care for elderly, dually eligible patients; BBA 1997 made it a permanent program and extended it to include Medicare

Provider Sponsored Organization (PSO); Provider Service Network (PSN):   health plans organized by providers who act to some extent as the insurers

Quality Assurance Reform Initiative (QARI):   project initiated in 1993 that helped develop quality measures for the Medicaid program; the QARI project contributed to the subsequent development of QISMC

Quality Improvement System for Managed Care (QISMC): quality improvement system incorporating outcome measures and continuous quality improvement that provided the conceptual foundations and methodology for the Medicare managed care quality provisions of BBA 1997

Reconciliation: process by which Congress requires committees to make the changes in legislation and appropriations to conform with the limits, allocations, and instructions contained in the budget resolution

Rescission: action by the president and Congress that cancels part or all of a previously enacted budget authorization

Risk Adjuster: measure or technique used to adjust payments to compensate for health care expenses expected to result from differences in the health status of enrollees in separate health plans

Risk Contracts: under Medicare, an arrangement made in 1972 (TEFRA) that allows HMOs to be compensated on a "risk" or "incentive," basis, i.e., through periodic capitation payments, with some subsequent allowable cost adjustments

Rulemaking: process by which implementing regulations are developed within the executive branch agencies or by regulatory agencies

Sequester: deficit reduction procedure that requires offsetting changes if spending exceeds or revenue falls short of the amount needed to meet a deficit reduction target set for a given year

Skilled Nursing Facility: facility that meets certification requirements for skilled nursing and provides mostly inpatient nursing and rehabilitation services to patients discharged from hospitals

Supplementary Medical Insurance Program (SMI): covers Part B of Medicare—mostly physician and some outpatient services; unlike the Part A or Hospital Insurance program, SMI membership is at the option of the beneficiary and requires the payment of an annual premium

Tax Equity and Fiscal Responsibility Act of 1982: created a payment system for the TEFRA or "exempt" hospitals; mandated the development of a hospital inpatient prospective payment system; included various other provisions dealing with HMOs, Competitive Medical Plans, and Peer Review Organizations

Volume: amount or number of services supplied (in contrast to their price)

Voucher: fixed subsidy or grant, typically made to an individual or family head, and limited to the purchase of a specific good, such as food, education, or health care

Waiver: states may apply to the Medicaid program for a "waiver" of some of the general requirements of the Medicaid program in order to experiment with different methods of payment (HMOs) or service delivery; waivers are subject to approval by the secretary and must be in accord with a number of guarantees and protections prescribed by Medicaid legislation

Bibliography

Abraham, Laura Kaye (1993). *Mama Might Be Better Off Dead: The Failure of Health Care in America*. Chicago, IL: University of Chicago Press.

Altman, Stuart H., Uwe E. Reinhardt, and Alexander E. Shields (Eds.) (1998). *The Future U.S. Healthcare System: Who Will Care for the Poor and Uninsured*. Chicago, IL: Health Administration.

Ball, Robert M. (1993). "Report to the SSA Staff on the Implications of the Social Security Amendments of 1965," November 16, 1965. Reprinted by the National Academy of Social Insurance in *Reflections on Implementing Medicare*, Washington, D.C.

Ball, Robert M. (1995). "Perspectives on Medicare: What Medicare's Architects Had in Mind." *Health Affairs* 14(4):62–72.

Benda, Peter M. and Charles H. Levine (1999). "Reagan and the Bureaucracy: The Bequest, the Promise, and the Legacy." In Charles O. Jones (Ed.), *The Reagan Legacy: Promise and Performance*. Chatham, NJ: Chatham House.

Berenson, Robert A. (2001). "Medicare+Choice—Doubling or Disappearing?" www.healthaffairs.org, accessed December 20. Also related essays in this posting.

Berenson, Robert A., and Walter A. Zelman (1998). *The Managed Care Blues and How to Cure Them*. Washington, DC: Georgetown University Press.

Brown, Lawrence D. (1983). *Politics and Health Care Organization—HMOs as Federal Policy*. Washington, DC: Brookings Institution.

Butler, Stuart M. and Robert E. Moffit (1995). "The FEHBP as a Model for a New Medicare Program." *Health Affairs* 14(4):47–61.

Cain, Harry P. (1999). "Moving Medicare to the FEHBP Model, or How to Make an Elephant Fly." *Health Affairs* 18(4):25–39.

Center for Budget and Policy Priorities (1997). *Medicaid and Child Health Provisions of the Bipartisan Budget Agreement*. Washington, DC: Author.

Chasan-Sloan, Deborah M. (2001). "NOTE: Managed Care, the Poor, and the Constitution: Are Due Process Rights Ailing Under Medicaid Managed Care?" *Georgetown Journal of Poverty Law and Policy* 8:283–306.

Chassin, Mark R. (1997). "Assessing Strategies for Quality Improvement." *Health Affairs* 16(3):151–73.

Collender, Stanley E. (1995). *The Guide to the Federal Budget Fiscal 1996.* Lanham, MD: Rowman and Littlefield.

Collender, Stanley E. (1996). *The Guide to the Federal Budget Fiscal 1997.* Lanham, MD: Rowman and Littlefield.

Collender, Stanley E. (1997). *The Guide to the Federal Budget Fiscal 1998.* Lanham, MD: Rowman and Littlefield.

Coughlin, Teresa A., Leighton Ku, and Johnny Kim (2000). "Reforming the Medicaid Disproportionate Share Hospital Program." *Health Care Financing Review* 22(2):137–57.

Coughlin, Teresa A., and David Liska (1998). "Changing State and Federal Payment Policies for Medicaid Disproportionate-Share Hospitals." *Health Affairs* 17(3):118–36.

Council on Economic Impact of Health System Change (2001). *Conference on the Future of Managed Care,* May 18. Princeton, NJ: Author. Transcript, www.FedNet.net, p. 3.

Dallek, Geraldine (1998). *Consumer Protections in Medicare+Choice.* Washington, DC: Kaiser Family Foundation.

Davidson, Stephen M. and Joners, Stephen A. (eds.) 1998. *Remaking Medicaid: Managed Care for the Public Good.* San Francisco: Jossey-Bass.

Department of Health and Human Services (2000). *Report to Congress— Safeguards for Individuals with Special Healthcare Needs Enrolled in Medicaid Managed Care.* Washington, DC: Author.

Desmarais, Henry R. and Michael M. Hash (1997). "Financing Graduate Medical Education: The Search for New Sources of Support." *Health Affairs* 16(4):48–63.

Dionne, E. J. (1998). "Congressional Shakedown." *Washington Post,* September 7.

Dowd, Bryan, Robert Coulam and Roger Feldman (2000). "A Tale of Four Cities: Medicare Reform and Competitive Pricing." *Health Affairs* 19(5): 9–29.

Drew, Elizabeth (1996). *Showdown: The Struggle Between the Gingrich Congress and the Clinton White House.* New York: Simon & Schuster.

Eisenberg, John M. (1998)."Health Services Research In a Market-Oriented Health Care System" (with comment by Charles N. Kahn III). *Health Affairs* 17(1):98–108.

Ellis, Randall P. and Associates (1998). "Diagnosis-Based Risk Adjustment for Medicare Capitation Payments." *Health Care Financing Review* 17(3):101–28

Ellwood, Marilyn R. and Leighton Ku (1998). "Welfare and Immigration Reforms: Unintended Side Effects for Medicare." *Health Affairs* 17(3): 137–51.

Enthoven, Alain C. and Carol B. Vorhous (1997). "A Vision of Quality in Health Care Delivery." *Health Affairs* 16(3):44–57.

Etheredge, Lynn (1995a). *Re-Engineering Medicare from Bill-Paying Insurer to Accountable Purchaser.* Washington, DC: George Washington University, Health Insurance Reform Project.

Etheredge, Lynn (1995b). "The Evolution of a New Paradigm: Competitive Purchasing of Health Care." Paper prepared for conference on "The New Competition: Dynamics Shaping the Health Care Market," Washington, D.C., Nov. 16.

Etheredge, Lynn (1998). "The Medicare Reform of 1997: Headlines You Didn't Read." *Journal of Health Politics, Policy and Law* 23(3):573–79.

Etheredge, Lynn (1999a). "Purchasing Medicare Prescription Drug Benefits: A New Proposal." *Health Affairs* 18(4):7–19.

Etheredge, Lynn (1999b). "Three Streams, One River: A Coordinated Approach to Financing Retirement." *Health Affairs* 18(1):80–91.

Etheredge, Lynn (2000). "Medicare's Governance and Structure: A Proposal." *Health Affairs* 19(5):60–71.

Falkson, Joseph F. (1980). *HMOs and the Politics of Health Services Reform.* Chicago: American Hospital Association.

Feder, Judith M. (1977). *Medicare: The Politics of Federal Hospital Insurance.* Lexington, MA: D.C. Heath.

Feder, Judith, Larry Levitt, Ellen O'Brien, and Diane Rowland (2001). "Covering the Low-Income Uninsured: The Case for Expanding Public Programs." *Health Affairs* 20(1):27–39.

Feldman, Roger and Bryan Dowd (1998). "Structuring Choice under Medicare." in Robert D. Reischauer, Stuart Butler, and Judith Lave (Eds.), *Medicare: Preparing for the Challenge of the 21st Century.* Washington, DC: National Academy of Social Insurance.

Fenno, Richard E., Jr. (1997). *Learning to Govern: An Institutional View of the 104th Congress.* Washington, DC: Brookings Institution.

Fishman, Linda E. and James D. Bentley (1997). "The Evolution of Support for Safety-Net Hospitals." *Health Affairs* 16(4):30–47.

Fox, Peter D. (1997). "Applying Managed Care Techniques in Traditional Medicare." *Health Affairs* 16(5).44–57.

Fox, Peter (1998). "The Medicare Fee-for-Service System: Applying Managed Care Techniques." Pp. 185–206. in Robert D. Reischauer, Stuart Butler, and Judith Lave (Eds.), *Medicare: Preparing for the Challenge of the 21st Century.* Washington, DC: National Academy of Social Insurance.

Fox, Peter D., Lynn Etheredge, and Stanley B. Jones (1998). "Addressing the Needs of Chronically Ill Persons under Medicare." *Health Affairs* 17(2): 40–69.

Frank, Richard G., Chris Koyanagi, and Thomas G. McGuire (1997). "The Politics and Economics of Mental Health 'Parity' Laws." *Health Affairs* 16(4):108–19.

Fried, Bruce Merlin and Janet Ziegler (2000). *The Medicare+Choice Program: Is It Code Blue?* Washington, DC: ShawPittman.

Friedman, Emily (1995). "The Compromise and the Afterthought. Medicare and Medicaid after 30 Years." *Journal of the American Medical Association* 274(3, July 19):278–82.

Friedman Thomas (2000). *New York Times*, "Original Sin," November 10, p. 33.

Frist, Bill (1995). "The Future of Medicare: One Senator's Vision." *Health Affairs* 14(4):31–46.

Fuchs, Victor (1999). "Health Care for the Elderly: How Much? Who Will Pay for It?" *Health Affairs* 18(1):11–21.

Fullerton, William D. (1996). "Politics of Federal Health Policy, 1964–75." *Health Care Financing Review* 18(2):169–77.

Gagel, Barbara (1995). "Health Care Quality Improvement Program: A New Approach." *Health Care Financing Review* 16(4).15–24.

Gillespie, Ed and Bob Schellhas (1994). *Contract With America*. New York: Times Books.

Gingrich, Newt (1995). *To Renew America*. New York: HarperCollins.

Ginsburg, Paul B. and John R. Gabel (1998). "Tracking Health Care Costs: What's New in 1998?" *Health Affairs* 17(5):141–46.

Ginsburg, Paul B. and Jeremy D. Pickreign (1996). "Tracking Health Care Costs." *Health Affairs* 15(3):140–49.

Ginzberg, Eli (Ed.) (1994). *Critical Issues in U.S. Health Care Reform*. Boulder, CO: Westview.

Gold, Marsha (2001). "Medicare+Choice: An Interim Report Card." *Health Affairs* 20(4):120–38.

Gold, Marsha, et al. (1997). "Disabled Medicare Beneficiaries in HMOs." *Health Affairs* 16(5):149–62.

Goldsmith, Jeff (1994). "Perspective: Impact of Technology on Health Care." pp. 80–81. *Health Affairs* 13(3):80-81.

Goodman, John C. and Gerald Musgrave (1992). *Patient Power: Solving America's Health Care Crisis*. Washington, DC: Cato Institute.

Gormley, William T., Jr., and Cristina Boccuti (2001). "HCFA and the States: Politics and Intergovernmental Leverage." *Journal of Health Politics, Policy and Law* 26(3):557–80.

Gosfield, Alice (1997). "Who Is Holding Whom Accountable for Quality." *Health Affairs* 16(3):126–40.

Gruber, Jonathan and James Poterba (1995). "Tax Subsidies to Employer-Provided Health Insurance," Working Paper 5147, June, National Bureau of Economic Research, Cambridge, MA.

Guenther, Gary (2001). *Tax Subsidies for Health Insurance for the Uninsured: An Economic Analysis of Selected Policy Issues for Congress*. Washington, DC: Congressional Research Service.

Havighurst, Clark C. (2000). "American Health Care and the Law—We Need to Talk." *Health Affairs* 19(4):84–106.

Havighurst, Clark C. (2001). "Consumers Versus Managed Care: The New Class Actions." *Health Affairs* 20(4):8–27.

Health Affairs (2000). "Special Section: Medicare's Experience with Competitive Pricing," *Health Affairs* 19(5):9–59.

Health Care Financing Administration (1994). *Health Care Financing Administration—Strategic Plan.* Washington, DC: USGPO.

Heclo, Hugh (1978). "Issue Networks and the Executive Establishment." In Anthony King (Ed.), *The New American Political System.* Washington, DC: American Enterprise Institute.

Hegner, Richard E. (1997). *Dual Eligibility for Medicaid and Medicare: Options for Creating a Continuum of Care.* Washington, DC: George Washington University, National Health Policy Forum.

Holahan, John (2001). *Restructuring Medicaid Financing: Implications of the NGA Proposal.* Washington, DC: Kaiser Family Foundation.

Holahan, John, Teresa Coughlin, Leighton Ku, David Heslam, and Colin Winterbottom (1993). "Understanding the Recent Growth in Medicaid Spending." In Rowland, Feder, and Salganicoff (Eds.), *Medicaid Financing Crisis: Balancing Responsibilities, Priorities, and Dollars.* Washington, DC: AAAS Press.

Holahan, John, Stephen Zuckerman, Alison Evans, and Suresh Rangarajan (1998). "Medicaid Managed Care in 13 States." *Health Affairs* 17(3): 43–63.

Hurley, Robert F. and Michael McCue (1998). *Medicaid and Commercial HMOs: An At Risk Relationship.* Princeton, NJ: Center for Health Strategies.

Iglehart, John K. (1997). Interview, "Changing with the Times: The Views of Bruce C. Vladeck." *Health Affairs* 16(3):58–71.

Iglehart, John K. (1999). Interview, "Bringing Forth Medicare+Choice: HCFA's Robert A. Berenson." *Health Affairs* 18(1):144–49.

Institute of Medicine (1996). *Improving the Medicare Market: Adding Choice and Protections.* Washington, DC: National Academy Press.

Institute of Medicine (2001). *Crossing the Quality Chasm—A New Health System for the 21st Century.* Washington, DC, National Academy Press.

Johnson, Haynes and David S. Broder (1996). *The System: The American Way of Politics at the Breaking Point.* Boston, MA: Little, Brown.

Kaiser Commission on Medicaid and the Uninsured (2001). *Medicaid and State Budgets: An October 2001 Update.* Washington, DC: Author.

Kahn, Charles N., III, and Hanns Kuttner (1999). "Budget Bills and Medicare Policy: The Politics of the BBA." *Health Affairs* 18(1):37–47,

Kerwin C. M. (1999). *Rulemaking: How Government Agencies Write Laws and Make Policy,* 2d ed. Washington, DC: CQ.

Kondratos, Anna, Alan Weil, and Naomi Goldstein (1998). "Assessing the New Federalism: An Introduction." *Health Affairs* 17(3):17–24.

Lambrew, Jeanne (2001). *Section 1115 Waivers in Medicaid and the State*

Children's Health Insurance Program: An Overview. Washington, DC: Kaiser Commission on Medicaid and the Uninsured.

Levitt, Katherine, Helen C. Lazenby, and Lekha Sivarajan (1996). "Health Care Spending in 1994: Slowest in Decades." *Health Affairs* 15(2):130–44.

Levitt, Katherine, et al. (2000). "Health Spending in 1998: Signals of Change." *Health Affairs* 19(1):124–38.

Lewin, Marion Ein and Jones, Stanley B. (1996). "The Market Comes to Medicare: Adding Choice and Protections." *Health Affairs* 15(4):57–61.

Lindblom, C. E. (1950). "The Science of 'Muddling Through.'" *Public Administration Review* 19:79–99.

Long, Norton E. (1954). "Public Policy and Administration: The Goals of Rationality and Responsibility." *Public Administration Review* 14:22–30.

Marmor, Theodore R. (1998). "Forecasting American Health Care: How We Got Here and Where We Might Be Going." *Journal of Health Politics, Policy and Law* 23(3):557–71.

Marmor, Theodore R. (2000). *The Politics of Medicare,* 2d ed. Hawthorne, NY: Aldine de Gruyter.

Marmor, Theodore R. (2001). "How Not to Think About Medicare Reform." *Journal of Health Politics, Policy and Law* 26(1):107–17.

Marmor, Theodore R. and Jonathan Oberlander (1998). "Rethinking Medicare Reform" (with comments by Henry J. Aaron, Robert Reischauer, and Stuart M. Butler). *Health Affairs* 17(1):52–74.

Mashaw, Jerry L. (1996). "Reinventing Government and Regulatory Reform: Studies in the Neglect and Abuse of Administrative Law." *University of Pittsburgh Law Review* 57(2):405–22.

Matherlee, Karen (2000). *The Federal-State Medicaid Match: An Ongoing Tug-of-War over Practice and Policy.* Washington, DC: George Washington University, National Health Policy Forum.

McGlynn, Elizabeth A. (1997). "Six Challenges in Measuring the Quality of Health Care." *Health Affairs* 16(3):7–21.

Mechanic, David and Donna D. McAlpine (2000). "Mission Unfulfilled: Potholes on the Road to Mental Health Parity." *Health Affairs* 19(1):7–21.

Medicare Payment Advisory Commission (1998). *Report to the Congress: Medicare Payment Policy.* Washington, DC: MedPAC (published annually in March).

Medicare Payment Advisory Commission (1999). *Report to the Congress: Medicare Payment Policy.* Washington, DC: MedPAC.

Medicare Payment Advisory Commission (2000). *Report to the Congress: Medicare Payment Policy.* Washington, DC: MedPAC.

Medicare Payment Advisory Commission (2001). *Report to the Congress: Medicare Payment Policy.* Washington, DC: MedPAC.

Mendelson, Daniel N. and Ellen Miller Salinsky (1997). "Health Information Systems and the Role of State Government." *Health Affairs* 16(3): 106–19.

Moon, Marilyn (1993). *Medicare Now and in the Future.* Washington, DC: Urban Institute Press.

Moon, Marilyn (1999). "Will the Care Be There? Vulnerable Beneficiaries and Medicare Reform." *Health Affairs* 18(1):107–17

Moon, Marilyn (2000). "Medicare Matters: Building on a Record of Accomplishments." *Health Care Financing Review* 22(1):23–34.

Moon, Marilyn and Davis, Karen (1995). "Preserving and Strengthening Medicare." *Health Affairs* 14(4):31–46.

Moore, Judith D. (2000). *SCHIP in the Formative Years, An Update,* Issue Brief No. 759. Washington, DC: George Washington University, National Health Policy Forum.

Myers, Robert J. (1970). *Medicare.* Homewood, IL: Irwin.

Newhouse, Joseph P., Melinda Beeukes Buntin, and John D. Chapman (1997). "Risk Adjustment and Medicare: Taking a Closer Look." *Health Affairs* 16(5):26–43.

Newhouse, Joseph P. and Gail R. Wilensky (2001). "Paying for Graduate Medical Education: the Debate Goes On." *Health Affairs* 20(2):136–58.

Nichols, Len M. and Linda J. Blumberg (1998). "A Different Kind of 'New Federalism'?" *Health Affairs* 17(3):25–42.

Oberg, Charles N. and Cynthia Polich (1998). "Medicaid: Entering the Third Decade." *Health Affairs* 9(3):83-96.

Oberlander, Jonathan B. (1997). "Managed Care and Medicare Reform." *Journal of Health Politics, Policy and Law* 22(2):595–631.

Pear, Robert E. (2000a). "Demands to Review Medicare Mailings by H.M.O's." *New York Times,* March 19, p. i28.

Pear, Robert (2000b). "G.O.P. Postponing Vote in the House on Patients' Rights." *New York Times*, July 26, p. A-1.

Pear, Robert (2001a). "HMO's Flee Medicare Despite Rise in Payments." *New York Times*, December 4, p. A16.

Pear, Robert (2001b). "Bush Strikes Deal on a Bill Defining Rights of Patients." *New York Times*, August 2, p. A1.

Peterson, Mark A. (ed.) (1998) *Health Markets? The New Competition in Medical Care.* Durham, NC: Duke University.

Peterson, Mark A. (1997). "The Limits of Learning: Translating Analysis into Action." *Journal of Health Politics, Policy and Law* 22(4):1077–1114.

Phillips, Kevin (1994). *Arrogant Capital: Washington, Wall Street, and the Frustration of American Politics.* Boston: Little, Brown.

Physician Payment Review Commission (1995). *Annual Report to Congress.* Washington, DC: Author.

President's Advisory Commission on Consumer Protection and Quality in the Health Care Industry (1998). *Quality First: Better Health Care for All Americans.* Washington, DC: USGPO.

Prospective Payment Assessment Commission (1995). *Report and Recommendations to the Congress.* Washington, DC: Author.

Prospective Payment Assessment Commission (1997). *Report and Recommendations to the Congress*. Washington, DC: Author.

Reischauer, Robert D., Stuart Butler, and Judith Lave (Eds.) (1998). *Medicare: Preparing for the Challenge of the 21st Century*. Washington, DC: National Academy of Social Insurance.

Rich, Robert F. and William D. White (Eds.) (1996). *Health Policy, Federalism, and the American States*. Washington, DC: Urban Institute Press.

Robinson, James C. (2001). "The End of Managed Care." *Journal of the American Medical Association* 285(20):2622–28.

Rodwin, Marc A. (1996). "Consumer Protection and Managed Care: The Need for Organized Consumers." *Health Affairs* 15(3):110–23.

Rodwin, Marc A. (1999). "Backlash as Prelude to Managing Managed Care." *Journal of Health Politics, Policy and Law* 24(5):1115–26.

Rosenbaum, Sara (2000). *The Olmstead Decision: Implications for Medicaid*. Washington, DC: Kaiser Commission on Medicaid and the Uninsured.

Rosenbaum, Sara and Julie Darnall (1998). *Medicaid Managed Care: An Analysis of the HCFA's Notice of Proposed Rule Making*. Washington, DC: George Washington University, Center for Health Policy Research.

Rosenbaum, Sara, Rafael Serrano, Michele Magar, and Gillian Stern (1997). "Civil Rights in a Changing Health Care System." *Health Affairs* 16(1): 90–105.

Rowland, Diane, Judith Feder, and Alina Salganicoff (Eds.) (1993). *Medicaid Financing Crisis: Balancing Responsibilities, Priorities, and Dollars*. Washington, DC: AAAS Press.

Rowland, Diane and Rachel Garfield (2000). "Health Care for the Poor: Medicaid at 35." *Health Care Financing Review* 22(1):23–34.

Safire, William (1993). *Safire's New Political Dictionary*. New York: Random House.

Sangl, Judith A. and Linda F. Wolf (1996). "Role of Consumer Information in Today's Health Care System." *Health Care Financing Review* 18(1):1–8.

Schick, Allen (1995). *The Federal Budget: Politics, Policy, and Process*. Washington, DC: Brookings Institution.

Schlesinger, Arthur, Jr. (2001) "Democracy in Wartime." *New York Times*, October 3, p. A23.

Schneider, Andy, Victoria Strohmeyer, and Risa Ellberger (2000). *Medicaid Eligibility for Individuals with Disabilities*. Washington, DC: Kaiser Commission on Medicaid and the Uninsured.

Schoenman, Julie A. (1999). "The Impact of the BBA on Medicare Payments for Rural Areas." *Health Affairs* 18(1):244–54.

Schwartz, William B. (1994). "In the Pipeline: A Wave of Valuable Medical Technology." *Health Affairs* 13(3):70–79.

Simon, Herbert A. (1955). "A Behavioral Model of Rational Choice." *Quarterly Journal of Economics* 69:99–118.

Skocpol, Theda (1996). *Boomerang: Clinton's Health Security Effort and the Turn Against Government in U.S. Politics*. New York: W.S. Norton.

Smith, David G. (1992). *Paying for Medicare: the Politics of Reform*. Hawthorne, NY: Aldine de Gruyter.

Smith, Sheila, Mark Freeland, et al. (1998). "The Next Ten Years of Health Spending: What Does the Future Hold." *Health Affairs* 17(5):128–140.

Sorel, Georges (1912). *Reflections on Violence,* transl. T. E. Hulme. New York: B. W. Huebsch.

Sorian, Richard and Judith Feder (1999). "Why We Need a Patient's Bill of Rights." *Journal of Health Politics, Policy and Law* 24(5):1137–44.

Sparer, Michael S. (1998). "Devolution of Power: An Interim Report Card." *Health Affairs* 17(3):7–16.

Stanton, Thomas H. (2001). "Medicare Fraud-And-Abuse Enforcement." *Health Affairs* 20(4):28–42.

Stephanopoulos, George (1999). *All Too Human: A Political Education*. Boston: Little, Brown.

Stevens, Robert and Rosemary Stevens (1974). *Welfare Medicine in America— A Case Study of Medicaid*. New York: Free Press.

Studdert, David M., William M. Sage, Carole Roan Gresenz, and Deborah R. Hensler (1999). "Expanded Managed Care Liability: What Impact on Employer Coverage?" *Health Affairs* 18(6):7–27.

Thompson, Frank and John DiIulio, Jr. (Eds.) (1998). *Medicaid and Devolution: A View from the States*. Washington, DC: Brookings Institution.

Thorpe, Kenneth E. (1997). "Incremental Approaches to Covering the Uninsured Children: Design and Policy Issues." *Health Affairs* 16(4):64–78.

Toner, Robin (2001a). "Major Battle Looms Over Medicare." *New York Times,* February 11, p. I–34.

Toner, Robin (2001b). "A Stubborn Fight Revived." *New York Times,* December 20, p. A–34.

U.S. Congress (1993). *Medicaid Source Book: Background Data and Analysis.* Report prepared by the Congressional Research Service for the Subcommittee on Health and the Environment of the Committee on Energy and Commerce, Cmte. Print 103-A, 103rd Congress, 1st session.

U.S. Congress (1995a). Saving Medicare and Reconciliation Issues, Hearings before the Subcommittee on Health of the Committee on Ways and Means, 104th Congress, 1st Session, July 19, 20, 25.

U.S. Congress (1995b). Senate, Budget Reconciliation Recommendations of the Committee on Finance, S Prt. 104-34, Committee on Finance, 104th Congress, 1st session, Oct.

U.S. Congress (1995c). Transformation of the Medicaid Program, Hearings before the Subcommittee on Health and Environment of the Committee on Commerce, 104th Congress, 1st session, 3 parts, June 8, 15, 21, 22, July 26, and Aug. 1.

U.S. Congress (1997a). Medicare HMO Payment Policies, Hearing before the Subcommittee on Health of the Committee on Ways and Means, 105th Congress, 1st session, February 25. [One of an informative series of hearings on a broad range of Medicare reform issues held to prepare members and staff for the Balanced Budget Act of 1997.]

U.S. Congress (1997b). Senate, Budget Reconciliation Recommendations of the Committee on Finance, S. Prt. 105-29, Committee on Finance, 105th Congress, 1st session, June.

U.S. Congress (1997c). The Balanced Budget Act of 1997—Conference Report to Accompany HR 2015, Rpt. 105-217, 105th Congress 1st session, July 30.

U.S. Congress (1997d). The Balanced Budget Act of 1997—Report of the Committee on the Budget to Accompany HR 2015, Rpt. 105-149, 105th Congress, 1st session, June 24.

U.S. Congress (1999). Senate, Medicare Reform, Hearings before the Committee on Finance, 106th Congress, 1st session, April 28 and May 5, 12, 26, 27.

U.S. Congress (2000). Background Material and Data on Programs within the Jurisdiction of the Committee on Ways and Means, (Green Book), WMCP 106-14, Committee on Ways and Means, 106th Congress, 2nd session, Oct. 6.

U.S. Congress, House of Representatives (1995). Balanced Budget Act of 1995—Conference Report to Accompany HR 2491, Pts. 1 & 2, Rpt. 104-350, 104th Congress, 1st session, Nov. 15.

U.S. Congress, Senate (1970). *Medicare and Medicaid—Problems, Issues, and Alternatives,* Staff Report to the Committee on Finance, 91st Congress, 1st session, February 9. Washington, DC: USGPO.

U.S. General Accounting Office (1995a). *Antifraud Technology Offers Significant Opportunity to Reduce Health Care Fraud,* GAO/AIMD-95-77 (Washington, DC: USGPO.

U.S. General Accounting Office (1995b). *Medicare—Excessive Payments for Medical Supplies Continue Despite Improvements,* GAO/HEHS-95-171. Washington, DC: USGPO.

U.S. General Accounting Office (1996a). *Health Insurance for Children—Private Insurance Continues to Deteriorate,* GAO/HEHS-96-129. Washington, DC: USGPO.

U.S. General Accounting Office (1996b). *Private Payer Strategies Suggest Options to Reduce Rapid Spending,* GAO/T-HEHS-96-138. Washington, DC: USGPO.

U.S. General Accounting Office (1997). *Weaknesses in Medicare Transaction System—Success Depends Upon Correcting Critical Managerial and Technical Weaknesses,* GAO/AIMD-97-78. Washington, USGPO.

Vladeck, Bruce C. (1999). "The Political Economy of Medicare." *Health Affairs* 18(1):22–36.

Waite, Linda J. (1996). "The Demographic Face of America's Elderly." *Inquiry* 33(3):220.

Walsh, Elsa (1997). "Kennedy's Hidden Campaign." *New Yorker* (March 31): 66–81.

Weaver, R. Kent (1987). "The Politics of Blame: Public Policy and Avoidance Behavior." *Current* 296(Oct.):11–15.

Weissert, Carol S. and William G. Weissert (1996). *Governing Health: The Politics of Health Policy*. Baltimore, MD: Johns Hopkins University Press.

White, Joseph (1999). "Uses and Abuses of Long-Term Medicare Cost Estimates." *Health Affairs* 18(1):63–79.

Whitelaw, Nancy A. and Gail L Warden (1999). "Reexamining the Delivery System as Part of Medicare Reform." *Health Affairs* 18(1):132–43.

Wiener, Jonathan P. and Associates (1996). "Risk-Adjusting Medicare Capitation Rates Using Ambulatory and Inpatient Diagnoses." *Health Care Financing Review* 17(3):77–99.

Wiener, Joshua M. and David G. Stevenson (1998). "State Policy on Long-Term Care for the Elderly." *Health Affairs* 17(3):81–100.

Wilensky, Gail R. (1997). "Pursuing Quality: A Public Policy View." *Health Affairs* 16(3):77–81.

Wilensky, Gail R. and Joseph P. Newhouse (1999). "Medicare: What's Right? What's Wrong? What's Next?" *Health Affairs* 18(1):92–106.

Zarabozo, Carlos (1999). "Explosion in the Medicine Chest." *Health Care Financing Review* 20(3):1–13.

Zelman, Walter A. (1996). *The Changing Health Care Market Place—Private Ventures, Public Interests*. San Francisco, CA: Jossey Bass.

Zelman, Walter A. and Robert A. Berenson (1998). *The Managed Care Blues and How to Cure Them*. Washington, DC: Georgetown University Press.

Zubkoff, Michael (Ed.) (1976). *Health: A Victim or Cause of Inflation?* New York: Milbank Memorial Fund.

Index

Bipartisanship, 8, 9, 31, 54, 62, 149,
    341, 370
  in 1997, 175, 194, 196, 202, 213
  Senate and, 167, 173
Blame avoidance, shifting, 81
Block grant proposals, 39, 48, 52, 54,
    63, 149
  excluded in 1997, 200
  Reagan administration and, 54
Blue Cross/Blue Shield, 80, 99, 101,
    128
Blue Dog coalition, 84, 89–90,
    140 n54
  budget proposals, 89–90, 124, 135,
    185
Boehner, John, 123, 183, 225
Boren Amendment, 27–29, 48, 61,
    200, 202, 212, 219
Bowles, Erskine, 131, 176, 182, 226–
    227
Budget deficits, 44, 50, 153, 175
  Pete Domenici and, 50
  (*see also specific legislation to reduce*)
Budget proposals
  Blue Dog coalition, 89–90, 123, 135,
    202, 212, 219
  Clinton budget, in 1995, 5, 84–88,
    124, 131
    and CBO scoring, 127, 130, 134
    in 1997, 178–179
  Daschle, 124, 150
Budget reconciliation process
  campaign mode and, 72
  fiscal discipline and, 4, 371–372
  instrument of change, 71, 126, 190,
    371–372
  mobilization, partisan and, 42–43
Budget resolution of 1996, 148
  three-part strategy, 153–154
  Medicaid-welfare link severed, 152–
    155
Bureau of Policy Development, 249,
    255

Burke, Edmund, 53
Burney, Ira, 57, 86
Bush, George H. W., 82, 178, 182
  and 1990 budget summit, 82
Bush, George W., 2–4, 340, 342, 347
  patients' right bill and, 340–342
  tax cuts, 6
Bush (George W.) administration, 2,
    311–316, 330
Buto, Kathy, 246, 251, 253–55,
    258–260, 264
Byrd Rule, 111, 122, 143 n135
Byrnes Bill (Medicare Part B), 14

Cade, David, 302
Campaign mode, 3, 6, 31–33
  budget reconciliation and, 42–43
  Senate and, 49, 122
Capitation payments, 19, 94, 377
Capped entitlement, 48–49, 54
Carriers (Medicare), 15, 16
Carter administration, 18, 78
Case management, 193, 356
  PACE, 191, 203
Center for Beneficiary Services (CBS),
    266–267, 269–270, Appen-
    dix B
Center for Health Plans and Provider
    Operations (CHPP) 266–
    267
Center for Medicare and Medicaid Ser-
    vices (CMS), 312, 315
Centers of Excellence, 194, 356
Chafee, John, 62–65, 119–121, 210,
    213, 216, 218–219, 222
Chafee-Breaux bill (extending Medic-
    aid), 219–220, 229
Chafee-Lieberman proposal (patients'
    rights bill), 337
Chafee-Rockefeller amendment
    (expanding Medicaid), 6,
    213, 216–218
Chang, Deborah, 298